Fundamentals of Computational Neuroscience

T0073673

Fundamentals of Computational Neuroscience
Third Edition

Thomas P. Trappenberg

Dalhousie University

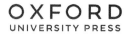

OXFORD
UNIVERSITY PRESS

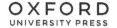

OXFORD
UNIVERSITY PRESS

Great Clarendon Street, Oxford, OX2 6DP,
United Kingdom

Oxford University Press is a department of the University of Oxford.
It furthers the University's objective of excellence in research, scholarship,
and education by publishing worldwide. Oxford is a registered trade mark of
Oxford University Press in the UK and in certain other countries

© Oxford University Press 2023

The moral rights of the author have been asserted

First Edition published in 2002
Second Edition published in 2010
Third Edition published in 2023
Impression: 1

All rights reserved. No part of this publication may be reproduced, stored in
a retrieval system, or transmitted, in any form or by any means, without the
prior permission in writing of Oxford University Press, or as expressly permitted
by law, by licence or under terms agreed with the appropriate reprographics
rights organization. Enquiries concerning reproduction outside the scope of the
above should be sent to the Rights Department, Oxford University Press, at the
address above

You must not circulate this work in any other form
and you must impose this same condition on any acquirer

Published in the United States of America by Oxford University Press
198 Madison Avenue, New York, NY 100106, United States of America

British Library Cataloguing in Publication Data
Data available

Library of Congress Control Number: 2022943170

ISBN 978–0–19–286936–4

DOI: 10.1093/oso/9780192869364.001.0001

Printed in the UK by
Ashford Colour Press Ltd, Gosport, Hampshire

Links to third party websites are provided by Oxford in good faith and
for information only. Oxford disclaims any responsibility for the materials
contained in any third party website referenced in this work.

Preface

Computational neuroscience is still a young and dynamically developing discipline, and some choice of topics and presentation style had to be made. This text introduces some fundamental concepts, with an emphasis on basic neuronal models and network properties. In contrast to the common research literature, this book is trying to paint the larger picture and tries to emphasize some of the concepts and assumptions for simplifications used in the scientific technique of modelling.

Computational neuroscience and Artificial Intelligence (AI) are close cousins. The term AI is said to be invented at the Dartmouth workshop in 1956 with many famous participants including psychiatrist Ross Ashby, the neurophysiologist Warren McCulloch who created one of the first mathematical neuron models, and Arthur Samuel, one of the pioneers in reinforcement learning. Computational models of neural systems such as models of neurons are much older, but connecting learning and cognitive systems created excitement over the possibility to better understand mind. The invention of learning machines has revolutionized many applications as recently seen in the dramatic progress of machine vision and natural language processing through deep learning.

While there has been much recent progress in machine learning, researchers in this area often wonder how the brain works. It sometimes seems that scientific progress oscillates between computational neuroscience and machine learning. For example, the progress of neural networks and statistical learning theory in the later 1980s and early 1990s was followed by enormous activities in computational neuroscience in the 1990s and early 2000s. For the last decade, deep learning has occupied an explosive growth in machine learning and data science, and now the time seems ripe for more renewed interest in looking more closely at the brain for inspirations to go deeper. This is fuelled by the increasing realization of limitations of deep learning, in particular with the challenge of learning semantic knowledge with limited data and the ability to transfer knowledge to situations that are not directly represented in the learning set.

In this new edition of my book, I tried to incorporate many of the recent lessons from deep learning. While there are excellent books on deep learning, our emphasis here is their connection to brain processing. An important aspect is thereby the concepts of representational learning and computation with uncertainties. Also, I now included gated recurrent neural networks that are becoming an important fundamental mechanisms when thinking about brain processing. While we will not be able to dive into all the recent progress, I hope that the text will guide further specific studies and research. Furthermore, it was important for me to streamline the existing text. I hope that I improved the readability of some of the text and even removed parts that seem less relevant to study the most basic fundamentals.

The themes included in this book are chosen to provide some path through the different levels of description of the brain. Chapter 1 provides a high-level overview and some fundamental questions about brain theories, a brief discussion about the role of modelling, and some basic neuroscience facts that are useful to keep in mind for later use. We also review the essential scientific programming in Python and the basic mathematical and statistical concept used in the book. Chapters 2–4 focus on basic mechanisms and modelling of single neurons or population averages. This starts from a fairly detailed discussion of changes in the membrane potentials through ion channels, spike generations, and synaptic plasticity, with increasingly abstractions in the following chapters. Chapters 5–7 describe the information-processing capabilities of basic networks, including feedforward and competitive recurrent networks. The last part of the book describes some examples of combining such elementary networks as well as some examples of more system-level models of the brain.

Most models in the book are quite general and are aimed at illustrating basic mechanisms of information processing in the brain. In the research literature, the basic elements reviewed in this book are often combined in specific ways to model specific brain areas. Our hope is that the study of the basic models in this book will enable the reader to follow some of the recent research literature in computational neuroscience.

While we tried to emphasize some important concepts, we did not want to give the impression that the chosen path is the only direction in computational neuroscience. Therefore, we sometimes mention concepts without extensive discussion. These comments are intended to increase the reader's awareness of some issues and to provide some keywords to facilitate further literature searches. Also, while some examples of specific brain areas are mentioned in this book, a comprehensive review of models in computational neuroscience is beyond the scope of this text. We do not claim that this book covers all aspects of computational neuroscience nor do we claim it to be the only approach to this area, but we hope that it will contribute to the discussion.

Mathematical formulas

This book includes mathematical formulas and concepts. We use mathematical language and concepts strictly as practical tools and to communicate ideas in contrast to using such formalism for mathematical proofs. We thereby tried to balance detailed mathematical notations with readability and communicating the basic concepts. From readers with less extensive training in such formal systems I ask for patience. We did not try to avoid mathematical formulations since such notations allow a brevity in communication that would be lengthy with plain written language. The chosen level of mathematical descriptions are mainly intended to be translated directly into programs and other quantitative evaluations.

There is no reason to be afraid of formulas, and it is important to see beyond the symbols and to understand their meaning. Many mathematics notations are invented to simplify descriptions. This includes the use of vectors and matrices, which will drastically shorten the specification of network models. We provide review chapters in the first part of the book to review such notations. We recommend some tutorials on such materials to allow students to move beyond these technicalities in the main text.

Most models in this book describe the change of a quantity with time, such as the change of a membrane potential after synaptic input or synaptic strength values over time during learning. Equations that describe such changes are called differential equations. A comprehensive knowledge of the theory of differential equations is not required for understanding this book. However, discussing the consequences of specific differential equations and simulating them with computer programs is at the heart of this book. I hope our treatment will encourage a new look into a topic that sometimes seems overwhelming when treated in specialized classes. We will specifically become familiar with a simple yet telling example of a differential equation, that of a leaky integrator. A basic knowledge of the numerical approaches to solving differential equations is essential for this book and many other dynamic modelling approaches. Thus, we also include a review of differential equations and their numerical integration.

Another mathematical theory, that of random numbers, is also reviewed in the third chapter. The language of probability theory is very useful in computational neuroscience and should be taught in such a course. In neuroscience (as in other disciplines), we often get different values each time we perform a measurement, and random numbers describe such situations. We often think of these circumstances as noise, but it is also useful to think about random variables and statistics in terms of describing uncertainties. Indeed, it can be argued that learning and reasoning in uncertain circumstances is a fundamental requirement of the brain. We will argue that mental functions can be viewed as probabilistic reasoning.

Programming examples

While this book includes a few examples of powerful analytical techniques to give the reader a flavour of some of the more elaborate theoretical studies, not every neuroscientist has to perform such calculations themselves. However, studying some of the general ideas behind these techniques is essential to be able to get support from those who specialize in such techniques. In particular, it is instructive when studying this book to perform some numerical experiments yourself. We therefore included an introduction to a modern programming environment that is very much suited for many of the models in neuroscience. Writing programs and creating advanced graphics can be learned easily within a short time, even without extensive prior programming knowledge.

The programs in this book are now provided in Python to improve accessibility and due to Python's increasing importance in machine learning and data science. While it was challenging to balance a scientist's approach of making minimalist and clean examples with common programming approaches, I hope that I found some balance. Comments in programs are often a good idea in complex software packages. However, the situation is different here. The programs are purposefully kept short and the expectation is that each line should be read and understood entirely. For example, we think that comments like `# assigning value b to variable a` to describe the code `a = b` should not be necessary. Instead, the reader should strive to be able to read the code directly. Comments in the program were therefore deliberately avoided except to explain some variable names to keep the variable names short, and some comments to structure the code. Many people have different styles of coding, and the style here tried deliberately to strive for compactness and simplicity. While it might be a new language for some, trying to understand each line in a program will help to master programming in a short time.

References

This book does not provide a historical account of the development of ideas in computational neuroscience. Indeed, extensive references have been avoided where possible to concentrate on describing fundamental ideas. This is hence more consistent with course textbooks. References to the original research literature are only provided when following corresponding examples closely. The text is very much aimed at providing a starting place for further studies, and search engines will now easily provide further directions.

Acknowledgements

Many friends and colleagues have contributed over the years to this book I am specifically thankful to Farzaneh Sheikhnezhad Fard, Alan Fine, Steve Grossberg, Alexander Hanuschkin, Geoffrey Hinton, Abraham Nunez, Kai Trappenberg, Nami Trappenberg, Jason Satel, Michael Schmitt, Dominic Standage, Fumio Yamazaki, and Si Wu.

Contents

I

Background

1 Introduction and outlook

This introductory chapter is outlining the big picture. We define the scope of the computational neuroscience discussed in this book and outline some basic facts of brain organization and principles that we encounter in later chapters. This chapter includes a discussion on the role of scientific modelling in general and in neuroscience specifically. In addition, we outline a high-level theory of the brain as a predictive model of the world, and we outline some principles that will guide much of the discussions in this book.

1.1 What is computational neuroscience?

Computational or theoretical neuroscience uses distinct techniques and asks specific questions aimed at advancing our understanding of the nervous system. A brief definition might be:

> Computational neuroscience is the theoretical study of the brain used to uncover the principles and mechanisms that guide the development, organization, information processing and mental abilities of the nervous system.

Most papers in computational neuroscience journals follow one of two quite different principle directions. One direction is the use of computational methods to analyses data such as sorting spikes or to quantitatively test hypothesis. In this context, methods from AI (Artificial Intelligence) such as machine learning techniques are now often included as tools for data analytics. We will encounter such techniques, specifically that of neural networks and deep learning. However, our focus here is less on describing data analytics methods but rather to build models of brain functions to understand its processing capabilities. The type of computational neuroscience described in this book is hence mostly synonymous with theoretical neuroscience in that we develop and test hypotheses of the functional mechanisms of the brain.

We often use computer simulations in our studies, though 'computational' highlights more broadly our interested in the computational and information-processing aspects of brain functions. A main focus in this book is hence the development and evaluation of brain models, or models of specific functions of the brain. These are important to summarize knowledge, to quantify theories, and to test computational hypotheses. We focus thereby on fundamental mechanisms and mechanistic foundations which seem to be underlying brain processes. We also try to highlight some emerging principles of brain-style information processing. This book does claim a comprehensive theory of the mind. However, we hope that learning these fundamentals will be an important part of further developments.

Fundamentals of Computational Neuroscience. Third edition. Thomas P. Trappenberg,
Oxford University Press. © Oxford University Press 2023. DOI: 10.1093/oso/9780192869364.003.0001

1.1.1 Embedding within neuroscience

Computational neuroscience is a specialization within neuroscience. Neuroscience itself is a scientific area with many different aspects. Its aim is to understand the nervous system, in particular the *central nervous system* and the spine that we call the brain. The brain is studied in diverse disciplines such as physiology, psychology, medicine, computer science, and mathematics. Neuroscience emerged from the realization that interdisciplinary studies are vital to further our understanding of the brain. While considerable progress has been made in our understanding of brain functions, there are many open questions that we want to answer. What is the function of the brain and how does it achieve its task? What are the biological mechanisms involved? How is it organized? What are the information-processing principles used to solve complex tasks such as perception? How did the brain evolve? How does it change during the lifetime of organisms? What is the effect of damage to particular areas and the possibilities of rehabilitation? What are the origins of degenerative diseases and possible treatments? These are questions asked by neuroscientists in many different subfields, using a multitude of different research techniques.

Many techniques are employed in neuroscience to study the brain. Those techniques include genetic manipulations, recording of cell activities in cultured cells, brain slices, optical imaging; non-invasive functional imaging, psychophysical measurements; and computational simulations, to name but a few. Each of these techniques is complicated and laborious enough to justify a specialization of neuroscientists in particular techniques. Therefore, we speak of neurophysiologists, cognitive scientists, and anatomists. It is, however, vital for any neuroscientist to develop a basic understanding of all major techniques, so he or she can comprehend and utilize the contributions made within these specializations. Computational neuroscience is a relative new area of neuroscience with increasing importance. It fills an important role in quantifying theories based on the increasing amount of experimental discoveries. A basic comprehension of the contribution that computational neuroscience can make is becoming increasingly important for all neuroscientists.

Within computational neuroscience we often use computers, although other areas of neuroscience use computers. Our main reason for using computers is that the complexity of models in this area is often beyond analytical tractability. For such models we have to employ carefully designed numerical experiments to be able to compare the models to experimental data. However, we do not need to restrict our studies to this tool. Some models are analytically tractable or might be deliberately simplified to be analytically tractable. Such models often provide a deep and more controlled insight into the features of certain mechanisms and the reasons behind numerical findings.

Although computational neuroscience is theoretical by its very nature, it is important to bear in mind that models must be gauged on experimental data; they are otherwise useless for understanding the brain. Only experimental measurements of the real brain can verify 'what' the brain actually does. In contrast to the experimental domain, computational neuroscience tries to speculate 'how' the brain operates. Such speculations are developed into hypotheses, realized into models, evaluated analytically or numerically, and tested against experimental data. Also, models can often be used to make further predictions about the underlying phenomena.

1.2 Organization in the brain

Mental functions such as perception and learning motor skills are not accomplished by single neurons alone. These functions are an emerging property of specialized networks with many neurons that form the nervous system. The number of neurons in the central nervous system is estimated to be on the order of 10^{12}, and it is demanding to explore such vast systems of neurons. Therefore, rather than trying to rebuild the brain in all its detail on a computer, we aim to understand the principal organization of brains and how networks of neuron-like elements can support and enable particular mental processes. Integration of neurons into networks with specific architectures seem to be essential for such skills. We will explore the computational abilities of several principal architectures of neural networks in this book.

A thorough knowledge of the anatomy of the brain areas we want to model is essential for any research that attempts to understand brain functions. However, although recent research has revealed many important facts about neural organization, it is still often difficult to specify all the components of a model on the basis of anatomical and physiological data alone, and plausible assumptions have to be made to bridge gaps in the knowledge. Even if we can draw on known details, it is often useful to make simplifying assumptions that enable computational tractability or the tracing of principal organizations sufficient for certain functionalities. It is beyond the scope of this book to describe all the details of neuronal organization, and more specialized books and research articles have to be consulted for specific brain areas. The aim of the following section is to outline a large variety of facts mainly to raise awareness of the many factors of structures and organizations in the brain. In computational neuroscience we have a constant struggle between incorporating as many details as possible while keeping models simple to illuminate the principles behind brain functions. We hope that this section will encourage more specific studies of brain anatomy.

1.2.1 Levels of organization in the brain

Models in computational neuroscience can target many different levels of descriptions. This in itself is a consequence of the fact that the nervous system has many levels of organization on spatial scales ranging from the molecular level of a few Angstrom ($1\mathring{A} = 10^{-10}$m), to the whole nervous system on the scale of over a metre. Biological mechanisms on all these levels are important for the brain to function.

Different levels of organization in the nervous system are illustrated in Fig. 1.1. An important structure in the nervous system is the neuron, which is a cell that is specialized for signal processing. Depending on external conditions, neurons are able to generate electric potentials that are used to transmit information to other cells to which they are connected. Mechanisms on a subcellular level are important for such information processing capabilities. Neurons use cascades of biochemical reactions that have to be understood on a molecular level. These include, for example, the transcription of genetic information which influences information-processing in the nervous system. Many structures within neurons can be identified with specific functions. For example, mitochondria are structures important for the energy supply in the cell, and synapses mediate information transmission between cells. The complexity of a single neuron, and even isolated subcellular mechanisms, makes computational studies essential for the development and verification of hypotheses. It is possible today to simulate morphologically reconstructed neurons in great detail, and there has been much progress in understanding important mechanisms on this level.

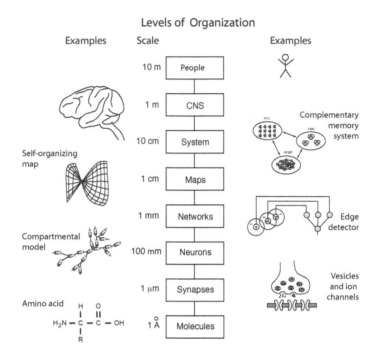

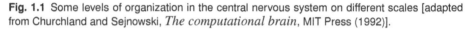

Fig. 1.1 Some levels of organization in the central nervous system on different scales [adapted from Churchland and Sejnowski, *The computational brain*, MIT Press (1992)].

However, single neurons certainly do not tell the whole story. Neurons contact each other and thereby compose networks. A small number of interconnected neurons can exhibit complex behaviour and enable information-processing capabilities not present in a single neuron. Understanding networks of interacting neurons is a major domain in computational neuroscience. Networks have additional information-processing capabilities beyond that of single neurons, such as representing information in a distributed way. An example of a basic network is the edge detector formed from a centre-surround neuron as proposed by Hubble and Wiesel. The illustrated levels above the level labelled 'Networks' in Fig. 1.1 are also composed of networks, yet with increasing size and complexity. An example on the level termed 'Maps' in Fig. 1.1 is a self-oganizing topographic map, which is part of an important discussion in this book.

The organization does not stop at the map level. Networks with a specific architecture and specialized information-processing capabilities are composed into larger structures that are able to perform even more complex information-processing tasks. System-level models are important in understanding higher-order brain functions. The central nervous system depends strongly on the dynamic interaction of many specialized subsystems, and the interaction of the brain with the environment. Indeed, we will see later that active environmental interactions are essential for brain development and function.

Although an individual researcher typically specializes in mechanisms of a certain scale, it is important for all neuroscientists to develop a basic understanding and appreciation of the functionalities of different scales in the brain. Computational neuroscience can help the investigations at all levels of description, and it is not surprising that computational neuroscientists investigate different types of models at different levels of description. Computational methods have long contributed to cellular neuroscience, and computational cognitive neuroscience is now a rapidly emerging field. The contributions of computational neuroscience are, in particular, important to understand non-linear interactions of subprocesses. Furthermore, it is important to comprehend the interactions between different levels of description, and computational methods have proven very useful in bridging the gap between physiological measurements and behavioural correlates.

1.2.2 Large-scale brain anatomy

The nervous system is distributed throughout the whole body. Some of the peripheral nervous system include sensors such as touch sensors or sensors for auditory signals. Some of those sensors like the eyes are in themselves already highly sophisticated neural systems, and the brainstem already processes sensory signals to produce fast responses such as reflexes. Of course, it is clear that more complex information processing can be achieved with the added complexity of the central nervous system that we usually call the brain (Fig. 1.2). The brain itself has a lot of structure in itself, such as subcortical midbrain areas that include structures that we will mention like the basal ganglia or the thalamus. Even within the cortex we can easily distinguish areas of the paleocortex and archicortex, which include structures like the amygdala, the secondary olfactory cortex, and the hippocampal formation. These cortical structures have mostly three or four layers of cortex compared to the six layers of the neocortex that coverse the outside of the mammalian brain. As the name indicates, the neocortex seems phylogenetically newer than the archicortex and the paleocortex, meaning that the neocorrtex developed later during evolution.

While the neocortex looks more homogeneous, regions of the neocortex are commonly divided into four lobes as illustrated in Fig. 1.2B, the occipital lobe at the rear of the head, the adjacent parietal lobe, the frontal lobe, and the temporal lobes at the flanks of the brain. Further subdivisions can be made, based on various criteria. For example, at the beginning of the twentieth century the German anatomist Korbinian Brodmann identified 52 cortical areas based on their cytoarchitecture, the distinctive occurrence of cell types and arrangements, which can be visualized with various staining techniques. Brodmann labelled the areas he found with numbers, as shown in Fig. 1.2B. Some of these subdivisions have since been refined, and letters following the number are commonly used to further specify some part of an area defined by Brodmann. Brodmann's cortical map is, however, not the only reference to cortical areas used in neuroscience. Other subdivisions and labels of cortical areas are based, for example, on functional correlates of brain areas. These include behavioural correlates of cortical areas as revealed by brain lesions or functional brain imaging, as well as neuronal response characteristics identified by electrophysiological recordings.

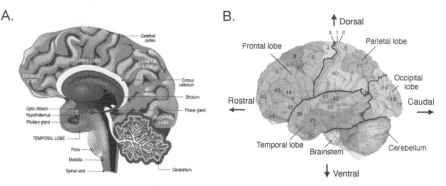

Fig. 1.2 Outline of the lateral view of the human brain including the neocortex, cerebellum, and brainstem. The neocortex is divided into four lobes. The numbers correspond to Brodmann's classification of cortical areas. Directions are commonly stated as indicated in 1.2B.

It is, of course, of major interest to establish functional correlates of different cortical areas, a challenge that drives many physiological studies. We might speculate that the diverse functional specialization within the neocortex found with electrophysiological measurements is reflected in major structural differences among the different cortical areas to support specialized mental functions. It is therefore remarkable to realize that this is not the case. Instead, it is found that different areas of the neocortex have a remarkably common neuronal organization. All neocortical areas have anatomically distinguishable layers as discussed below. The differences in the cytoarchitecture, which have been used by Brodmann to map the cortex, are often only minor compared to the principal architecture within the neocortex, and these variations cannot account solely for the different functionalities associated with the different cortical areas.

The neocortex is different in this respect to older parts of the brain, such as the brainstem, where structural differences are much more pronounced. This is reflected in a variety of more easily distinguishable nuclei. We can often attribute specific low-level functions to each nucleus in the brainstem. In contrast to this, it seems that the cortex is an information-processing structure with more universal processing abilities that we speculate enable more flexible mental abilities. It is therefore most interesting to investigate the information-processing capabilities of neuronal networks with a neocortical architecture.

1.2.3 Hierarchical organization of cortex

A common feature of neocortex is that there are primary sensory areas in which basic features of sensory signals are represented, while other areas seem to support more complex representations or mental tasks. Let us highlight this common view of neocortex with the example of vision. The primary visual area that receives mayor input from the eyes lies in the caudal end of the occipital lobe and is called V1. Information is then transmitted to other visual areas in the occipital lobe before splitting into two major processing streams, the dorsal stream along a parietal to frontal pathway, and the ventral stream along the temporal lobe. It has been argued that the dorsal stream is specifically adapted to spatial processing, whereas the ventral stream is well equipped for object recognition. We will investigate a model of such what-and-where processing later in the book. The main point here is that brain scientists try to identify functional specific areas and connections between these areas.

In order to understand how different brain areas work together it is important to establish the anatomical and functional connectivity between brain areas in more detail. Anatomical connections are not easy to establish as it is extremely difficult to follow the path of stained axons through the brain in brain slices (including the branches that can often have different pathways). This is a daunting task, though it has been done in isolated cases. There are other methods of establishing connectivities in the brain. These include the use of chemical substances that are transported by the neurons to target areas or from target areas to the origin. Functional connectivity patterns, in which we are particularly interested when studying how brain areas work together, can also be established with simultaneous stimulations and recordings in different brain areas. Such experiments show correlations in the firing patterns of neurons in different brain areas if they are functionally connected. Also, some large-scale functional brain organizations can be revealed by brain-imaging techniques such as functional magnetic resonance imaging (fMRI), which can highlight the areas involved in certain mental tasks. Such studies established clearly that different brain areas do not work in isolation. On the contrary, many specialized brain areas have to work together to solve complex mental tasks.

Some scientists, such as Van Essen and colleagues, have long tried to compile experimental data into connectivity maps similar to the one shown in Fig. 1.3. The specific example was produced by Claus C. Hilgetag, Mark A. O'Neill, and Malcolm P. Young. The researchers used a neuroinformatics approach. Neuroinformatics is specifically concerned with the collection and representation of experimental data in large databases to which modern data mining methods can be applied. Hilgetag and colleagues considered an algorithm that would evaluate many possible configurations, and they found a large set of possible connectivity patterns in the visual cortex satisfying most of the experimental constraints. Each box in Fig. 1.3 represents a cortical area that has been distinguished from other areas on different grounds, typically anatomical and functional. The solid pathways between these boxes represent known anatomical or functional connections. The order from bottom to the top indicates roughly the hierarchical order in which these brain areas are contacted in the information-processing stream, from primary visual areas establishing some basic representations in the brain to higher cortical areas that are involved in object recognition and the planning and execution of motor actions. The authors also took the two basic visual processing pathways in their representation into account, plotting brain areas of the dorsal stream on the left side and the ventral stream on the right side. Note that there are also interactions within these pathways.

Interestingly, most solutions of the numerical optimization problem have displayed some consistent hierarchical structures. All solutions found violated some of the experimental constraints (dashed line in Fig. 1.3), which is probably based on the inaccuracy of some of the experimental results. Also, the connections indicated are not unidirectional. It is well established that a brain area that sends an axon to another brain area also receives back-projections from the structures it sends to. Such back-projections are often in the same order of magnitude as the forward projections. Interesting examples, not included in Fig. 1.3, are so-called corticothalamic loops. The subcortical

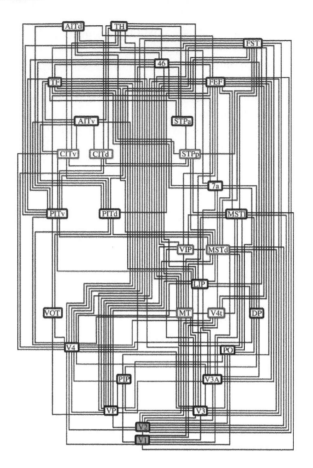

Fig. 1.3 Example of a map of connectivity between cortical areas involved in visual processing [reprinted with permission from C. Hilgetag, M. O'Neill, and M. Young, *Philosophical Transactions of the Royal Society of London B* 355: 71–89 (2000)].

structure called the thalamus was initially viewed as the major relay station through which sensory information projects to the cortex. However, it is becoming increasingly clear that the notion of a pure relay station is too simple as there are generally many more back-projections from the cortex to the thalamus compared to the forward projections between the thalamus and the cortex. Some estimates even indicate a number of back-projections that exceed the forward projections tenfold. The specific functional consequences of back-projections between the thalamus and the cortex as well as within the cortex itself are still not well understood. However, such structural features are consistent with reports of the influence of higher cortical areas on cell activities in primary sensory areas, for example, attentional effects in V1.

In the last decade there have been increasingly elaborate attempts to produce a more detailed wiring diagram of the brain, as so called connectome. One of the first full mapping of all neurons and connection has been done for a roundworm called Caenorhabditis elegans. This animal had therefore become one of the best-studied model systems in neuroscience. The European Blue Brain Project attempts to map the mouse brain, and there are also attempts to map the human brain. A visualization of white matter connections from 20 subjects is shown in Fig. 1.4

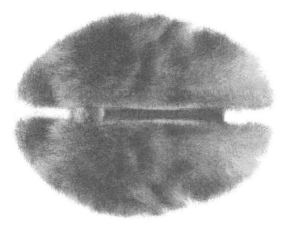

Fig. 1.4 Example of a group-level connectome of human white matter. [A. Horn, D. Ostwald, M. Reisert, F. Blankenburg (November 2014). *'The structural-functional connectome and the default mode network of the human brain'. NeuroImage* 102(1): 142-{51].

1.2.4 Rapid data transmission in the brain

From the system level view of the brain it seems that there are many stages of processing in the brain so that achieving even basic tasks like object recognition could take a considerable time. An good illustration of how quickly information can be transmitted through the brain is provided by the research of Simon Thorpe and colleagues. They showed that human subjects are able to discriminate the presence or absence of specific object categories, such as animals or cars, in visual scenes that are presented for very short times, as short as 20 ms. The percentage of correct manual responses, which consisted of releasing a button only when an animal was present in a complex image that was presented for 20 ms, is shown for 15 subjects in Fig. 1.5A plotted against the mean reaction time for each subject. The experiment shows some trade-off between reaction time and recognition accuracy, but the important point to note here is the high level of performance for such short presentations of the images.

The ability to recognize objects with these short presentation times is not the only astonishing result in these experiments. The authors also recorded skull EEGs during the experiments. The event-related potential, averaged over frontal electrodes, is shown in Fig. 1.5B, separated for image presentations with and without animals. The average response is not different for the first 150 ms, but becomes markedly different thereafter. The response of the frontal cortex therefore already indicates a correct answer after 150 ms. This is remarkable because for such categorization tasks we know that neural activity has to pass through several layers of brain areas. Each neuron in the processing stream necessary for the categorization path must thus be able to process and pass on information in time intervals of the order of only 10–20 ms or so.

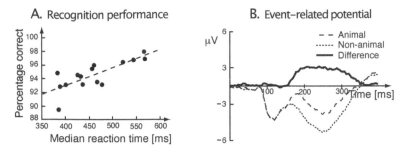

Fig. 1.5 (A) Recognition performance of 15 subjects who had to identify the presence of an animal in a visual scene (presented for only 20 ms) versus their mean reaction time. (B) Event-related potential averaged over frontal electrodes across the 15 subjects [redrawn from Thorpe, Fize, and Marlow, *Nature* 381: 520–2 (1996)].

1.2.5 The layered structure of neocortex

Staining of cell bodies or neurites reveals a generally layered structure of the neocortex, as illustrated in Fig. 1.6. We include here some brief comments on experimental staining techniques to clarify assumptions and limitations of such techniques, since these techniques are often crucial for estimating parameters on which models are based. Many different staining techniques can be used to identify neurons or parts thereof. Some staining techniques, such as the Nissl stain, colour only the cell body and cannot be used to investigate dendritic or axonal organizations. The Golgi stain, based on a silver solution, can be used to visualize more parts of the neuron than those accessible by Nissl staining. When viewing illustrations of such stained tissues it is important to know that only a small percentage of neurons, on the order of only 1–2%, are stained by the Golgi staining method, and different neurons can have different receptivities to this stain. The appearance of neocortical slices visualized by different staining techniques is illustrated in Fig. 1.6A.

In addition to these traditional dyes there is now a variety of other staining techniques including direct intracellular dye injections reaching most parts of a neuron, anterograde staining that utilizes dyes that are taken up by the cell body and transported down the axons, and retrograde staining that utilizes dyes that are taken up by the terminal endings of axons and transported back to the cell body. The former two staining techniques can be used to identify the projection range of neurons, and the latter is useful to highlight the neurons that project into a particular brain area. Mastering such techniques and applying them carefully to get estimates of neuronal populations and dendritic or axonal organizations is a specialization within neuroscience on which computational neuroscientists rely heavily in order to develop biologically faithful models.

Historically, the neocortex is divided into six layers labelled with Roman numerals from I to VI, although more than six layers, commonly 10 including the white matter, can be identified and are included into the historical labelling scheme by further subdivisions. Layer IV is thereby subdivided into IVA, IVB, and IVC, and layer IVC is further subdivided into layers IVCα and IVCβ. The extent, or thickness, of the layers varies throughout the neocortex up to a point where some layers are difficult to identify if not absent. Examples of stained slices from different areas within the

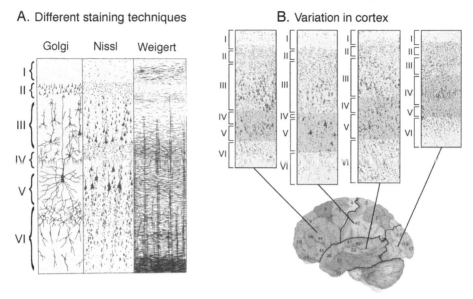

Fig. 1.6 Examples of stained neocortical slices showing the layered structure of the neocortex. (A) Illustration of different staining techniques [adapted from Heimer, *The human brain and the spinal cord*, Springer, 2nd edition (1995)]. (B) Different sizes of cortical layers in different areas [adapted from Kandel, Schwartz, and Jessell, *Principles of neural science*, McGraw-Hill, 4th edition (2000)].

neocortex are shown in Fig. 1.6B. The visual appearance in the stained slices defining the layers is dependent on different populations of cell bodies and neurites. Layer I is easily distinguishable as it is mainly lacking in cell bodies and consists mainly of neurites. The other layers are marked by the domination of different cell types.

The soma of several neuronal types can be found in each neocortical layer, although the distribution can be used to mark the layers to some extent. As mentioned above, layer I is nearly completely lacking in cell bodies and consists mainly of neurites. Pyramidal cells can be found in most other layers of the neocortex. Layers II and III consist predominantly of small pyramidal cells, although the cells in layer III tend to be larger than those in layer II. Stellate neurons seem, in particular, concentrated around layer IV. In the upper part of this layer (IVA and IVB) one can find a mixture of medium-sized pyramidal cells and stellate cells, whereas the deeper layer (layer IVC) seems to be dominated by stellate neurons. Large pyramidal cells are found predominantly in layer V. A variety of cell types can be found in the deepest layer, layer VI. This includes Martinotti cells and also cells that have elongated cell bodies and are sometimes used to mark this layer. Such cells are sometimes called fusiform neurons.

1.2.6 Columnar organization and cortical modules

The neuronal organization in the neocortex discussed so far is mainly based on anatomical evidence. There is, in addition, an important functional organization in the neocortex revealed by electrophysiological recordings. These experiments have shown that neurons in a small area of the cortex respond to similar features of an input stimulus. Hubel and Wiesel have investigated such organization in the primary visual (or striate) cortex. Neurons in this cortical area respond to visual bars moving in particular directions. More precisely, neurons in a small cortical column perpendicular to the layers and separated by around 30–100 μm respond to moving bars with a specific retinal position and orientation. These regions are called orientation columns. Separate from these arrangements are ocular dominance columns, cortical sections that respond preferentially to input from a particular eye (see Fig. 1.7A). The relations of orientation columns and ocular dominance columns are illustrated schematically in Fig. 1.7B. Neurons in small columns in other parts of the cortex also tend to respond to similar stimulus features. For example, cortical columns in the somatosensory cortex each respond to specific sensory modalities such as touch, temperature, or pain. The distribution of neurons with specific response characteristics is hence not purely random in the cortex, but there seems to be some form of organization.

A. Ocular dominance columns

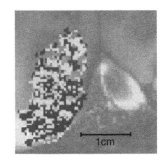

B. Relation between ocular dominance and orientation columns

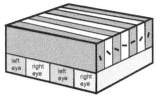

C. Topographic map of the visual field in primary visual cortex

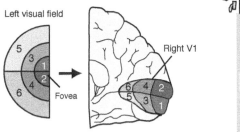

D. Somatosensory map

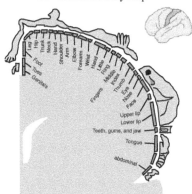

Fig. 1.7 Columnar organization and topographic maps in the neocortex. (A) Ocular dominance columns as revealed by fMRI studies [from K. Cheng, R.A. Waggoner, and K. Tanaka, *Human ocular dominance columns as revealed by high-field functional magnetic resonance imaging, Neuron* 32: 359–74, (2001)]. (B) Schematic illustration of the relation between orientation and ocular dominance columns. (C) Topographic representation of the visual field in the primary visual cortex. (D) Topographic representation of touch-sensitive areas of the body in the somatosensory cortex. [(C) and (D) adapted from Kandel, Schwartz, and Jessell, *Principles of neural science*, McGraw-Hill, 4th edition (2000).]

Hubel and Wiesel called a collection of orientation columns representing a complete set of orientations a hypercolumn. They showed that adjacent hypercolumns in the striate cortex respond to visual input from adjacent retinal areas as illustrated in Fig. 1.7C. Central regions of the visual field are represented by a larger cortical area than peripheral areas. The mapping between the visual field and the cortical representation is therefore not area-preserving; the central visual area is over-represented, a feature that is called cortical magnification. However, the map preserves the relationships between adjacent points but not the area. Such maps are commonly labelled as topographic in the related literature. We will use this term in a general sense, meaning any map of a feature space with some systematic relations between points (features) on the map. For example, a tonotopic map, which is a map of sound representations, is topographic when adjacent frequencies are represented at adjacent locations in the map. A hypercolumn itself is a topographic map as it contains an ordered representation of orientation, and there are many more examples of such maps in cortex and in subcortical areas. One other example is illustrated in Fig. 1.7D, that of the somatosensory cortex which represents tactile input from different body parts. This cortical area represents again more sensitive areas with larger cortical areas. Chapter 8 explores mechanisms that can explain how such cortical organization can be formed though experience.

It is conceptually important that neurons in a small areas of the cortex respond to similar sensory stimuli as we can use this to simplify models of cortical organization and functions. For many models in this book it is therefore sufficient to represent the neurons in a certain area as a single unit, as discussed further in Chapter 5. With such population neurons it is then much easier to explore various brain mechanisms, such as the formation of topographic organizations or the transformation of representations.

1.2.7 Connectivity between neocortical layers

The connectivity pattern within the layered structure of neocortex is becoming increasingly important for computational models. Neurons in layer IV seem to receive a particularly large number of afferents through the white matter from subcortical and other cortical areas. This layer is therefore often viewed as an input layer. Layer V has many large pyramidal cells with axons extending into the white matter. This layer seems therefore to contribute largely to the output of cortical processing. As the white matter is the main pathway between remote cortical areas and, in particular, between cortical and subcortical areas, it is obvious to suggest that the information flowing through the white matter is, to a large extent, responsible for global information transmission in the brain. In contrast, pyramidal cells in layers II and III are thought to be largely responsible for long-range cortico-cortical tangential (lateral) connections. Martinotti cells in the deep layers of the neocortex have axons extending into layer I. These could be responsible for information transfer between adjacent cortical modules from which pyramidal neurons in the upper layers receive synaptic input. Stellate neurons, on the other hand, seem to be more local in their neuritic sphere. The smooth stellate cells are therefore candidates for inhibitory interneurons. Their role in the stabilization of cortical processing is an important issue that we will discuss in later sections of this book.

An outline of connectivity patterns within a small column of the neocortex is

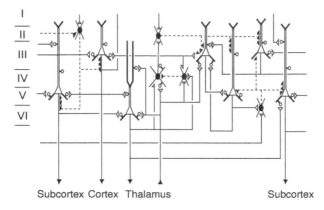

I
II
III
IV
V
VI

Subcortex Cortex Thalamus   Subcortex

Fig. 1.8 Schematic connectivity patterns between neurons in a cortical layer. Open cell bodies represent (spiny) excitatory neurons such as the pyramidal neuron and the spiny stellate neuron. Their axons are plotted with solid lines that end at open triangles that represent the axon terminal. The dendritic boutons are indicated by open circles. Inhibitory (smooth) stellate neurons have solid cell bodies and synaptic terminals, and the axons are represented by dashed lines [adapted from Douglas and Martin, in *Synaptic organization of the brain*, Shepherd (ed.), Oxford University Press (1990)].

summarized in Fig. 1.8. This scheme is, of course, only a rough approximation of the many details that are known experimentally. More detailed computational studies have still to be performed to understand the functional role of such organizations in more detail. An example of a model which incorporates laminar circuits is shown in Fig. 1.9. Grossberg and colleagues have now related such laminar models to many physiological and psychological findings, extending and unifying much of their earlier work. It is thereby interesting to note that, even on this level, cortical areas do not work in isolation. In the example shown it is important to consider the combined layered network of cortical area V1 and V2. Grossberg and collegaues showed that the deep layers (4–6) support thereby item storage, normalization of signals, and contrast enhancement, and that superficial layers (2/3) support grouping of information across processing channels, important factor in forming higher-order representations.

1.2.8 Cortical parameters

It is not feasible, and not a major scientific focus, to extract a detailed wiring diagram of the brain. Even an estimation of cortical parameters, such as the number of neurons in a cortical area, the number of connections and their physiological strength, the composition of an area with neuronal types, etc., is often not easy to extract experimentally. In addition, most of the experimental estimations can only be made for particularly favourable cases from which we have to generalize. The generalizations of such experimental studies are often obscured by considerable variations of such numbers within different cortical areas and between different species. Also, the estimation of such parameters varies considerably with different experimental techniques. You might therefore ask yourself how we can build biologically faithful network models of the brain without the necessary experimental support.

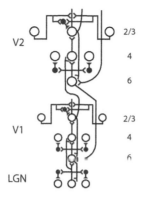

Fig. 1.9 Example of laminar model for the early visual system which attributes specific information processing abilities to the laminar circuits. [With permission from S. Grossberg, see Grossberg, *Spatial Vision* 12: 163–86 (1999).]

The answer is that we have to approach the study of brain networks from different angles. We will study in this book primarily general network architectures and study the general computational capabilities of such networks. These studies reveal, as we will see throughout the book, that many computational abilities of the networks do not depend critically on specific details and are hence present in a large variety of networks within certain classes. Furthermore, we will discuss mechanisms that guide the development and fine tuning of networks to achieve specific computational tasks. We therefore approach the study of the brain from the perspective of extracting general principles that guide the organization of the brain as well as revealing the computational consequences of classes of structurally related networks.

To explain brain functions we have, of course, to concentrate on the classes of networks that are consistent with brain networks. Predictions of models therefore have to be tested carefully with experiments on the real brain. Biologically faithful models can also be guided by experimental estimations of general cortical organization. In Table 1.1 we summarize some rough estimates of neocortical parameters that are good to be aware of when discussing biologically faithful network models. The values presented only indicate an order of magnitude, which is good to keep in mind when developing very general models, and we will see that it is already instructive to study models with some very crude approximations of cortical organization. More specific estimates for specific cortical areas that are modelled should, of course, be taken into account for more specific studies.

How much of the detail of neocortical organization is necessary to explain certain brain functions is difficult to assess and has to be considered for each specific question. Some specifics are certainly essential for very detailed explanations, while we can gain a lot of insight into some information-processing principles in the brain from very general organizational principles. There are also good reasons to believe that the brain itself has to work within general architectures in contrast to very detailed specific architectures coded, for example, genetically. A generally accepted hypothesis is that the brain architecture is based on genetically coded organizational principles on which self-organization mechanisms and experience-based learning act to fine-tune

Table 1.1 Some rough estimates of neocortical parameters [see for example Abeles, *Corticonics: neural circuits of the cerebral cortex*, Cambridge University Press (1991)]

Variable	Value
Neuronal density	40,000/mm^3
Neuronal composition:	
Pyramidal	75%
Smooth stellate	15%
Spiny stellate	10%
Synaptic density	8×10^8/mm^3
Synapses per neuron	1000–20,000
Distribution of synaptic types on pyramidal cell	
Inhibitory synapses	10%
Excitatory synapses from remote sources	45%
Excitatory synapses from local sources	45%
Asynchronous gain (relative synaptic efficiency)	0.003–0.2
Time duration of spike	$\sim$ 1 ms
Velocity of spike (myelinated axon of 0.02 mm diameter)	120 m/s
Length of axon	few mm to $\sim$ 1 m
Synaptic cleft	20 nm
Synaptic transmission delay due to diffusion	0.6 ms

the organization to achieve accurate and flexible behaviour.

1.3 What is a model?

Modelling is an integral part of many scientific disciplines, and neuroscience is no exception. The more complex a system is, the more we have to make simplifications and build example systems to provide insights into aspects of the complex system under investigation. The term 'model' appears frequently in many scientific papers, and describes a vast variety of constructs. Some papers present a single formula as a model, some papers fill several pages with computer code, and some describe with words a hypothetical system. We need to understand what a model is, and, in particular, what the purposes of models are.

It is important to distinguish a model from a hypothesis or a theory. Scientists develop hypotheses of the underlying mechanisms of a system that have to be tested against reality. In order to test a specific feature of a hypothesis, we build a model that can be evaluated. Sometimes we try to mimic real systems under artificial means, in order to be able to test the systems by different conditions, or to make measurements that would not be possible in a 'real' system. A model is hence a simplification of a system in order to test particular aspects of the system or hypothesis. A brief explanation of a model, which is useful to remember throughout this book and in research, is:

> A model is an abstractions of a real-world system to demonstrate particular
> features of, or investigate specific questions about, the system. Or, in more

scientific terms, a model is a quantification of a hypothesis to investigate the hypothesis.

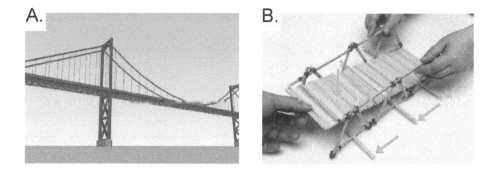

Fig. 1.10 (A) A computer model of a building which gives a three-dimensional impression of the design [image courtesy of 3dwarehouse.sketchup.com]. (B) A physical model of a bridge that can be used to test the statics [image courtesy of wikiHow.com].

A good example of this is the use of models in the field of architecture and structural engineering. Small-scale paper models of buildings, or computer graphics (Fig. 1.10) generated with sophisticated three-dimensional graphics packages, can be used to get a first impression of the physical appearance and aesthetic composition of a design. Or we can build a model to test some statics of a design. A model has a particular purpose attached to it and has to be viewed in this light. A model is not a recreation of the 'real' thing. The paper model of a house cannot be used to test the stability of the construction, a purpose for which a building engineer uses different models. In such models, it is important to scale down physical properties of the building materials regardless of the physical appearance, such as the colour of the building.

1.3.1 Phenomenological and explanatory models

In science, we typically represent experimental data in the form of graphs, and then seek to describe these data points with mathematical functions (Fig. 1.11). An example of this is the 'modelling' of response properties (tuning curves) of neurons in the lateral geniculate nucleus (LGN), which can be fitted with a specific class of functions called Gabor functions by adjusting the parameters of these functions. Gabor functions are therefore said to be 'models' of the receptive fields in the LGN. Of course, this phenomenological model does not tell us anything about the biophysical mechanisms underlying the formation of receptive fields and why cells respond in this particular way, so such a 'model' seems rather limited. Nevertheless, it can be useful to have a functional description of the response properties of LGN cells. Such parametric models are a shorthand description of experimental data that can be used in various ways. For example, if we want to study a model of the primary visual cortex, to which these cells project, then it is much easier to use the parametric form of LGN responses as input to the cortical model, rather than including further complicated models of the earlier visual pathway in detail.

As scientists, we want to find the roots of natural phenomena. The explanations

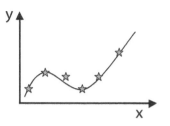

Fig. 1.11 The graph shows some data points, plotted with star symbols, such as data derived from experimental measurements. Also shown is a model represented by the line, and this curve fits the data reasonable well. The curve can be derived from a simple mathematical formula that fits the data points (phenomenological model), or result from more detailed models of the underlying system.

we are seeking are usually deeper than merely parameterizing experimental data with specific functions. Most of the models in this book are intended to capture processes that are thought of as being the basis of the information-processing capabilities of the brain. This includes models of single neurons, networks of neurons, and specific architectures capturing brain organizations. Models are used to study specific aspects of a hypothesis or theory, but can also help to interpret experimental data.

A major role of models in science is to illustrate principles underlying natural phenomena on a conceptual level. Sometimes the level of simplification and abstraction is so crude that scientist talk about toy models, although this terminology undermines slightly the importance of such models in science. The simplifications made in such models might be necessary to employ analytical methods to analyse such models at a depth that is not possible in more realistic models. The educational importance of these toy models should not be underestimated, in particular, in demonstrating principal mechanisms of natural phenomena. It is easy to complicate things, but the real scientific challenge is to simplify theoretical concepts.

The current state of neuroscience, often still exploratory in nature, frequently makes it difficult to find the right level of abstraction to properly investigate hypotheses. Some models in computational neuroscience have certainly been too abstract to justify claims derived from them. On the other hand, there is a great danger in keeping too many details that are not essential for the scientific argument. Models are intended to simplify experimental data, and thereby to identify which details of the biology are essential to explain particular aspects of a system. Modelling the brain is not a contest in recreating the brain in all its details on a computer. It is questionable how much more we would comprehend the functionality of the brain with such complex and detailed models. Models must be carefully constructed, and reasonable simplification is the result of careful scientific investigations and insight into natural processes. It is not always possible to justify all assumptions adequately, but it is important to at least clarify which assumptions have been made and to argue about them. The purpose of models is to better comprehend the functionality of complex systems, and simplicity should be a major guide in designing appropriate models. This philosophy is sometimes called the principle of parsimony, also known as Occam's razor. Basically, we want the model as simple as possible, while still capturing the main aspects of data that the model should capture. We will see this principle in action throughout this book, and discuss the issue specifically in conjunction with machine learning in Chapter 6.

1.3.2 Models in computational neuroscience

Where do we start when trying to explain brain functions? Do we have to re-build the brain in its entirety with computational techniques in order to understand it? Currently, many neuroscientists are collaborating in an ambitious project, called the Blue Brain Project, to implement in a computer, with as much detail as possible, neocortical circuits. This type of detailed project can show us which emergent phenomena can be expected in the brain, or where gaps in our knowledge require further investigation. However, even if it was be possible to simulate a whole brain on a computer, with all the details from biochemistry to large-scale organization, this would not explicitly mean that we have better explanations of brain functions. What we are looking for, at least in this book, is a better comprehension of brain mechanisms on explanatory levels. It is therefore important to learn about the art of abstraction, making suitable simplifications to a system without abolishing the important features we want to comprehend.

The level that is most appropriate for the investigation and explanatory abstraction depends on the scientific question. For example, epileptic seizures are known to be caused by synchronization of whole brain areas, and an understanding of brain dynamics on a systems level is important to comprehend such disorders. This should, of course, not exclude the search for causes on much smaller scales. We know that Parkinson's disease is caused by the death of dopaminergic neurons in the substantia nigra, and the role of dopamine in the initiation of motor actions is important to comprehend the full scale of impairments, and to develop better methods of coping with such conditions. The causes of the cell death of dopaminergic neurons are still not known, and it is important to find the reasons, possibly on a genetic level in this case, to enable a real treatment of Parkinson's disease. Therefore, various levels must be investigated, and we have to learn to make connections between the different levels in order to follow how the low-level circumstances, such as mechanisms on a genetic level or biochemical processes in neurons, can influence the characteristics of large-scale systems, such as behaviour of an organism.

1.4 Is there a brain theory?

It is often said that the brain is the most complex system that we know of in nature, and understanding how it works is a large, if not impossible, task. It is true that understanding how the brain works seems difficult when trying to reverse engineer it. However, reverse engineering a system can even be difficult for systems that we created in the first place. For example, imagine measuring the varying states of a transistor in a computer while the computer is running a word processor. Such measurements give important clues from which it should be possible to discover regularities when certain operations are repeated on the computer. Also, such measurements make it possible to discover important principles that must be at work in the digital computer system, such as the discrete nature of information representations. However, it seems a daunting task to recreate a computer program such as a word processor from these data, even if we were able to analyse a large number of measurements of many parts of the computer at the same time. The direct reverse engineering of the brain from data seems even more challenging, given the biological nature of the object. However, we can use the data to understand the principles of brain processing, and we can then use this knowledge to build brain-style information-processing systems. This approach is taken this book.

Correspondingly, there has been some shift in the research approach of the neuroscience community. The past decades have been an era in neuroscience marked by a flood of explorations. Recordings with micro-electrodes from single cells contributed significantly to this exploration, and searching for response properties of neurons is at least as exciting as it must have been for explorers such as Marco Polo to discover new lands. New brain-imaging techniques, such as functional magnetic resonance imaging (fMRI), make it possible to monitor living brains of subjects performing specific mental tasks. Explorations of brain functions with such techniques have been essential in advancing our knowledge in neuroscience. However, while a mountain of data has been gathered for brain functions, using a multitude of techniques, we are now slowly entering a new phase in neuroscience, that of formulating more quantitative hypotheses of brain functions. This shift in the focus of neuroscience research demands some more specific experimental analysis and more dedicated tests of such hypothesis. It is increasingly important to formulate a quantitative hypotheses, and possible alternatives, in such a way that the hypothesis can be tested experimentally.

This new era of neuroscience sounds a lot like quantitative scientific areas such as chemistry or physics, and while a quantitative analysis will generate new breakthroughs in our understanding of brain functions, the ultimate question is if there can be a brain theory. We could take the position that in order to understand the brain we need to understand all of the structural details and the current state of a particular brain. This is no different in other scientific areas such as physics. For example, to completely describe the physics of an individual aeroplane we have to know the precise location and form of each nut and bolt and all other structural details up to the amount of dirt on the wings and the details of the air it is flying through. Another example is that of a pot of boiling water, which consists of a lot of individual molecules in a very dynamic state. Measuring all the microscopic details in the last two examples seems impossible. Yet, we have a fairly good understanding of the process of boiling water and why an aeroplane can fly. This was not possible overnight but is the result of dedicated scientific research over the past few centuries. Important for the success in physics, chemistry, and other scientific disciplines, was the realization of the right level of description or the right level of abstraction of a problem. For example, we learned to describe the average behaviour of the molecules in an ideal gas, which gave us the fundamentals of thermodynamics and ultimately led to a better understanding of the mechanisms of flowing air that enables engineers to construct more efficient aeroplane. We know today about the essential quantum nature of atomic and subatomic interactions, but a description of Mount Everest on this level is not reasonable. There are geological theories of mountain formation that are more appropriate than employing quantum theory to these questions.

There is no reason to conjecture that the brain cannot be tractable with similar scientific rigour to that developed in other disciplines. The brain is certainly more complex than a gas of weakly interacting atoms. However, there are very fundamental questions that we can attack; for example, how a network stores memories that can be recalled in an associative way. Indeed, we have made considerable progress with this question, considering our understanding of associative networks discussed in this book. Another fundamental question is why the brain is relatively stable, while still being able to adapt to novel environments. Brain theories of this kind are now emerging, and some of these theories will be discussed in this book. It may be too early to talk about a single brain theory, but there is no reason to suspect that theories will advance our understanding of brain functions. Indeed, I think that major breakthroughs have already been made, which need to be brought to a wider audience. The goal of this book is to contribute to this endeavour.

1.4.1 Emergence and adaptation

Standard computers, such as PCs and workstations, have one or more central processors. Each processor is rather complex, with specialized hardware and microprograms implementing a variety of functions, such as loading data into registers, adding, multiplying, and comparing data, as well as communicating with external devices. These basic functions can be executed by instructions, which are binary data loaded into a special interpreter module. Complicated data processing can be achieved by writing, often lengthy, programs, which are instructions representing a collection of the basic processor functions. When solving a task with a computer, we have to instruct the machine to follow precisely all the steps that we determined beforehand would solve a particular problem. The sophistication of computers basically reflects the ingenuity of the programmer.

In contrast, information processing in the brain is very different in several respects. The brain employs simpler processing elements than computers, but lots of them. To explore information processing in networks of neurons, we will mainly use very simple abstractions of real neurons, which we call nodes to stress this drastic simplification. These fundamental processing units can be implemented in hardware, or simulated on a standard computer; for the discussions in this book this does not make a difference. We keep the functionality of nodes as simple as possible for the sake of employing lots of them, typically hundreds, thousands, or even more. The usage of many parallel working processors has motivated the term parallel distributed processing in this area. However, with this term one is tempted to think that the processes are independent because only processes that are independent can be processed on different processors in parallel. In contrast to this, a major ingredient of information processing in the brain is the interaction of neurons, and the interaction of neurons is accomplished by assembling them into large networks.

It is the interaction of nodes that enables processing abilities not present in single nodes. Such capabilities are good examples of emergent properties in rule-based systems. Emergence is the single most defining property of neural computation, distinguishing it from parallel computing in classical computer science, which is mainly designed to speed up processing by distributing independent algorithmic threads. Interacting systems can have unique properties beyond the mere multiplication of single processor capabilities. It is these types of abilities we want to explore and utilize with neural networks. These system properties are labelled as emergent to stress that we did not encode these properties directly into the system. To better appreciate this, we distinguish the description of a system on two levels, the level of basic rules defining the system, and the level of description aimed at understanding the consequences of such rules. In the study of neural networks we are interested in understanding the consequences of interacting nodes.

Scientific explanations were dominated in the past by the formulation of a set of principles and rules that govern a system. A system can be defined by a set of rules, like in a game. In science, we assume that natural systems are governed by a finite set of rules. The search for these basic rules, or fundamental laws as they are called in this case, was the central scientific quest for centuries. It is not easy to determine such laws, but enormous progress has been made nevertheless. Newton's laws defining classical mechanics, or the Maxwell equations of electromagnetism are beautiful examples of fundamental laws in nature. We do not have a theory of the brain on this level, and some have argued that we might never find a simple set of rules explaining brain functions. However, in many scientific disciplines we are beginning to realize that even with a given set of rules we might still not have a sufficient understanding of the underlying systems. This is analogous to the idea that knowing the rules of the card game Bridge is not sufficient to be a good Bridge player.

Rules define a system completely, and it can therefore be argued that all the properties of a system are encoded in the rules. However, we have to realize that even a small set of rules can generate a multitude of behaviours of the systems, which might be difficult to understand from the basic rules due to the presence of emergent properties. A different level of description might then be more appropriate. For example, thermodynamics can describe appropriately the macroscopic behaviour of systems of many weakly interacting particles, even though the systems are governed by other microscopic rules. On the other hand, there are emergent properties in Newtonian systems that are not well described by classical thermodynamics, such as turbulent fluids. A deeper understanding of emergent properties is becoming a central topic in the science of the twenty-first century.

The importance of emergent properties in networks of simple processing elements is not the only extension of traditional information-processing approaches that we think are crucial for understanding brain functions. Another important ingredient is that the brain is an example of an adaptive system. In our context, we define adaptation as the ability of a system to adjust its response to external stimuli in dependence of the environment states and the expectations of the system. Humans are a good example of systems that have mastered adaptive abilities and learning. Adaptation and learning is an area that has attracted a lot of interest in the engineering community. The reason for this is that learning systems, which are systems that are able to change their behaviour based on examples in order to solve information-processing demands, have the potential to solve problems where traditional algorithmic methods have not been able to produce sufficient results. Adaptation has two major virtues. One is, as just mentioned, the promise to solve information-processing problems for which explicit algorithms are not yet known. A second virtue is our aim to build systems that can cope with continuously changing environments. A lot of research in the area of neural networks is dedicated to the understanding of learning. Engineering applications of neural networks are not bound by biological plausibility. In contrast to this, we concentrate in this book on biologically plausible learning mechanisms that can help us to comprehend the functionality of the brain.

1.4.2 Levels of analysis

David Marr and Tomaso Poggio realized the usefulness of distinguishing between different levels of description when explaining processes, which Marr later explains beautifully in his posthumously published book *Vision*. One issue that Marr raised in his book was that different people need different kinds of explanations. Explanations of brain functions that are satisfactory for a non-specialist can be insufficient for a physiologist or psychologist who is trying to make sense of specific observations in his or her expriments. A computer engineer may require different types of explanations of brain functions again, to be able to implement specific information-processing algorithms. Marr also stressed the difference between understanding computers and understanding computation. Knowing how bits are represented and transformed in a computer is far from understanding high-level applications such as the World Wide Web.

Besides these important considerations for any explanatory theory, Marr made an important distinction between different levels of analysis. These are summarized in Marr's book as:

1. **Computational theory:** What is the goal of the computation, why is it appropriate, and what is the logic of the strategy by which it can be carried out?
2. **Representation and algorithm:** How can this computational theory be implemented? In particular, what is the representation for the input and output, and what is the algorithm for the transformation?
3. **Hardware implementation:** How can the representation and algorithm be realized physically?

The most abstract and general level, that of a computational theory, is concerned with what a process is trying to achieve, and what the principal approach to the solution is. In his book, Marr discusses the example of a cash register, which is adding up the price of goods brought to the checkout counter. This explanation answers the question of what the cash register is doing, but we need also to ask why the cash register is doing it (adding the numbers) in this specific way. The answer to this question is that the rules of adding numbers, rather than multiplying them, encapsulates what we think is appropriate for this process; that prices of individual goods should just add up, independent, for example, of the order in which the goods are presented. Marr assigns great importance to this level and explains in his book:

> To phrase the matter in another way, an algorithm is likely to be understood more readily by understanding the nature of the problem being solved than by examining the mechanism (and hardware) in which it is embodied.

Having a clear theory of what the brain, or specific brain processes, are trying to accomplish can be a powerful research guide and needs to be considered more in neuroscientific research.

The next level of description is concerned with how the computation, specified on the computational level, is realized on an algorithmic level. Marr considered brain research as an information-processing problem, and he clearly was aware of the duality between representing and processing information. That is, in order to process information, this information has first to be represented in a specific form. For example, numbers can be represented in binary form or with Roman numbers. Representations are important since the specific algorithm used for implementing a process usually depends on the representation. Many different representations are possible, and there are usually many algorithms for each type of representation which can accomplish the task. Different representations can drastically influence algorithms, and different algorithms can have quite different properties, such as robustness or efficiency. Theories in computational neuroscience have strongly focused on representations, on which specific algorithms are built. It should also be mentioned that there are examples that use the arguments in the opposite direction, such as deriving representations from constraints on algorithms, such as robustness. Clearly, the brain must use specific representations, and specific algorithms, and it is the goal of computational neuroscience to help find them.

As a side note, in the definition of this representational and algorithmic level, Marr speaks specifically of input and output representations, and the process of transforming, or mapping, input to output. We will soon discuss why this mapping view is not adequate for brain functions. In a later section of his book, Marr discusses the difficulty in finding invariant features from changing data. This is an example that is difficult in a mapping framework but which can be resolved easily in the computational theory of the brain presented below. But this criticism should not distract from the importance of this level of explanation.

The third level of Marr's scheme is concerned with the physical realization of the algorithms and representation. This is the level to which neuronal biophysics and physiology can speak most directly. Again, there might be several possible physical realizations of a specific algorithm, and we want to understand the physical realizations in the brain. This level of explanation does not only back up the level of explanations above, but is also important in its own right for specific interventions. The different levels are weakly related, and inspiration and constrains from different levels of analysis can guide research on other levels.

Since this book is intended to be an introductory guide, we follow mainly a bottom-up approach, through learning first about some physical properties of the nervous system, how information is represented in the brain, and some algorithmic theories of solving specific problems. A broad knowledge of such issues is necessary for any advanced work in neuroscience. However, as Marr suggested, it is important to guide research more specifically through computational theories. We therefore outline in the following section a broad computational theory of the brain to which we return in more detail in the final chapter.

1.5 A computational theory of the brain

1.5.1 Why do we have brains?

One of the first questions we might want to ask is why we have a brain at all. While this question has likely been asked and answered in many different ways, the take of Daniel Wolpert is particularly illuminating. Wolpert studies sensorimotor control; how brains are able to supervise appropriate movements in a complex sensory world. He notes that plants live stable lives without a brain and he also tells the story of a little sea creature, called the sea squirt, which is hatched with a small nervous system and swims through the ocean until it settles down on some rock, after which it digests its brain. Hence, it seems that animals need a brain to move.

We can go further and ask why we want to move and why it seems that increasingly complex brains are developed even though we there are much simpler creatures that move. Moving around can help to find food and sexual partners to enable survival of its species and to make evolutionary progress. Mathematically, we view this as maximizing an objective function. With this view, we can imagine that nervous systems developed into more and more sophisticated systems that help to achieve the evolutionary objectives of moving organisms. The human brain is thereby, arguably, the most developed example of such evolved systems, even inventing machines to travel. Thus, a more formal answer to what the brain is doing might be:

> The brain produces goal-directed behaviour to maximize our probability of survival.

If individual brains exist to maximize the organism's survival capacity, then why could it happen that a teenager gets drunk and falls off a cliff? The reason is that maximizing survival probability acts on a population, not on an individual level. The brain implements a specific strategy for each individual, which itself may not be perfect but necessary to explore new solutions. Experimenting with the unknown is essential for finding new, and ultimately better, solutions, so that the adventurous behaviour of a teenager can ultimately help our society.

1.5.2 The anticipating brain

In order for the brain to produces goal-directed behaviour to maximize our probability of survival, or in short, for the brain to make good decisions, we argue that there are two principle strategies. One is to build a reactive system that learns from previous rewards in the environment. Such habitual learning and decision-making is widespread in adaptive agents including humans. If we touch a hot stove we learn fast to avoid this in the future without deliberative effort. Such a system is central in fast decision-making and is sometimes called System 1.

The other strategy, that of system 2, is to build a model of the world that can be used to calculate good decisions. Such a deliberative system is of course much more complex and requires a much more elaborate information-processing system. Such a system is likely much more complex to learn, and decisions have to be calculated and therefore require more mental effort and are likely more time consuming. However, a huge advantage is that such a system is able to generalize better to more novel situations with causal relations.

Both systems must be able to function with uncertainties. This is important as the real world has either hidden causes or is too complex to comprehend or too difficult to sense in all its details. We will encounter more concrete discussions of the different decision systems in Chapter 11, and we stress some of the probabilistic underpinnings throughout the book. Here we outline some important ingredients for building both systems and the view of the brain as an anticipatory decision system.

Mechanistically, we can start describing brain as a decisions system that senses the world and then produce appropriate actions to achieve some objectives. In a sensorimotor sense, this would be to ask how a agent can produce goal directed movements that enables a creature to react to specific environmental situations. The brain helps in this task by analysing sensory representations of the environment and mapping them to appropriate motor actions. We will show in Chapter 7 that feedforward neural networks can learn very complex mapping functions. The study of sensory-motor mappings has been important in neuroscientific investigations. However, rather than concentrating on fairly direct response functions, our aim in this book is to understand sophisticated human actions enabled by the brain, and ultimately the entire human mind. The central thesis outlined here is that sophisticated human thought processes cannot be achieved by simple feedforward mapping systems, but require sophisticated feedback systems.

To illustrate the importance of feedback systems further, let us take a concrete example. Imagine that we go into a concert hall to listen to a symphony. After entering the concert hall, we easily recognize that there are chairs. These chairs certainly look different to chairs at home, but people usually have no problem recognizing them as chairs, even in a very brief moment. One can do this even with very brief image presentations. We discussed already above studies by Simon Thorpe who showed that visual stimuli of very short duration, are enough to enable the categorization of some of the content of visual stimuli. How is this possible?

Visual scene analysis is quite challenging from a information-processing percep-tive. The human eye contains around 130 million photoreceptors, so that a visual snapshot on the retina would have 15 MB (megabytes) of data, and this is if we only consider binary responses of each photoreceptor. While this is roughly the magnitude of modern digital cameras, it is puzzling that we cannot achieve any comparable scene analysis with modern computer systems, despite the fact that computers are more than a million times faster; a computer can easily compute several billion instructions per second, or one instruction in less than a nanosecond (ns), which is very fast compared to the millisecond (ms) time scale of a neuron. The often-suggested answer, that the brain is a large parallel computer, is not sufficient, since only a small number of steps can be processed in the brain in a reasonable time between sensation and perception/response. For example, a common guide for neural processing time is around 10 ms per synaptic stage, such that only 10 to 100 processing steps can be assumed for a task in which humans form percepts or start reacting to stimuli. The problem is that we don't know an algorithm that can work with so few steps. Even basic steps in traditional image processing, such as segmenting an image to separate objects from the background, can take thousands of computational steps.

How, then, can the fast perception of the brain be achieved? Our thesis here is that fast perception can only be achieved though advanced knowledge, and that the human brain functions as a predictive or anticipatory memory system. In short, the idea is that we already have a rich knowledge of our commonly encountered environment, and that we can extrapolate this knowledge quickly to individual circumstances. Thus, the brief version of our computational theory can be outlined as:

> The brain is an anticipating memory system that learns to represent expectations
> of the world, which can be used to generate goal-directed behaviour.

For example, people generally know about objects such as chairs and possibly con-cert halls. Thus, when entering the concert hall, the analysis of the visual scene becomes tractable. Central to this thesis is that the brain implements some form of top-down processing, in addition to bottom-up processing for acquiring environmental evidence. We will discuss some bottom-up systems, as described by feedforward networks, also called perceptrons, that can capture some form of object recognition. However, we will also argue that this form is insufficient to explain human-like information-processing. The brain is not like most machines that simply react predictably to external commands, it is a more sophisticated system with an internal dynamics that can interact with the environment. For this we need top-down processing and an active engagement of the system with the environment. This makes the brain dependent on its history and current states.

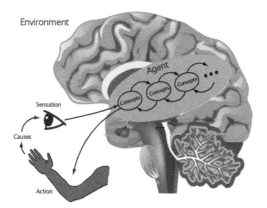

Fig. 1.12 Basic outline of a high-level model of the brain describing a fundamental hypothesis of brain processing as an active, anticipatory, hierarchical memory system.

An outline of some important components of such an anticipating system is shown in Fig. 1.12. It is essential that the agent acts in an environment through sensations and actions. Causes in the environment, such as objects or sequences of events, cause specific sensations for organism. These sensations activate learned representations in a hierarchical organization within the organism. While the first level of processing is aimed at closely matching peripheral sensations, each additional level is trained to represent increasingly abstract concepts learned from the environment by minimizing the prediction error at each level. Such a layered hierarchical representation is often called deep. Concepts are learned, and self-organize, through actions that the organism takes in the environment.

While concepts on different levels can change over time, activations of higher-level concepts will also influence expectations of activating specific lower-level concepts. The anticipating system tries to match sensations through activating appropriate concepts on different hierarchical levels. This anticipation of sensations via top-down influences is crucial for the operational capabilities of organisms. Such anticipation can solve the time constraints in perception mentioned above, since not all information has to be processed bottom-up to activate the hypothesis of which objects are in the environment. The complexity of perception is solved by learning during development. The concepts can be modified on an ongoing basis through minimizing the expectation error of sensory experiences and corresponding internal activation. This is the concept of predictive coding. Karl Friston summarized these ideas in the free energy principle.

The brain is thereby viewed as a model of the world in form of a density function, and minimizing the difference between this model density and the real world is a variational free energy in the information theoretic sense. Such high-level theories of the brain are important to comprehend the bigger picture.

While most of our discussion in this book will touch mainly on the basic mechanisms and principles, one can go further and consider active learning. It is important for the development of an anticipating organism to act in its environment. For example, objects can be touched and rotated to verify whether concepts activated by initial sensations conform with the additional information. This active hypothesis testing can dramatically reduce the learning problem by focusing on relevant data. Organisms can actively explore the environment, which is crucial in forming concepts in the brain. Thus, the action–perception loop outlined in Fig. 1.12 is an integral part of understanding the mind as stressed by the embedded cognition community.

1.5.3 Deep sparse predictive coding and the uncertain brain

In the last several years there has been a surge of breakthroughs in the area of machine learning, which can be considered to be a subarea of Artificial Intelligence (AI). The biggest recent breakthroughs are thereby based on deep learning which is basically the application of feedforward neural networks with many layers or recurrent neural networks with gated memories. These techniques have opened a lot of technical applications, and they also shed light on theoretical questions of building predictive leaning machines. This area is therefore a rich source for theoretical underpinnings of the neuroscience of adaptive systems. There are now a lot of resources for studying this rapidly expanding field, and I have refrained from delving too deep into this to keep the focus on the relation with brain and cognitive processing. Such deep networks are not equivalent to a brain. However, they encapsulate aspects of brain processing that have been recognized to fill important roles in brain processing. We want to summarize here some of them from the outset to keep the further discussions focused.

Central to the success of deep learning models is their ability to learn from many data hierarchical representations of mapping sensory representations to higher-level concepts. This is certainly an important aspect to consider when discussing brain structures and tasks that have to be mastered by the brain. Due to the availability of some very large labelled data sets, in particular ImageNet, it was possible to demonstrate that such deep networks can learn to achieve high performance in visual recognition tasks. While this demonstration has sparked new technical applications, for us this is important as it demonstrates the general ability and challenges of large hierarchical networks. Interestingly, deep networks have also been shown to correlate with a lot of aspects of hierarchical visual representation in the brain. The principle of hierarchical representational learning is therefore an important principle for neuroscience.

Of course, when comparing a specific machine learning network with the brain beyond the principle insight of representational learning, a well-recognized challenge is that the real world is much more complex and that we humans can learn with far less samples compared to such supervised learning models. Furthermore, it is also well recognized that the flexibility of a human mind is far superior to machine learning solutions that are generally very specialized to specific tasks such as giving an image a label. There is now a lot of recent progress in understanding how self-supervised learning can eliminate the need for large labelled data. Recent self-supervised representational learning methods are built around the idea of training a deep network on variations of samples. This idea of learning to minimize prediction errors in the networks representation resembles somewhat the predictive coding idea which we will elaborate later. In this discussion it will also be central that the learned representations and resulting brain activity is sparse. Sparse coding is therefore another principle that has been advanced for many years in neuroscience.

Much of the book looks into the mechanistic realization of a world model in the brain. This includes how neurons can generate spikes and how such spikes can be used to process information and change synaptic efficacies that are thought to physically realize learning. This includes also the organization and information processing in neural networks such as the representational learning discussed so far. This approach can currently say less to the description of the mind with its ability of symbolic processing. This domain of cognitive science is a whole other level of modelling the brain. While a detailed treatment of cognitive models is beyond the scope of this book, we will discuss some fundamentals that might be able to bridge this gap between symbolic and subsymbolic brain processes.

Discussing some fundamentals of some form of symbolic reasoning, it is important to include from the beginning another aspect of modelling the world that seems to be another fundamental principle to be included in theories of the brain. This aspect and challenge for the brain is that of uncertainty in the world. It thereby does not matter if there are fundamental stochastic processes that cannot be predicted (irreducible indeterminacy), or the uncertainty represents limitation of observations or hidden processes (epistemological limitations). Sensory measurements can be uncertain for many reasons. A big factor is that sensory representations of an object in the world might be ambiguous due to similarities between objects. And sensors are also changing with time so that the same object can elicit different responses. Many processes in nature, including brain processes, are inherently noisy. This is reflected by the fact that the outcomes of repeated measurements are often fluctuating. Regardless of the origin of uncertainty, the introduction of the mathematical construct of random variables, and the corresponding formal system of probability theory, was a major advancement in science and a useful language for theoretical neuroscience.

If we accept that probabilistic modelling is essential for advanced models that we believe the brain represents, there is one final principle that we want to highlight as important for further progress in understanding the brain and maybe even advancing machine learning itself. This principle is causal modelling. It is clear that a lot of human reasoning has some form of structure that we perceive as causal. Causality is traditionally not well represented in probability theory, which has often focused on applications of correlations. We will argue that building causal model are superior to more general probabilistic models. Such models can be formalized with Bayesian causal models that we will briefly introduce in Chapter 12. Those models often start based on symbolic entities that represent semantic knowledge, and bridging the gap between learning semantic knowledge and causal reasoning is an area of current scientific debates.

2   Scientific programming with Python

Python is the programming language that we use to illustrate a lot of the concepts discussed in this book. Python is a high-level programming language, and we will use this strictly as a scientific tool. We will be walking through a program that contains most of the commands and constructs used in this book.

2.1   The Python programming environment

This brief introduction to scientific programming with Python puts the emphasis on mathematical operations used in this book. This includes working with vectors and matrices based on the NumPy library. Python is a high-level programming language similar to Matlab and R that has gained increasing popularity. The main reason we use Python in this book is that it is freely available and now provides considerable support for an increasing number of areas such as machine learning, statistics, computer vision, and psychophysics. We assume some familiarity with programming concepts and concentrate on a quick introduction to the specific environment and supporting libraries used in this book.

The programs in this book are based on Python 3, and we assume that all relevant packages are installed. At this point we need the NumPy and the Matplotlib libraries as well as a programming environment such as `Jupyter` or `Spyder`. Comprehensive documentation and tutorials for Python and related tools are available at `https://www.python.org`.

We start here using a programming environment called Jupyter. More specifically, we will be using the Jupyter Notebook in this chapter that allows us to write code with a simple editor and display comments and outputs in the same file. Jupyter is accessed through the browser and contains form fields in which code and comments can be added. These fields can then be executed and the feedback from print commands or figure plots are displayed after each block within the same document. This makes it very useful in documenting brief code and small exercises. An example program in the Jupyter environment is shown on the left in Fig. 2.1.

Jupyter files have the extension `.ipynb` that can be loaded in the browser environment. The Jupyter notebook program has an interface to launch the Python interpreter and to run individual sections or all the code. The header with comments is produced by executing a text cell. This is useful to produce some documentations. Also, the notebook can be distributed with the output that can facilitate communications about code. The numbers on the left shows a consecutive number of calls to the interpreter. In the shown example, the first program cell was run first to load the libraries, and then the second cell was run twice; this is why a [3] is displayed in front of this cell.

Fundamentals of Computational Neuroscience. Third edition. Thomas P. Trappenberg,
Oxford University Press. © Oxford University Press 2023. DOI: 10.1093/oso/9780192869364.003.0002

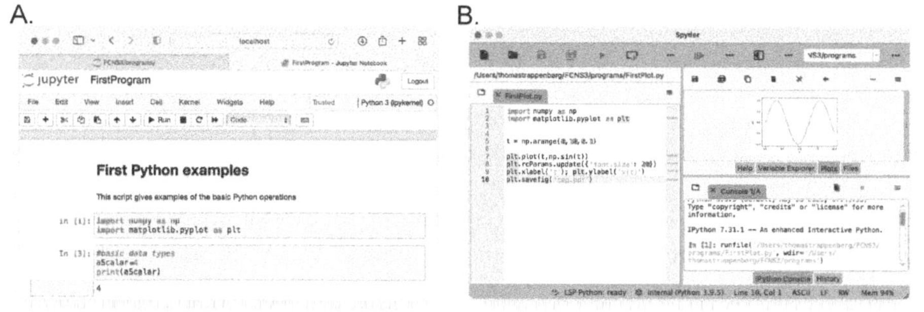

Fig. 2.1 (A) An example of a Python program within the Jupyter notebook and (B) the Spyder programming environment.

When the program is running, an [∗] is displayed. The second cell produces the output 4, which is displayed after the cell.

In later sections we simply provide the python programs as .py files. It is then easier to use other programming environments of your choice, including copying the code into a Jupyter notebook. An example of a more advanced environment with more traditional programming support is Spyder. This tool includes an editor, a command window, and further programming support such as displays of variables and debugging support. This program mimics more traditional programming environment such as the ones found in Matlab and R. An example view of Spyder is shown on the right in Fig. 2.1. On the left in this environment is the editor window that contains a syntax-sensitive display to write the programs, and on the bottom right is the console to launch line commands such as executing and interpreting the code. The example program plots a sine curve, which is also displayed. As Python is an interpreted language, it is possible to work with the programs in an interactive way, such as running a simulation and than plotting results in various ways. The Spyder development environment is recommended for bigger projects.

2.2 Basic language elements

2.2.1 Basic data types and arrays

As a general purpose programming language, Python contains basic programming concepts such as basic data types, loops, conditional statements, and subroutines. We will briefly review the associated syntax with examples that are provided in file FirstProgram.ipynb. In addition to such basic programming constructs, all high-level programming languages such as Python are supported by a large number of libraries that enable a wide array of programming styles and specialized functions. We are here mainly interested in basic scientific computing, in contrast to system programming, and for this we need multidimensional arrays. We therefore base almost all programs in this book on the NumPy library. NumPy provides basic support of common scientific constructs and functions such as trigonometric functions and random number generators. Most importantly, it provides support for N-dimensional arrays. NumPy has become the standard in scientific computing with Python. We will use this well-established constructs to implement vectors, matrices and higher dimensional arrays. We sometimes also use the SciPy library which builds on the NumPy library with more scientific functions such as numerical integration routines and statistics.

An established way to import the NumPy library in our programs is to map them to the name space 'np' with the command `import numpy as np`. In this way, the specific methods or functions of NumPy are accessed with the prefix `np`. In addition to importing NumPy, we always import a plotting library as plotting results will be very useful and a common way to communicate results. We specifically use the popular PyPlot package of the Matploitlib library. Hence, we nearly always start our program with the two lines

Listing 2.1 FirstProgram.ipynb (part 1)

```
1  import numpy as np
2  import matplotlib.pyplot as plt
```

Let us walk through the program in the Jupyter environment called `FirstProgram`. These lines of code are intended to show the syntax of the basic programming constructs that we need in this book. We start by demonstrating the basic data types that we will be using frequently. We are mainly concerned with numerical data, of which a scalar is the simplest example,

Listing 2.2 FirstProgram.ipynb (part 2)

```
1  # basic data types
2  aScalar = 4
3  print(aScalar)
```

>> 4

We here show the code as well as the response of running the program with the `print()` function. Comment lines can be included with the hash-tag symbol #. The type of the variables are dynamically assigned in Python. That is, a variable name and corresponding memory space is allocated the first time a variable with this name is used on the left-hand side of an assignment operator '='. In this case it is an interger value, but we could also assign a real-valued variable with `aScalar=4.0`.

Most of the time we will be working on a large collection of data so that we need a concept to access the data collection. In Python, there are several forms of lists. For example, a basic one-dimensional list is given in the basic Python stack by enclosing a comma-separated list in square brackets such as

Listing 2.3 FirstProgram.ipynb (part 3)

```
1  aList = [1,2,3]
2  print(aList)
```

>> [1, 2, 3]

Such lists are useful for collecting data. However, since we need to perform well-defined mathematical operations on lists of data, it is useful to introduce a more versatile construct of such data collections in forms of a NumPy array.

Before proceeding, it might be good to review some of the naming conventions. A basic data structure for a collection of data is called an 'array' in computer science. In contrast to these simple data structure concepts, the mathematical concepts of a vector or matrix are different in that they include well-defined mathematical operations on these data structures. Thus, the mathematical concept of a vector is a one-dimensional array on which some operations are defined, such as adding two vectors with the same dimension by adding their components, or multiplying a vector with a scalar by multiplying each component of the vector with a scalar. Similar, a matrix is a two-dimensional construct with correspondingly defined operation. We can even generalize this to higher dimensions, and such mathematical constructs are called tensors. It is convenient to view a vector or matrix operation just as a special case of the general tensor operations.

To create a NumPy array we use the NumPy function `array()`. For example, a 1-dimensional Python list can be turned into a NumPy vector like,

Listing 2.4 FirstProgram.ipynb (part 4)

```
1  aVector = np.array([1,2,3])
2  print(aVector)
3  print(aVector[0], aVector[-1])
4  print(aVector[1:3])
```

```
>> [1 2 3]
   1 3
   [2 3]
```

As shown in the second print statement, we can access an element of the array with indices in square brackets. The first element in an array has the index 0. Hence, the print command returns the value 1. It is useful to think about this index as the offset from the first element. The index -1 accesses the last element in the vector. The third print command shows how to access a range of indices. Unfortunately, there is no distinction between a row vector and a column vector in NumPy, so this needs some more careful considerations when a distinction is necessary. We return to this point in a moment.

Similar to defining a vector with NumPy, a two-dimensional array with the appropriate definition of mathematical operations is called a matrix and can be defined and accessed with NumPy like,

Listing 2.5 FirstProgram.ipynb (part 5)

```
1  aMatrix = np.array([[1,2,3],[4,5,6]])
2  print(aMatrix)
3  print(aMatrix[1,2])
```

```
>> [[1 2 3]
   [4 5 6]]
   6
```

The notation indicates that a two-dimensional array is considered in the Python syntax as a one-dimensional list of one-dimensional lists. Note how individual array elements are accessed; the first index specifies the position in the column, and the second index specifies the position in the row. This is equivalent to the common mathematical notation for matrices. With this we can revise the notation for the vectors above by defining a row vector as

Listing 2.6 FirstProgram.ipynb (part 6a)

```
1  aVector = np.array([[1,2,3]])
```

This can then be converted into a column vector with the help of the transpose operation

Listing 2.7 FirstProgram.ipynb (part 6b)

```
1  print(aVector.T)
```

```
>> [[1]
    [2]
    [3]]
```

After defining such NumPy arrays we can apply mathematical function on these NumPy arrays. For example, some element-wise operations on matrices are

Listing 2.8 FirstProgram.ipynb (part 7)

```
1  matrix2 = np.array([[5,5,6],[7,8,9]])
2  result1 = aMatrix * matrix2   # element-wise
3  result2 = aMatrix ** 3   # element-wise exponentiation:
4  result3 = aMatrix > 3   # find the indices where (matrix > 3)
5  print(result1,result2,result3)
```

```
>> [[ 5 10 18]
    [28 40 54]]
   [[ 1 8 27]
    [ 64 125 216]]
   [[False False False]
    [ True True True]]
```

A basic matrix multiplication, also called a dot product or inner product, is implemented as function `np.dot(a,b)` and in Python 3 also as operator @,

Listing 2.9 FirstProgram.ipynb (part 8)

```
1  result = aMatrix @ matrix2.T
2  print(result)
```

```
>> [[ 33 50]
    [ 81 122]]
```

We have thereby included the transpose operation through the operator specification '.T'. Such operator specification are common in object-oriented programming constructs.

We are often in need of accessing subsets of data in arrays and also merging arrays. To access a subset of an array we can first generate an index vector called `idx` below, which specifies the indices we want to process such as the first and second element in the second row of the matrix, called aMatrix, defined earlier

Listing 2.10 FirstProgram.ipynb (part 9)

```
1 idx = ([[1],[0,2]])
2 print(aMatrix[tuple(idx)])
```

>> [4 6]

Another useful example is to make a vector with a list,

Listing 2.11 FirstProgram.ipynb (part 10)

```
1 x=np.arange(10)
```

which is the same as array(range(10)), and to extract every second element of a vector,

Listing 2.12 FirstProgram.ipynb (part 11)

```
1 x = np.arange(10)    # same as array(range(10))
2 print(x[::2])
```

>> [0 2 4 6 8]

The array indexing is the same as x[0:-1:2] because the default boundaries for the first and second limits is the first and last element. Merging two arrays is done with the NumPy concatenate() method,

Listing 2.13 FirstProgram.ipynb (part 12)

```
1 result = np.concatenate((aMatrix,matrix2),axis=0)
2 print(result)
```

>> [[1 2 3]
    [4 5 6]
    [5 5 6]
    [7 8 9]]

A useful command to check the size and orientation of a matrix is

Listing 2.14 FirstProgram.ipynb (part 13)

```
1 result.shape
```

>> (4, 3)

As already mentioned, the first index specifies the row going downwards and the second index specifies the column going to the right. We sometimes want to reorder the elements of an array which can be done with a reshape function,

Listing 2.15 FirstProgram.ipynb (part 14)

```
1 print(result.reshape(2,6))
```

```
>> [[1 2 3 4 5 6]
   [5 5 6 7 8 9]]
```

So far, we have discussed the basic numerical data types that we need. Besides these numerical data types, there are of course, others such as characters. Text data is simply enclosed in parenthesis like.

Listing 2.16 FirstProgram.ipynb (part 15)
```
1 text = 'Hello World!'
2 print(text)
```

```
>> Hello World!
```

2.2.2 Control flow

In the following, we show three fundamental programming constructs, that of loops, conditional statements, and functions. To loop through some code, one can use the following construct,

Listing 2.17 FirstProgram.ipynb (part 16)
```
1 for i in range(4):
2     print(i)
```

```
>> 0      1
   2
   3
```

which starts at i=0 and goes in steps of one until i=3. Note that Python is sensitive to the code position; the indented code represents the block of statements executed inside the loop. A conditional statement takes the form

Listing 2.18 FirstProgram.ipynb (part 17
```
1 if scalar <1:
2     print("true")
3 else:
4     print("false")
```

```
>> false
```

Single or double quotes can be used in the print statement. Again note the indentation to specify the block of code for each condition.

2.2.3 Functions

This book tries to use minimal examples that do not require advanced code structuring techniques such as object oriented-programming, although those techniques are available in Python. A basic code reuse technique is the definition of a function. In Python this can be done with the following template. To structure code better, specifically to define some code that can be reused, we have the option to define functions like

Listing 2.19 FirstProgram.ipynb (part 18)

```
1  def func(arg1, arg2=10):
2      arg = arg1+arg2
3      arg1 = arg1+100
4      return arg;
5  a = 1
6  print(func(2), func(a,2), a)
```

>> 12 3 1

Simple variables are passed by value in Python, but more complex objects might be referred by reference. It is therefore wise to be careful when changing the content of calling variables in the functions. The function can be called with an argument, and we showed in the example how to provide a default argument.

It is also useful to define an inline version of a function, such as defining logistic sigmoid function

Listing 2.20 FirstProgram.ipynb (part 19)

```
1  logist = lambda x: 1 / (1 + np.exp(−x))
```

We will use this inline function below to plot it.

2.2.4 Plotting

Plotting graphs for data is a useful scientific tool, and we will be using the the popular scientific plotting library Matplotlib `http://matplotlib.org/`, specifically the pyplot package that provides a slightly simpler interface within the matplotlib package. We imported this library already at the beginning of the code. Using this library, an example of a basic line plot is given in the following code, and the resulting graph is shown in Fig. 2.2.

Listing 2.21 FirstProgram.ipynb (part 20)

```
1  t = np.arange(−10,10,0.1)
2  plt.plot(t,logist(t))
3  plt.rcParams.update({'font.size': 28})
4  plt.xlabel('t'); plt.ylabel('x(t)')
```

Note that it is always a good idea to include labels for the axis. If you need to include the figure in paper, then use the command

Listing 2.22 FirstProgram.ipynb (part 21)

```
1  plt.savefig('fileName.pdf')
```

2.2.5 Timing the program

Some of the programs might need some time to run, and it might be necessary to estimate the time of running with some smaller examples and measuring the time. This

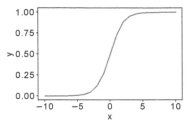

Fig. 2.2 Example of a plot for the logistic (sigmoid) function $f(x) = \frac{1}{1+e^{-x}}$ with the Matplotlib library.

can be done by importing the time package and usinf the `clock()` function in the following way.

Listing 2.23 FirstProgram.ipynb (part 22)

```
1  import time
2  tic = time.time()
3  toc = time.time()
4  print(toc - tic)
```

>> 8.678436279296875e-05

2.3 Code efficiency and vectorization

Machine learning is about working with large collections of data. Such data are kept in data bases, spreadsheets, or simply in text files, but to work with them we load them into arrays. Since we define operations on such arrays, it is better to treat these arrays as vectors, matrices, or generally as tensors. Traditional programming languages such as C and Fortran require us to write code that loops over all the indices in order to specify operations that are defined on all the data. For example, as provided in the program `MatrixMultiplication.ipynb`, let us define two random $n \times n$ matrices with the NumPy random number generator for uniformly distributed numbers,

Listing 2.24 MatrixMultiplication.ipynb (fragment)

```
1  a = np.random.rand(n,n)
2  b = np.random.rand(n,n)
```

and a matrix of zeros with the same size,

Listing 2.25 MatrixMultiplication.ipynb (fragment)

```
1  c = np.zeros((n,n))
```

We can than write the code of adding two numbers with an explicit loop over all indices as

Listing 2.26 MatrixMultiplication.ipynb (fragment)

```
1  for i in range(n):
2      for j in range(n):
3          c[i][j]=a[i][j]+b[i][j]
```

In high-level programming languages like Python, Matlab, and R, it is common to write such operations in a compact form like

$$c=a@b$$

It is now common to call this style of programming a vectorized code. Such a vectorized code is not only much easier to read, but it is also essential to write efficient code. The reason for this is that the system programmers can implement such routines very efficiently, and this is difficult to match with the more general but inefficient explicit index operation.

To demonstrate the efficiency issue, let us measure the time of operations for a matrix multiplication. We start as usual by importing the standard NumPy, the Matplotlib, and also the time libraries.s We then define a method called `matmulslow` that implements a matrix multiplication with an explicit iteration over the indices,

Listing 2.27 MatrixMultiplication.ipynb (fragment)

```
1  def matmulslow(a,b):
2      m = a.shape[1]
3      c=np.zeros((m,m))
4      for i in range(m):
5          for j in range(m):
6              for k in range(m):
7                  c[i,j] = c[i,j]+a[i,k]*b[k,j]
8      return c;
```

and a fast version of this operation in the method `matmulfast` which call the NumPy method `dot`,

Listing 2.28 MatrixMultiplication.ipynb (fragment)

```
1  def matmulfast(a,b):
2      return a@b
```

We then evaluate the time these routines take with the following test code,

Listing 2.29 MatrixMultiplication.ipynb (fragment)

```
1   size = np.array([])
2   time1 = np.array([])
3   time2 = np.array([])
4   for n in range(10,130,10):
5       print(n)
6       size = np.append(size,n)
7       a = np.random.rand(n,n)
8       b = np.random.rand(n,n)
9       c = np.zeros((n,n))
10
11      timestart = time.time()
12      c = matmulslow(a,b)
13      time1 = np.append(time1,time.time()-timestart)
14
15      timestart = time.time()
16      c = matmulfast(a,b)
17      time2 = np.append(time2,time.time()-timestart)
```

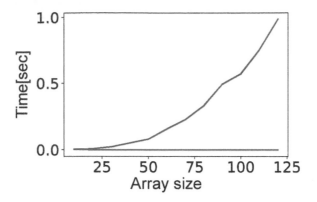

Fig. 2.3 Execution time of a matrix multiplication for different sizes of the matrices. The red line show the execution times for a element-wise implementation, whereas the blue line shows the execution times of the vectorized version with the build-in function. Using build-in functions is much more efficient than component-wise programming of this matrix multiplication.

The resulting time graph is shown in Fig. 2.3. This not only shows that the time difference can be substantial for larger arrays, but that the scaling is very different. Some concern that interpreted computer languages are slow comes from the inefficient implementations of programmers not used to this style of programming. It is often the most challenging part for experienced programmers of C-like languages to adopt to this vectorized code, but such a programming style is essential to produce efficient code.

3 Math and Stats

This chapter outlines here some of the mathematical and probabilistic concepts used in this book. We are hereby mainly users of a language, that of mathematical notations, that will enable us to describe concepts with great detail that can be translated directly into simulation programs. Thus, we are using a useful scientific language rather than delving into the science of these concepts.

3.1 Vector and matrix notations

We frequently use vector and matrix notation in this book as it is extremely convenient for specifying array operations. It is a shorthand notation for otherwise lengthy-looking formulas, and formulas written in this notation can easily be entered into Python as we have seen in the previous chapter. We consider three basic data types:

1. Scalar:
$$a \text{ for example } 41 \tag{3.1}$$

2. Vector:
$$\mathbf{a} \text{ or component-wise } \begin{pmatrix} a_1 \\ a_2 \\ a_3 \end{pmatrix} \text{ for example } \begin{pmatrix} 41 \\ 7 \\ 13 \end{pmatrix} \tag{3.2}$$

3. Matrix:
$$\mathbf{a} \text{ or component-wise } \begin{pmatrix} a_{11} & a_{12} \\ a_{21} & a_{22} \\ a_{31} & a_{32} \end{pmatrix} \text{ for example } \begin{pmatrix} 41 & 12 \\ 7 & 45 \\ 13 & 9 \end{pmatrix} \tag{3.3}$$

We used characters in bold fonts to indicate both a vector and a matrix; the difference is usually apparent from the circumstances. A matrix is just a collection of scalars or vectors. We talk about an $n \times m$ matrix where n is the number of rows and m is the number of columns. A scalar is thus a 1×1 matrix, and a vector of length n can be considered an $n \times 1$ matrix. A similar collection of data is called array in computer science. However, a matrix is difference because we also define operations on these data collections. The rules of calculating with matrices can be applied to scalars and vectors.

We define how to add and multiply two matrices so that we can use them in algebraic equations. The sum of two matrices is defined as the sum of the individual components

$$(\mathbf{a} + \mathbf{b})_{ij} = \mathbf{a}_{ij} + \mathbf{b}_{ij}. \tag{3.4}$$

For example, $\mathbf{a}$ and $\mathbf{b}$ are 3×2 matrices, then

Fundamentals of Computational Neuroscience. Third edition. Thomas P. Trappenberg, Oxford University Press. © Oxford University Press 2023. DOI: 10.1093/oso/9780192869364.003.0003

$$\mathbf{a} + \mathbf{b} = \begin{pmatrix} a_{11} + b_{11} & a_{12} + b_{12} \\ a_{21} + b_{21} & a_{22} + b_{22} \\ a_{31} + b_{31} & a_{32} + b_{32} \end{pmatrix} \tag{3.5}$$

Matrix multiplication is defined as

$$(\mathbf{a} * \mathbf{b})_{ij} = \sum_k \mathbf{a}_{ik} \mathbf{b}_{kj}. \tag{3.6}$$

The matrix multiplication is hence only defined as multiplication matrices **a** and **b** where the number of columns of the matrix **a** is equal to the number of rows of matrix **b**. For example, for two square matrices with two rows and two columns, their product is given by

$$\mathbf{a} * \mathbf{b} = \begin{pmatrix} a_{11}b_{11} + a_{12}b_{21} & a_{11}b_{12} + a_{12}b_{22} \\ a_{21}b_{11} + a_{22}b_{21} & a_{21}b_{12} + a_{22}b_{22} \end{pmatrix} \tag{3.7}$$

A handy rule for matrix multiplications is illustrated in Fig. 3.1. Each component in the resulting matrix is calculated from the sum of two multiplicative terms. The rule for multiplying two matrices is tedious but straightforward and can easily be implemented in a computer. A matrix multiplication when using numpy arrays is specified with the '@' symbol instead of a '*' symbol. The later would specify a component-wise multiplication for same size arrays.

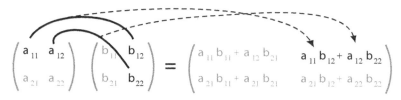

Fig. 3.1 Illustration of a matrix multiplication. Each element in the resulting matrix consists of terms that are taken from the corresponding row of the first matrix and column of the second matrix. Thus in the example we calculate the highlighted element from the components of the first row of the first matrix and the second column of the second matrix. From these rows and columns we add all the terms that consist of the element-wise multiplication of the terms.

Another useful definition is the transpose of a matrix. In mathematical notations, there is usually a prime (') or an superscript (t) attached to a matrix. In Python, this operation is applied by attaching the operator '.T' to a matrix. Taking the transpose of a matrix means that the matrix is rotated 90 degrees; the first row becomes the first column, the second row becomes the second column, etc. For example, the transpose of the example in 3.3 is

$$\mathbf{a}' = \begin{pmatrix} 41 & 7 & 13 \\ 12 & 45 & 9 \end{pmatrix} \tag{3.8}$$

The transpose of a vector transforms a column vector into a row vector and vice versa.

As already mentioned, matrices were invented to simplify the notations for systems of coupled algebraic equations. Consider, for example, the system of three equations

$$41x_1 + 12x_2 = 17 \tag{3.9}$$
$$7x_1 + 45x_2 = -83 \tag{3.10}$$

$$13x_1 + 9x_2 = -5. \tag{3.11}$$

This can be written as

$$\mathbf{ax} = \mathbf{b} \tag{3.12}$$

with the matrix $\mathbf{a}$ as in the example of 3.3, the vector $\mathbf{x} = (x_1 \ x_2)'$, and the vector $\mathbf{b} = (17 \ -83 \ -5)'$. Solutions of such equation systems can be formulated by using matrix notation, and many corresponding routines are implemented in MATLAB.

3.2   Distance measures

We are often confronted with comparing two vectors. It is straightforward comparing two vectors to decide if they are the same by inspecting the equivalence of each component. However, if they are different we would like to put a value, d, on the difference that gives us some measure of how different they are. There are many possible different definitions of such a difference measure, although we should impose some obvious restrictions on such measures:

- The value should be $d = 0$ if the vectors are the same. We do not allow negative values because we wish to interpret this value as a distance.
- The value should be positive, $d > 0$, if they are not the same.
- The distance from vector $\mathbf{a}$ to $\mathbf{b}$ should be the same as from $\mathbf{b}$ to $\mathbf{a}$.

We sometimes have to evaluate the distance between two binary vectors $\mathbf{a}$ and $\mathbf{b}$, in which the components have only two possible values for example $a_i, b_i \in \{0, 1\}$. A common value for the distance of such vectors is obtained by counting how many components (bits) are different. This measure is called the Hamming distance, d^h. If we normalize this value to the number of components of the vector, N, then we get a value between 0 and 1. This normalized Hamming distance can be calculated using the formula

$$d^h(\mathbf{a}, \mathbf{b}) = \frac{1}{N} \sum_i a_i(1 - b_i) + (1 - a_i)b_i. \tag{3.13}$$

However, it is not obvious how to generalize this measure to vectors with real numbered components as we would have to judge the amount of the difference among the components, using their possible values, which we might not know a priori. One possible definition is to use the normalized dot product between vectors. The dot product, or inner product, of two column vectors $\mathbf{a}$ and $\mathbf{b}$ is given by

$$\mathbf{a}'\mathbf{b} = \sum_i a_i b_i. \tag{3.14}$$

We used the transpose of the second vector so that this is only a special case of a matrix multiplication with a row vector $\mathbf{a}'$ and a column vector $\mathbf{b}$. In a geometrical interpretation of vectors (see Fig. 3.2) this number is proportional to the cosine of the angle between the two vectors,

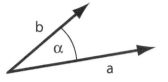

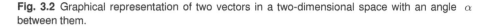

Fig. 3.2 Graphical representation of two vectors in a two-dimensional space with an angle α between them.

$$\mathbf{ab}' = ||\mathbf{a}|| \, ||\mathbf{b}'|| \cos(\alpha), \tag{3.15}$$

where $||\mathbf{a}||$ is the length or norm of vector $\mathbf{a}$. The Euclidean norm of the vector is defined as

$$||\mathbf{a}|| = \sqrt{\sum_i a_i^2}, \tag{3.16}$$

which can also be written with the help of a dot product as

$$||\mathbf{a}|| = \sqrt{\mathbf{a}'\mathbf{a}}. \tag{3.17}$$

The cosine of the angle α between two vectors is a number between -1 and 1 that is only zero when the vectors are pointing in the same direction. The absolute value of this number is therefore a possible definition of the similarity of two vectors,

$$d^{\text{dot}} = \left| \frac{\mathbf{ab}'}{||\mathbf{a}|| \, ||\mathbf{b}'||} \right|. \tag{3.18}$$

Other definitions, such as taking the square of the normalized dot product, are also valid. Another definition that is sometimes used as measure of the distance between two vectors with positive real numbered components $a_i, b_i \in \mathbf{R}^+$ has the form of the Pearson correlation coefficient from statistics, namely

$$d^{\text{Pearson}} = \frac{||\mathbf{ab}|| - ||\mathbf{a}|| \, ||\mathbf{b}||}{\sqrt{(||\mathbf{a}^2|| - ||\mathbf{a}||^2) \, (||\mathbf{b}^2|| - ||\mathbf{b}||^2)}}. \tag{3.19}$$

We call this distance measure the Pearson distance.

3.3 The δ-function

The δ-function is a very convenient notation to describe discrete events in a continuous format. One can think of it as a density function that is zero except for its arguments for which it is infinite, and the integral over the δ-function is one; that is,

$$\int_{-\infty}^{\infty} \delta(x = x_1) \mathrm{d}x = 1. \tag{3.20}$$

It is usually used as an integration kernel with other functions as in

$$\int_{-\infty}^{\infty} \delta(x_1) f(x) \mathrm{d}x = f(x_1). \tag{3.21}$$

In a strict mathematical context it is only defined as an operation over a function, and this is why it is sometimes called a functional. We will use it here mainly to specify discrete events and for using this in numerical simulations as we demonstrate in the following section.

3.4 Numerical calculus

3.4.1 Differences and sums

We are often interested how a variable, such as the membrane potential or population rate of cell assemblies, change with time. Let us call this quantity $x(t)$ for now, where we indicated that it changes with time. The change of this variable from time t to time $t' = t + \Delta t$ is then

$$\Delta x = x(t + \Delta t) - x(t). \tag{3.22}$$

The quantity Δt is the finite difference in time, which we will call the time step in the following. For a continuously changing quantity we could also think about the instantaneous change value, $\mathrm{d}x$, by considering an infinitesimally small time step. Formally,

$$\mathrm{d}x = \lim_{\Delta t \to 0} \Delta x = \lim_{\Delta t \to 0} (x(t + \Delta t) - x(t)). \tag{3.23}$$

The infinitesimally small time step is often written as $\mathrm{d}t$. Calculating with such infinitesimal small quantities is covered in the mathematical discipline of calculus, but on the computer we have always finite differences and we need to consider very small time steps to approximate continuous formulation. With discrete time steps, differentials become differences and integrals become sums

$$\mathrm{d}x \to \Delta x \tag{3.24}$$

$$\int \mathrm{d}x \to \Delta x \sum \tag{3.25}$$

Note the factor of Δx in front of the summation in the last equation. It is easy to forget this factor when replacing integrals with sums. The following demonstrates this discretization for a differential equation.

3.4.2 Numerical integration of an initial value problem

The time dynamics of several models in this book are defined with differential equations that specify the change of a quantity $\mathrm{d}x$ for an infinitesimal time step $\mathrm{d}t$. This change is specified by a function $f(x, t)$, which may depend on the quantity x and sometimes also explicitly by the time. Mathematically this is expressed by

$$\tau \frac{\mathrm{d}x}{\mathrm{d}t} = f(x, t), \tag{3.26}$$

which is a first-order differential equation with one independent variable and time constant τ. Sometimes, the derivative on the left hand side is written as

$$\frac{\mathrm{d}x}{\mathrm{d}t} = \dot{x}. \tag{3.27}$$

This is why we would use the name such as `xdot` in the programs. We outline here the principles of some numerical integration techniques for this simple case, but the methods can be generalized easily to more complex coupled differential equations and differential equations that contain higher-order differentials. We are concerned with calculating the values of the quantity $x(t)$ for specific times $t > t_0$ when the value of the quantity at time $t = t_0$ is known,

$$x(t_0) = x_0. \tag{3.28}$$

This is called an initial value problem. We often refer to the initial value problem in the text as numerical integration. However, numerical integration can also refer to other numerical tasks such as numerically approximating integrals like $\int_{x1}^{x2} f(x)\mathrm{d}x$, or to finding solutions of differential equations with other constraints.

3.4.3 Euler method

Digital computers can only represent discrete numbers and not infinitesimally small changes. We must therefore express the continuous dynamic given by eqn 3.26 in discrete time steps. We call this procedure discretization. The simplest form is to use small but finite time steps between two consecutive times t_1 and t_2. We write this time step as

$$\Delta t = t_2 - t_1. \tag{3.29}$$

The continuous process is recovered in the limit $\Delta t \to 0$, which we call the continuum limit. Numerical integration here is simply adding up changes at every time step. This is basically what the physical processes is doing which we want to describer except that we have to use finite time steps. The physical process is often given by specifying the change in a time step

$$\Delta x(t + \Delta t) = x(t + \Delta t) - x(t). \tag{3.30}$$

The differential eqn 3.26 is thus discretized simply as

$$\frac{\Delta x(t + \Delta t)}{\Delta t} = f(x(t), t). \tag{3.31}$$

We have assigned the value of the change specified on the right-hand side at time t to the change at time $t + \Delta t$, though we could have also chosen $f(x(t + \Delta t), t)$ as the right-hand side. The numerical values would then be a little bit different and the discrete systems are indeed a little bit different. However, we have to make all the following choices in the light of the continuum limit in which we should recover the same answers for the different methods. Substituting eqn 3.30 into eqn 3.31 gives

$$x(t + \Delta t) = x(t) + \Delta t f(x(t), t). \tag{3.32}$$

This equation simply states the meaning of a differential in a discrete situation. The value of variable x at the next time step is given by the value of the variable at the previous time step times plus Δt the change specified by the function f. This iterative method tracks the development of quantity x from an initial value to later times by summing up the changes. This simplest method of numerical integration, which extrapolates changes linearly, is known as the Euler method.

Let us illustrate this procedure with a simple yet important examples. In this example, the change of the quantify is proportional to the quantify itself. For example, in a population with a constant reproduction rate larger than 2, the number of offspring grows with the size of the population,

$$\tau\frac{dx}{dt} = x(t) \tag{3.33}$$

Now, before solving this differential equation numerically, we show that we can solve this analytically. Not all differential equations can be solved analytically, and we usually do not have to worry about this because we use directly numerical techniques. But we can use this knowledge of the analytical solution to discuss our numerical solution. Just reading the above equation, the function we are looking for is the function $x(t)$ who's value is proportional to its slope. This function is the exponential function,

$$x(t) = x(0)e^{\tau x} \tag{3.34}$$

which you can easily verify by taking the derivative. This differential equation can easily be solved analytically by the separation of variables, but this is not the subject of this book. Rather, the discrete version of this equation is

$$\tau\frac{\Delta x(t+\Delta t)}{\Delta t} = x(t). \tag{3.35}$$

The equivalent update equation for the initial value problem is

$$x(t+\Delta t) = x(t) + \frac{1}{\tau}\Delta t x(t). \tag{3.36}$$

The python implementation of solving this differential equation with three methods is given below for $\tau = 1$ and $x(0) = 1$.

Programs/ode1.py

```
1  # Example of numerical integration
2  import numpy as np
3  import matplotlib.pyplot as plt
4  from scipy.integrate import odeint
5
6  def xdot(x, t):
7      return x
8
9  x0 = 1 # initial conditions on at x=0
10 dt = 0.1 # time step
11 t = np.arange(0,3,dt) # integrate from 0 to 4
12
13 xEuler = np.array([x0])
14 for step in t:
15     xEuler = np.append(xEuler,
16             xEuler[-1]+dt*xdot(xEuler[-1],step))
17
18 xODEint = np.squeeze(odeint(xdot, x0, t))
19
20 xAna = x0 * np.exp(t) # analytic solution
21
22 plt.plot(t,xEuler[:-1],'r—'); plt.plot(t,xAna)
23 plt.xlabel('t'); plt.ylabel('xEuler, xAna')
```

We are first comparing the Euler solution xEuler with the analytical solution xAna. The Euler solution with a time step of $\Delta t = 0.1$ is shown in Fig.3.3A as red curve, while the analytical solution is shown in blue. While both curves show an exponential behaviour, the Euler solution is increasingly deviating from the analytical solution of the continuous system. At this point it is good to remember that the continuum solution should be recovered for $\Delta t \to 0$. Fig.3.3B shows the relative error $(xAna - xEuler)/xAna$ for two different levels of Δt. As expected, the error gets smaller with decreasing step size.

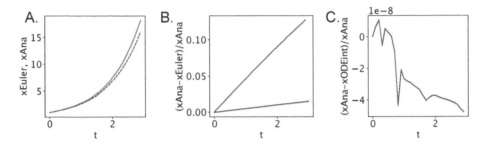

Fig. 3.3 (A) Analytical (blue curve) and Euler solution ($\Delta t = 0.1$, red dashed curve) with $\tau = 1$ for the initial value problem in eg. 3.33 (B) The relative difference between the analytic and Euler solution with $\Delta t = 0.1$ (red curve) and $\Delta t = 0.01$ (blue curve) (C) Relative between the analytic and the numerical solution with the LSODA1 implementation in odeint.

We will use the basic differential equation of an exponential function many times in this book, is particular in the form with a negative exponential. For example, let us consider an input signal with discrete events, like a spike train,

$$X(t) = \sum_{t'} \delta(t - t').$$ (3.37)

The differential equation like

$$\tau \frac{dx}{dt} = -x + X(t)$$ (3.38)

is often called a leaky integrator. This can be implemented with the following program.

Programs/LeakyIntegrator.py

```
1  import numpy as np
2  import matplotlib.pyplot as plt
3
4  tmax=10; dt=1; tau=2
5  X = np.zeros(tmax*int(1/dt));
6  a=np.array([1,3,8])/dt; X[a.astype(int)]=1
7
8  x = np.array([0]);
9  for t in range(0,tmax*int(1/dt)):
10     x = np.append(x,x[t]+dt*(-1/tau*x[t])+X[t])
11
12 plt.plot(x);
13 plt.xlabel('t in units of dt'); plt.ylabel('x(t)')
14 plt.savefig('li1.pdf')
```

This is again an implementation of the Euler method. Note that the amount of decay depends on the ratio of $\frac{tau}{dt}$ except the term $X(t)$ because this is made out of delta functions. The essence of a delta function is that it has the value of 1 in the smallest time interval, regardless of how small this time interval is. The solutions with two different time steps is shown in Fig. 3.4.

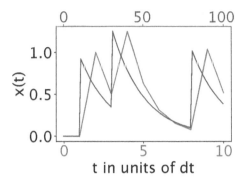

Fig. 3.4 Example of a leaky integrator with delta inputs at three times with `dt=1` (blue curve and scale) and `dt=0.1` (red curve and scale).

A quick note about program efficiency. It is of course the best to use analytical solutions when they exist. For example, in the leaky integrator we could just use the analytical solution between the spike times, and reset the x value at spike times. This typically increase speed and simulation accuracy. We will mostly not use such advanced techniques in our simulation as we want to focus on the principles behind the simulations and less on the precise numerical tricks.

3.4.4 Higher-order methods

In the Euler method just outlined we have taken the first derivative of the function f (the slope of the function) into account and have used this to extrapolate linearly to the value of x at the next time step $t + \Delta t$. This results in an integration error if the function is not linear between the integration points. We can improve the accuracy of the approximation in several ways. One is to take the curvature into account through the second or higher-order derivatives. We can formalize this by considering the Taylor expansion of the function around the time for which we want to estimate the value. The Taylor expansion is given by

$$x(t + \Delta t) = x(t) + \Delta t \frac{\mathrm{d}x}{\mathrm{d}t} + \frac{1}{2}(\Delta t)^2 \frac{\mathrm{d}^2 x}{\mathrm{d}t^2} + O\left((\Delta t)^3\right), \qquad (3.39)$$

where the last term stands for all possible higher-order terms. This equation with the first two terms is the Euler method (eqn 3.32) since the derivative is given by $f(x, t)$ as stated by eqn 3.26. If we consider the next order term in the Taylor expansion for our example, we get the approximation

$$x(t + \Delta t) = x(t) + (1 - x + t)\Delta t + \frac{1}{2}(1 - x)(\Delta t)^2, \qquad (3.40)$$

which adds a term proportional to $(\Delta t)^2$ to the previous expression. The second-order relative difference of the second-order solution to the exact solution is also shown in Fig. 3.3B as green curve. While this method is a little bit better for this example for intermediate extrapolation times, the error increases again for large times.

If we use higher-order terms we can further improve the approximations of the exact solution. This method requires that we know higher derivatives of the function f explicitly. In case they are difficult to calculate analytically, we can also estimate them numerically, although this introduces further numerical errors. This method is therefore not used directly but rather indirectly in the following way. If we use only the first derivative (slope) of the function at time t we assume that this is the same for subsequent times. If this is changing (for example, if the function has a curvature) then we use the slope at a time between t and $t + \Delta t$ as a better guess for the average slope in this interval. Thus, instead of using $f(x, t)$ in eqn 3.32 we should use

$$f(x, t) \rightarrow f(\tilde{x}, t + \alpha \Delta t), \tag{3.41}$$

where α is a parameter. The value $\tilde{x}$ should be the value of x at $t + \alpha \Delta t$, that is, $\tilde{x} = x(t + \alpha \Delta t)$, which we don't know a priori. We could, however, guess this using the first-order Euler method, that is,

$$\tilde{x} = x(t) + \alpha \Delta t f(x(t), t). \tag{3.42}$$

A common choice for the parameter α is $\alpha = 1/2$, in which case this method is called the midpoint method. This method cancels error terms of first order and corresponds therefore to a second-order method. The midpoint method requires two function calls, but no higher derivatives are needed. Note that we made several assumptions that might often be appropriate, but not always. Therefore, higher-order methods can usually improve the approximation of the solution $x(t)$, but this does not have to be the case in all circumstances.

Also, it is not necessary to stop at the second-order and midpoint approximation and it is possible (though tedious) to work out solutions for higher-order approximations. The method most commonly used for numerical integrations is thereby a fourth-order method known as the Runge–Kutta method, which is a direct generalization of the midpoint method. The conclusions we drew for the midpoint method still hold. This fourth-order method is often better than lower-order methods, although this cannot always be guaranteed.

Applying any of these numerical methods requires that we check that the results we get do not critically depend on the choice of the parameters such as the time step Δt. At the very least we should check that the numerical results do not change more than within a certain range that we demand of the solutions when modifying the time step parameter considerably (for example, double it and halve it). Many numerical solvers have already implemented such strategies with algorithms that change the time step as long as the variations in the results are lower than the error bound we give to the system. Such algorithms are called adaptive time step methods.

There are several other methods for numerical integration, each having different strengths and weaknesses in certain application domains. For example, the Runge–Kutta method breaks down if there are very sudden changes in the exact solution for which the linear interpolations used in the midpoint approach break down. The integrate module from the SciPy package provides several solvers through the function solve_ivp(). We will be using this recommended version in some programs, but we will also use the older function odeint(). This function uses the LSODA algorithm which is also implemented in solve_ivp(), but we also use odeint() that still uses LSODA internally and is a slightly elegant syntax for our example programs. Using this function to solve our initial value example of eq.3.33 is included in the program ode1.py shown before. The relative error to the analytical solution is shown in Fig. 3.3C. It is important to observe the scale of this error relative to the error in Fig. 3.3B.

3.5 Basic probability theory

This now reviews briefly review the basic properties of random numbers and the probabilistic framework. This includes a list of some probability density functions used in this book. This section is not about statistics, which is primarily concerned with hypothesis testing. Rather, we review here some concepts that provide a useful description framework of uncertainty as we will argue that brain functions are optimized for decision-making in uncertain environments.

3.5.1 Random numbers and their probability (density) function

The most important concept introduced in this section is that of random numbers, which are here denoted by capital letters to distinguish them from regular numbers written in lower case. A random variable, X, is a quantity that can have different values each time the variable is inspected, such as in measurements in experiments. This is fundamentally different to a regular variable, x, which does not change its value once it is assigned. A random number is thus a new mathematical concept, not included in the regular mathematics of numbers. A specific value of a random number is still meaningful as it might influence specific processes in a deterministic way. However, since a random number can change every time it is inspected, it is also useful to describe more general properties when drawing samples many times. The frequency with which numbers can occur is then the most useful quantity to take into account. This normalized frequency is captured by the mathematical construct of a probability.

We can formalize this with some compact notations. We speak of a discrete random variable in the case of discrete numbers for the possible values of a random number. A continuous random variable is a random variable that has possible values in a continuous range of numbers. There is, in principle, not much difference between these two kinds of random variables, except that the mathematical formulation has to be slightly different to be mathematically correct. For example, the probability function,

$$P(x) = P(X = x) \tag{3.43}$$

describes the frequency with which each possible value x of a discrete variable X occurs. Note that x is a regular variable which stands for one specific value, not a random variable that can change. The value of $P(x)$ gives the fraction of the times we get a value x for the random variable X if we draw many samples of the random variable. Note that probabilities are sometimes written as a percentage, but we will stick to the fractional notation. From this definition it follows that the frequency of having any of the possible values is equal to one, which is the normalization condition

$$\sum_x P(x) = 1. \tag{3.44}$$

In the case of continuous random numbers we have an infinite number of possible values x so that the fraction for each number becomes infinitesimally small. It is then appropriate to write the probability distribution function as $P(x) = p(x)\mathrm{d}x$, where $p(x)$ is the probability density function (pdf). The sum in eqn 3.44 then becomes an integral, and normalization condition for a continuous random variable is

$$\int_x p(x)\mathrm{d}x = 1. \tag{3.45}$$

We will formulate the rest of this section in terms of continuous random variables. The corresponding formulas for discrete random variables can easily be deduced by replacing the integrals over the pdf with sums over the probability function. It is also possible to use the δ-function, outlined in section 3 to write discrete random processes in a continuous form.

3.5.2 Moments: mean, variance, etc.

In the following we only consider independent random values that are drawn from identical pdfs, often labelled as iid (independent and identically distributed) data. That is, we do not consider cases where there is a different probabilities of getting certain numbers when having a specific number in a previous trial. The static probability density function describes, then, all we can know about the corresponding random variable.

Let us consider the arbitrary pdf, $p(x)$, with the following graph:

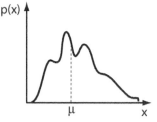

Such a distribution is called multimodal because it has several peaks. Since this is a pdf, the area under this curve must be equal to one, as stated in eqn 3.45. It would be useful to have this function parameterized in an analytical format. Most pdfs have to be approximated from experiments, and a common method is then to fit a function to the data. However, sometimes it is sufficient to know at least some basic characteristics of the functions. For example, we might ask what the most frequent value is when drawing many examples. This number is given by the largest peak value of the distribution. A more common quantity to know is the expected arithmetic average of those numbers, which is called the mean, expected value, or expectation value of the distribution, defined by

$$\mu = \int_{-\infty}^{\infty} xp(x)\mathrm{d}x. \tag{3.46}$$

In the discrete case, this formula corresponds to the formula of calculating an arithmetic average, where we add up all the different numbers together with their frequency.

The mean of a distribution is not the only interesting quantity that characterizes a distribution. For example, we might want to ask what the median value is for which it is equally likely to find a value lower or larger than this value. Furthermore, the spread of the pdf around the mean is also very revealing as it gives us a sense of how spread the values are. This spread is often characterized by the standard deviation (std), or its square, which is called variance, σ^2, and is defined as

$$\sigma^2 = \int_{-\infty}^{\infty} (x - \mu)^2 p(x)\mathrm{d}x. \tag{3.47}$$

This quantity is generally not enough to characterize the probability function uniquely; this is only possible if we know all moments of a distribution, where the nth moment about the mean is defined as

$$m^n = \int_{-\infty}^{\infty} (x - \mu)^n p(x)\mathrm{d}x. \tag{3.48}$$

The variance is the second moment about the mean. Higher moments specify further characteristics such as the kurtosis and skewness of the distribution. Moments higher than this have not been given explicit names. Knowing all moments of a distribution is equivalent in knowing the distribution precisely, and knowing a pdf is equivalent in knowing everything we could know about a random variable.

In case the distribution function is not given, moments have to be estimated from data. For example, the mean can be estimated from a sample of measurements by the sample mean,

$$\bar{x} = \frac{1}{n} \sum_{i=1}^{n} x_i, \tag{3.49}$$

and the variance either from the biased sample variance,

$$s_1^2 = \frac{1}{n} \sum_{i=1}^{n} (\bar{x} - x_i)^2, \tag{3.50}$$

or the unbiased sample variance

$$s_2^2 = \frac{1}{n-1} \sum_{i=1}^{n} (\bar{x} - x_i)^2. \tag{3.51}$$

A statistic is said to be biased if the mean of the sampling distribution is not equal to the parameter that is intended to be estimated. Knowing all moments uniquely specifies a pdf.

3.5.3 Examples of probability (density) functions

There is an infinite number of possible pdfs. However, some specific forms have been very useful for describing some specific processes and have thus been given names. Many of them are implemented in the `random` package of Numpy and in the stats module of SciPy. In the following we outline a short list of some frequently used distributions to give some examples and their corresponding Python code.

3.5.3.1 Uniform distribution

Equally distributed pseudo-random numbers in the interval $0 \leq x < 1$ are often generated by a routine called `rand()` in many programming languages. This is shown in the following listing that includes the code to plot a (normalized) histogram of 1000 samples that approximates the distribution.

Listing 3.1 From distributions.py

```
1  import numpy as np
2  import matplotlib.pyplot as plt
3  from scipy import stats
4
5  x = np.random.rand(1000)
6  n, bins = np.histogram(x)
7  plt.bar(bins[:-1]+0.05,n/1000,0.1)
8  plt.xlabel('x'), plt.ylabel('P(x)')
```

Uniform numbers in a different intervals is produced with the code

$$np.random.uniform(a,b,size=)$$

Uniform distributed numbers between $a \leq x < b$ re produced by

$$x = np.random.randint(a,b,size)$$

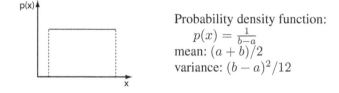

Probability density function:
$$p(x) = \frac{1}{b-a}$$
mean: $(a + b)/2$
variance: $(b - a)^2/12$

3.5.3.2 Normal (Gaussian) distribution

Another distribution we encounter frequently in the following is the Gaussian distribution. It is the limit of the binomial distribution for a large number of trials. This distribution depends on two parameters, the mean μ and the standard deviation σ, and the special case of $\mu = 0$ and $\sigma = 1$ is called the Normal distribution. Gaussian distributed random numbers can be drawn with `np.random.normal(mu, sig, size)`. The importance of the normal distribution stems from the central limit theorem outlined below.

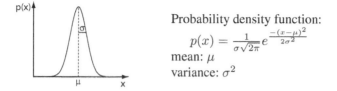

Probability density function:
$$p(x) = \frac{1}{\sigma\sqrt{2\pi}}e^{\frac{-(x-\mu)^2}{2\sigma^2}}$$
mean: μ
variance: σ^2

3.5.3.3 Bernoulli distribution

A Bernoulli random variable is a variable from an experiment that has two possible outcomes: success with probability p; or failure, with probability $(1 - p)$.

Probability function:
$$P(\text{success}) = p; P(\text{failure}) = 1 - p$$
mean: p
variance: $p(1 - p)$

3.5.3.4 Binomial distribution

The number of successes in n Bernoulli trials with probability of success p is binomially distributed. Note that the binomial coefficient is defined as

$$\binom{n}{x} = \frac{n!}{x!(n - x)!} \tag{3.52}$$

and is given by the Python function `np.random.binomial(n, p, size)`

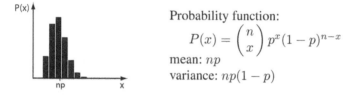

Probability function:
$$P(x) = \binom{n}{x}p^x(1 - p)^{n-x}$$
mean: np
variance: $np(1 - p)$

3.5.3.5 Multinomial distribution

Generalization of the binomial distribution where n trials can have k outcomes, each with different probabilities p_i. Such a random number can be grnerates with `random.multinomial(n, ps, size)`.

Probability function:
$$P(x_i) = n! \prod_{i=1}^{k}(p_i^{x_i}/x_i!)$$
mean: np_i
variance: $np_i(1 - p_i)$

3.5.3.6 Poisson distribution

This discrete distribution `random.poisson(lambda, size)` is frequently used to describe the number of rare but open-ended events and to model spike trains of cortical neurons. It is closely related to the exponential distribution given above. The parameter λ is equal to the mean and the variance.

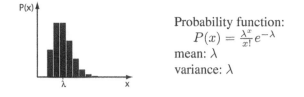

Probability function:
$$P(x) = \frac{\lambda^x}{x!} e^{-\lambda}$$
mean: λ
variance: λ

3.5.4 Cumulative probability (density) function and the Gaussian error function

The probability of having a value x for the random variable X in the range of $x_1 \leq x \leq x_2$ is given by

$$P(x_1 \leq X \leq x_2) = \int_{x_1}^{x_2} p(x)\mathrm{d}x. \tag{3.53}$$

Note that we have shortened the notation by replacing the notation $P_X(x_1 \leq X \leq x_2)$ by $P(x_1 \leq X \leq x_2)$ to simplify the following expressions. In the main text we often need to calculate the probability that a normally (or Gaussian) distributed variable has values between $x_1 = 0$ and $x_2 = y$. The probability of eqn 3.53 then becomes a function of y. This defines the Gaussian error function

$$\frac{1}{\sqrt{2\pi}\sigma} \int_0^y e^{-\frac{(x-\mu)^2}{2\sigma^2}} \mathrm{d}x = \frac{1}{2}\mathrm{erf}(\frac{y-\mu}{\sqrt{2}\sigma}). \tag{3.54}$$

This Gaussian error function (erf) for normally distributed variables (Gaussian distribution with mean $\mu = 0$ and variance $\sigma = 1$) is commonly tabulated in books on statistics. Programming libraries also frequently include routines that return the values for specific arguments. In MATLAB this is implemented by the routine `erf`, and values for the inverse of the error function are returned by the routine `erfinv`.

Another special case of eqn 3.53 is when x_1 in the equation is equal to the lowest possible value of the random variable (usually $-\infty$). The integral in eqn 3.53 then corresponds to the probability that a random variable has a value smaller than a certain value, say y. This function of y is called the cumulative density function (cdf; note that this is a probability function, not a density function),

$$P^{\mathrm{cum}}(x < y) = \int_{-\infty}^{y} p(x)\mathrm{d}x, \tag{3.55}$$

which we will utilize further below.

3.5.5 Functions of random variables and the central limit theorem

A function of a random variable X,

$$Y = f(X), \tag{3.56}$$

is also a random variable, Y, and we often need from know what the pdf of this new random variable is. Calculating with functions of random variables is a bit different to regular functions and some care has be taken in such situations. Let us illustrate how to do this with an example. Say we have an equally distributed random variable X as commonly approximated with pseudo-random number generators on a computer. The probability density function of this variable is given by

$$p_X(x) = \begin{cases} 1 & \text{for } 0 \leq x \leq 1, \\ 0 & \text{otherwise.} \end{cases} \quad (3.57)$$

We are seeking the probability density function $p_Y(y)$ of the random variable

$$Y = e^{-X^2}. \quad (3.58)$$

The random number Y is **not** Gaussian distributed as we might think naively. To calculate the probability density function we can employ the cumulative density function eqn 3.55 by noting that

$$P(Y \leq y) = P(e^{-X^2} \leq y) = P(X \geq \sqrt{-\ln y}). \quad (3.59)$$

Thus, the cumulative probability function of Y can be calculated from the cumulative probability function of X,

$$P(X \geq \sqrt{-\ln y}) = \begin{cases} \int_{\sqrt{-\ln y}}^{1} p_X(x) dy = 1 - \sqrt{-\ln y} & \text{for } e^{-1} \leq y \leq 1, \\ 0 & \text{otherwise.} \end{cases} \quad (3.60)$$

The probability density function of Y is the the derivative of this function,

$$p_Y(y) = \begin{cases} 1 - \sqrt{-\ln y} & \text{for } e^{-1} \leq y \leq 1, \\ 0 & \text{otherwise.} \end{cases} \quad (3.61)$$

The probability density functions of X and Y are shown below.

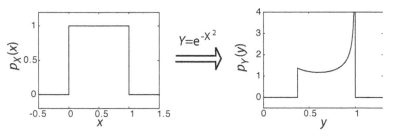

A special function of random variables, which is of particular interest it can approximate many processes in nature, is the sum of many random variables. For example, such a sum occurs if we calculate averages from measured quantities, that is,

$$\bar{X} = \frac{1}{n} \sum_{i=1}^{n} X_i, \quad (3.62)$$

and we are interested in the probability density function of such random variables. This function depends, of course, on the specific density function of the random variables

X_i. However, there is an important observation summarized in the central limit theorem that we can often utilize in this book. This theorem states that the average (normalized sum) of n random variables that are drawn from any distribution with mean μ and variance σ is approximately normally distributed with mean μ and variance σ/n for a sufficiently large sample size n. The approximation is, in practice, often very good also for small sample sizes. For example, the normalized sum of only seven uniformly distributed pseudo-random numbers is often used as a pseudo-random number for a normal distribution.

3.5.6 Measuring the difference between distributions

An important practical consideration is how to measure the similarity of difference between two density functions, say the density function p and the density function q. Note that such a measure is a matter of definition, similar to distance measures of real numbers or functions discussed in Appendix 3.2. However, a proper distance measure, d, should be zero if the items to be compared, a and b, are the same, its value should be positive otherwise, and a distance measure should be symmetrical, meaning that $d(a, b) = d(b, a)$. The following popular measure of similarity between two density functions is not symmetric and is hence not called a distance. It is called Kulbach–Leibler divergence and is given by

$$d^{\mathrm{KL}}(p, q) = \int p(x) \log(\frac{p(x)}{q(x)}) \mathrm{d}x \tag{3.63}$$

$$= \int p(x) \log(p(x)) \mathrm{d}x - \int p(x) \log(q(x)) \mathrm{d}x \tag{3.64}$$

This measure is zero if $p = q$ since $log(1) = 0$. This measure is related to the information gain or relative entropy in information theory.

3.5.7 Marginal, joined, and conditional distributions

When we have probability density functions of several variables, we can distinguish several cases. This is illustrated here in the case of two variables, while generalizations to more dimensions are straight forward. The most general information we can have about a process that depends on two random variables is the joined distribution,

$$p(x, y), \tag{3.65}$$

which is a two-dimensional function. The slice of this function, given the value of one variable, say y, is the conditional distribution,

$$p(x|y). \tag{3.66}$$

If we add over all realizations of y we get the marginal distribution,

$$p(x) = \int p(x, y) dy. \tag{3.67}$$

Two random variables x and y are called independent if

$$p(x, y) = p(x)p(y), \tag{3.68}$$

which is the same as saying

$$p(x|y) = p(x). \tag{3.69}$$

Note that we can decompose the joined distribution functions into the product of a conditional and a marginal distribution,

$$p(x, y) = p(x|y)p(y) = p(y|x)p(x), \tag{3.70}$$

which is sometimes called the product rule. If we divide this equation by $p(x)$, we get the identity

$$p(y|x) = \frac{p(x|y)p(y)}{p(x)}, \tag{3.71}$$

which is called Bayes's theorem. This theorem is important because it tells us how to combine a priori knowledge, such as the expected distribution of stimuli, $P(s)$, with some evidence as measured by a likelihood, $P(\mathbf{r}|s)$, to get the posterior distribution $P(s|\mathbf{r})$ from which the optimal estimate (in a statistical sense) of the stimulus can be calculated with eqn 8.31. $P(r)$ is the proper normalization so that the left-hand side is again a probability.

II

Neurons

4 Neurons and conductance-based models

Neurons are specialized cells that enable specific information-processing mechanisms in the brain. This chapter summarizes the basic functionality of neurons and outlines some of their fascinating biochemical processes. These include an outline of chemical synapses, the parametrization of the response of the postsynaptic membrane potential to synaptic events, the origin of action potentials and how they can be modelled using elegant differential equations introduced by Hodgkin and Huxley, generalizations of such conductance-based models, and compartmental models that incorporate the physical structure of neurons. The review in this chapter is intended to justify simplifications of following models and to mention some of the neuronal characteristics that may be relevant in future research.

4.1 Biological background

The central nervous system is primarily made up of two principal cell types, neurons and glial cells. Glial cells far outnumber neurons, and while glial cells have been seen as mainly providing supporting functions, there is increasing evidence of many more active processing functions of different types of glial cells. For example, the study of sophisticated processing mechanisms through neuron–glia interactions and signalling through glial networks is increasing. Glial cells can also regulate synaptic plasticity and possibly blood flow determined by synaptic activity. However, this chapter will concentrate on the information processing provided by neuronal networks. In order to describe the networks of neuron-like elements, we first have to gain some insight into the working of single neurons. Important issues include mechanisms of information transmission within single neurons and between neurons, and how the biologically complex neurons can be modelled sufficiently to answer specific scientific questions. The following review only mentions some of the sophisticated computational abilities of neurons, which some readers may want to study in more detail using the literature outlined at the end of this chapter. The review outlines briefly some of the computational approaches used to describe single neurons with biophysical and morphological details. The study of the biophysical machinery in single neurons is an active area within computational neuroscience. While most of the remainder of the book is based on strongly simplified models to investigate network properties, the main purpose of the discussion in this chapter is to gain an appreciation of the complexity in single neuron processes.

Neurons are biological cells and therefore have common features of other cells, including a cell body (also called a soma), a nucleus containing DNA, ribosomes assembling proteins from genetic instructions, and mitochondria providing energy for

Fundamentals of Computational Neuroscience. Third edition. Thomas P. Trappenberg, Oxford University Press. © Oxford University Press 2023. DOI: 10.1093/oso/9780192869364.003.0004

the cell. In contrast to other cells, neurons specialize in signal processing utilizing special electrophysical and chemical processes. Much progress has been made in unveiling some of those complex processes. Only some basic processes are reviewed here.

4.1.1 Structural properties

There are many different types of neurons, with differences in size, shape, or physiological properties. However, there are many general features of neurons, which are summarized here by describing a generic neuron, as illustrated in Fig. 4.1A, while outlining where variations are common. The major structural features are a cell body (or soma) and root-like extensions called neurites. The neurites are further distinguished into the receiving fibres of neurons, called dendrites from the Greek word dendron meaning tree, and one major outgoing trunk called an axon, which is the Greek word for axis.

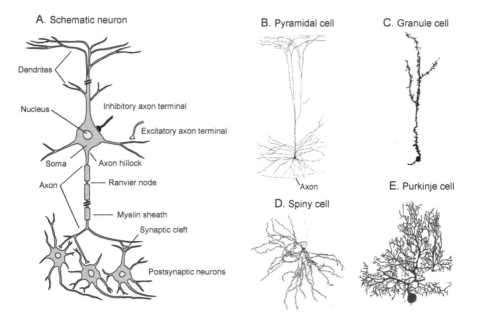

Fig. 4.1 (A) Schematic neuron that is similar in appearance to pyramidal cells in the neocortex. The components outlined in the drawing are typical for most major neuron types [adapted from Kandel, Schwartz, and Jessell, *Principles of neural science*, McGraw-Hill, 4th edition (2000)]. (B–E) Examples of morphologies of different neurons. (B) Pyramidal cell from the motor cortex [from Cajal, *Histologie du système nerveux de l'homme et des vertèbres*, Maloin, Paris (1911)], (C) Granule neuron from the olfactory bulb of a mouse [from Greer, *J. Comp. Neurol.* 257: 442–52 (1987)], (D) Spiny neuron from the caudate nucleus [from Kitai, in *GABA and the basal ganglia*, Chiara and Gessa (eds), Raven Press (1981)], (E) Golgi-stained Purkinje cell from the cerebellum [from Bradly and Berry, *Brain Research* 109: 133–51 (1976)].

The shape of neurons can vary considerably, and morphological criteria have been used as a scheme for classifying neurons. Some examples of shapes of neurons are illustrated in Fig. 4.1B–E. The most abundant neocortical neurons are categorized into pyramidal neurons and stellate neurons. Pyramidal neurons, of which an example is shown in Fig. 4.1B, are by far the most abundant neuronal type in the neocortex, accounting for as much as 75–90% of the neurons therein. They are characterized by a pyramid-shaped cell body with an axon usually extending from the base of the pyramidal cell body (basal base). The dendrites of the pyramidal cell can be divided into a far-reaching dendritic tree extending from the apical tip of the cell body into the upper layer of the cortex (discussed further in Chapter 5), and the basal dendrites with more local organizations. These neurons form contacts with other neurons with asymmetrical appearances and are thought to be excitatory.

The two other classes of neuronal types that are common in the neocortex have star-like appearances and are therefore called stellate neurons. Dendrites of spiny stellate neurons (as well as dendrites of pyramidal cells) are covered with many boutons, called spines. Typically, spiny stellate neurons have an excitatory effect on other cells. In contrast, the smooth stellate neurons are not covered with many spines and form inhibitory connections with other neurons that have a symmetrical appearance.

It should be clear that the division of neocortical neurons into pyramidal and stellate neurons is only a rough categorization of neuronal types in the neocortex. Other divisions can be made, although the distinction between different classes is often not easy to make on their spatial appearance alone. Some neurons that have been given other names include Martinotti cells, which are found mainly in the deeper layers of the neocortex and grow axons that extend commonly into the outer layer; basket cells, which are smooth stellate cells that synapse preferentially on the cell body of pyramidal cells; and chandelier cells, which synapse preferentially on the initial segment of pyramidal axons. Structural properties have computational consequences that must be explored. Later in this chapter we outline how cell morphologies can be incorporated in specific simulations of single neurons.

4.1.2 Information-processing mechanisms

Neurons can receive signals from many other neurons, called efferents, typically on the order of 10,000 neurons. Some neurons have many fewer incoming fibres such as motor neurons in the brainstem, and there are examples of cells receiving many more inputs, such as pyramidal cells in the hippocampus, which have been estimated to receive on the order of 50,000 inputs. The sending neurons contact the receiving neuron at specialized sites, either at the cell body or the dendrites. The English physiologist Charles Sherrington named these sites synapses. Various mechanisms are utilized to transfer information between the presynaptic neuron (the neuron sending the signal) and the postsynaptic neuron (the neuron receiving the signal). The general information-processing feature of synapses is that they enable signals from a presynaptic neuron to alter the state of a postsynaptic neuron, which eventually triggers the generation of an electric pulse in the postsynaptic neuron. This electric pulse, the important action potential, is usually initiated at the rooting region of the axon, the axon-hillock, and subsequently travels along the axon. Every neuron has one axon leaving the soma, although the axon can branch and send information to different regions in the brain. For example, some neurons spread information to neurons in neighbouring areas of the same neural structure with axon branches called axon collaterals, while other axons can reach through white matter to other brain areas. White matter contains no neuron bodies, only axons and oligodendrocytes, special glial cells that provide the myelin sheath for axons as described later. At the receiving site the axons commonly split into several fine branches, so-called arbors (Latin for tree), with axon terminals or axon boutons (French for buttons) forming part of the synapses to other neurons or muscles.

4.1.3 Membrane potential

The ability of a neuron to vary its intrinsic electric potential, the membrane potential, is important for the signalling capabilities of a neuron. The membrane potential, which we shall denote by V_m, is defined as the difference between the electric potential within a cell and its surroundings. The inside of a cell is neutral when positively charged ions (cations) are bound to negatively charged ions (anions). The origin of this potential difference comes from a different concentration of ions within and outside a cell. For example, the concentration of potassium (K^+) ions is around twenty times larger within a cell compared to the surrounding fluid. This concentration difference encourages the outflow of potassium by a diffusion process as long as the membrane is permeable to this ion. The neuronal membrane is, however, not permeable to the anions that typically bind to potassium, so the diffusion process leaves an excess of negative charge inside a neuron and an excess of positive charge in the surrounding fluid of the neuron.

The increasing electrical force resulting from the increased difference in the membrane potential will eventually be strong enough to match the force generated by the concentration difference of potassium within and outside of the cell. Hence, the electrical force will balance the diffusion process, and the neuron settles at an equilibrium state. The resulting potential is formally described by the Nernst equation which relates the work that is necessary to compensate for the diffusion gradient to the logarithm of the ratio of the concentrations, the absolute temperature, and some system-specific parameters. Calculating the equilibrium potential for potassium channels in a typical neuron results in a value around $E_K = -80$ mV, which is called the reversal potential for the channel. Only a very small percentage of K^+ ions have to leave the neuron in order cause the membrane potential. Similar processes for other ions, in particular sodium (Na^+) which has a concentration in the surroundings of a neuron exceeding the concentration within the neuron, eventually lead to the resting potential of a neuron, which is typically around $V_{rest} = -65$ mV.

Of course, it is probably more exciting and important to study how the membrane potential can be altered to transmit information. The membrane potential can be altered by a variety of mechanisms for which different neurons are specialized. For example, sensory neurons are specialized in converting external stimuli into electrical signals; examples include tactile neurons, which are sensitive to pressure, and photoreceptor neurons in the retina, which are sensitive to light. The information transmission between neurons, with which we are mainly concerned in this book, is achieved in a variety of ways. For example, electrical synapses or gap-junctions consist of special conducting proteins that allow a direct electromagnetic signal transfer between two neurons. However, the most common type of connection between neurons in the central nervous system is the chemical synapse, which will be described below.

4.1.4 Ion channels

The permeability of cell membranes to certain ions is achieved via ion channels. Ion channels are special types of proteins embedded in the membranes of cells (see Fig. 4.2). These proteins form pores that enable specific ions to enter or to leave cells. Common ions involved in such processes within the nervous system are sodium (Na^+), potassium (K^+), calcium (Ca^{2+}), and chloride (Cl^-). The ion channels that drive the resting potential of neurons are usually open all the time (see Fig. 4.2A). It is hence appropriate to call them leakage channels. We will shortly meet other types of ion channels that can open and close under various conditions.

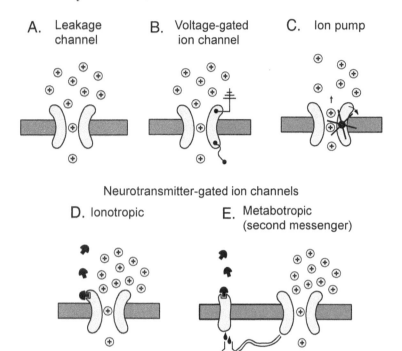

Fig. 4.2 Cartoonish illustrations of different types of ion channels. (A) Leakage channels are always open. (B) The opening of voltage-gated ion channels depends on the membrane potential. This is indicated by a little wire inside the neuron and a grounding wire outside the neuron. Such ion channels can, in addition, be neurotransmitter-gated (not shown in this figure). (C) Ion pumps are ion channels that transport ions against the concentration gradients. (D) An ionotropic neurotransmitter-gated ion channel opens when a neurotransmitter molecule binds to the channel protein, which, in turn, changes the shape of the channel protein so that specific ions can pass through. (E) A metabotropic synapse influences ion channels only through secondary messengers.

Information transmission within and between cells is largely based on ion channels. The following section describes these mechanisms in more detail, starting with a discussion of chemical synapses and followed by a discussion of the generation of action potentials in Section 4.3. In Section 4.5 we put the pieces together and describe the major functionality of neurons, using a compartmental model. The remainder of

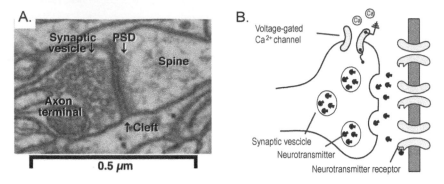

Fig. 4.3 (A) Electron microscope image of a synaptic terminal. The postsynaptic density (PSD) is a protein rich area in the dendrite terminal. Photo courtesy of Zeiss at https://blogs.zeiss.com/microscopy. (B) Schematic illustration of chemical synapses.

the chapter contains a brief discussion of extensions of the basic mechanisms, while the Chapter 5 concentrates on simplifications that enable us to study the behaviour of large networks of neurons.

4.2 Synaptic mechanisms and dendritic processing

4.2.1 Chemical synapses and neurotransmitters

Chemical synapses, are the workhorses of neuronal information transfer in the mammalian nervous system. An electron micrograph of a synaptic terminal is shown in Fig. 4.3A, and a schematic outlined in shown in Fig. 4.3B. These contact sites of neurons consist of a specialized extension on an axon, the axon terminal, and specific receiving sites on dendrites. Axon terminals of chemical synapses have the ability to synthesize special chemicals called neurotransmitters, concentrated and stored in synaptic vesicles. The arrival of an action potential triggers the probabilistic release of neurotransmitters. Released neurotransmitters drift across the synaptic cleft, a small gap of only a few micrometres ($1\mu m = 10^{-6}m$) between the axon terminal and the dendrite of the postsynaptic neuron.

Many different neurotransmitters have been identified in the nervous system. Common neurotransmitters in the central nervous system include small organic molecules such as glutamate (Glu) or gamma-aminobutyric acid (GABA). Dopamine (DA) is another neurotransmitter that has attracted a lot of attention for its role in motivation, attention, and learning. Synaptic transmission at neuromuscular junctions, important for initiating muscle movements, is primarily mediated by acetylcholine (ACh), and sensory nerves utilize a variety of other neurotransmitters.

Neurotransmitter-gated ion channels are special types of ion channels in postsynaptic dendrites that open and close under the regulation of neurotransmitters. Without the presence of the neurotransmitter the size of the pore is too small to let ions flow through it. These ion channels open when neurotransmitters bind to specific receiving sites of the ion channels, after which ions of the right size and shape can flow through them, changing the membrane potential of the cell in turn. The response in the membrane potential is called the postsynaptic potential (PSP). A larger quantity of neurotransmitter released by the presynaptic neuron can trigger a stronger response in the postsynaptic membrane potential, but this relationship does not have to be linear; twice the amount of neurotransmitter or twice the number of synapses involved in the overall synaptic event does not necessarily increase the membrane potential twofold.

The effects of neurotransmitters depend on the receptor type, so that the same neurotransmitter can have different effects in postsynaptic neurons. Receptors that are tightly coupled to an ion channel are called ionotropic and are illustrated in Fig. 4.2D. Such neurotransmitter-gated ion channels typically open rapidly after binding neurotransmitters. In contrast, metabotropic synapses, stylized in Fig. 4.2E, only influence ion channels through secondary messengers and are thus much slower and less specific.

4.2.2 Excitatory/inhibitory synapses

Different types of neurotransmitters and their associated ion channels have different effects on the state of receiving neurons. An important class of neurotransmitters opens channels that will allow positively charged ions to enter the cell. These neurotransmitters therefore trigger the increase of the membrane potential that drives the postsynaptic neurons toward their excited state. The process (and sometimes simply the synapse) is therefore said to be excitatory. Synaptic channels gated by the neurotransmitter Glu are a very common example of such excitatory synapses with different types of receptors. One fast ionotropic Glu receptor is called AMPAR because it can be activated with the synthetic chemical α-amino-3-hydroxy-5-methylisoxazole-4- propionic acid. Another Glu receptor is called NMDAR because it can be activated by the synthetic chemical N-methyl-D-aspartate; it is much slower and voltage dependent. The voltage dependence comes from the fact that these channels are blocked by magnesium ions (Mg^{2+}) in the neuron's resting state, even when Glu is bound. The Mg^{2+} ions can only be removed through depolarization of the membrane potential such as through back-propagating action potentials (BAPs) explained below. Only after the removal of magnesium can sodium and calcium, the two major ions that can pass through this channel, enter the neuron. In Chapter 6 we discuss the importance of these mechanisms for synaptic plasticity.

In contrast to excitatory synapses, some neurotransmitter-gated ion channels can drive the postsynaptic potential towards the resting potential or inhibit the effect of excitatory synapses. Such synapses are collectively called inhibitory. A prominent example of inhibitory synapses uses the neurotransmitter GABA with a fast receptor called $GABA_A$ and a slower receptor called $GABA_B$. The neurotransmitter DA has several receptor types, some of which are excitatory and some of which are inhibitory. Inhibition can be subtractive in the sense that it lowers the membrane potential. However, inhibition can also be divisive in the sense that it modulates the effect of excitation. For example, $GABA_A$ receptors have no effect on the membrane potential if the membrane potential is at rest, so it does not reduce the potential further. Inhibitory synapses close to the cell body can have such modulatory (multiplicative) effects on summed excitatory postsynaptic potentials (EPSPs). Such a form of inhibition is also called shunting inhibition.

4.2.3 modelling synaptic responses

As mentioned above, the variation of a membrane potential initiated from a presynaptic spike can be described as a postsynaptic potential (PSP). Excitatory synapses increase a membrane potential in what is called the excitatory postsynaptic potential (EPSP). In contrast, inhibitory postsynaptic potentials (IPSPs) are responses that lower the membrane potential. The form of IPSPs can often be modelled similar to EPSPs but with negative currents. We describe here only a generic implementation of ion-channel mediated PSP.

The experimentally measured time course of a PSP following a presynaptic event, in particular for fast excitatory AMPA receptors and inhibitory GABA receptors, can be parameterized by the function

$$V_{\mathrm{m}}^{\mathrm{non-NMDA}} = At\, e^{-t/t^{\mathrm{peak}}}, \tag{4.1}$$

where ΔV_{m} denotes the difference between the membrane potential and the resting potential, A is an amplitude parameter, and t^{peak} is the time for which this function reaches its maximal value. Synaptic responses of the above types are typically fast, with peak times around 0.5–2ms. The above function is sometimes called the alpha-function in neuroscience.

We can plot this function with the following Python program $\mathtt{Synapse.py}$. This is formally our first simulation program.

Programs/Synapse.py

```
1  # voltage over time for non-NMDA synapse
2  import numpy as np
3  import matplotlib.pyplot as plt
4
5  t = np.arange(0,10,0.1)
6  v = t*np.exp(-t/2)
7  plt.plot(t,v); plt.xlabel("t"); plt.ylabel("v")
```

In this function we did not include the typical synaptic delay of the PSP after the firing of a presynaptic neuron. This delay is caused by the time it takes for a neurotransmitter to be released in an axon terminal, the duration of the diffusion process of the neurotransmitter, and the time necessary to open the channels. All of these processes are typically fast (often less than 1 ms) and can be added directly in network simulations. Note that while we consider here synaptic delays as negligible, we will argue in Chapter 7 that latency between presynaptic and postsynaptic events, termed axonal delays, can be large and variable.

The alpha-function can be implemented with a basic model often used to describe chemical synapses. We thereby treat a segment of dendrite as a simple compartment that is a leaky capacitor (a capacitor with a constant resistor) together with a neurotransmitter-gated resistor, as illustrated in Fig. 4.4A. Each resistor is also supplied with a battery representing the concentration difference of ions within and outside the cell (Nernst potentials). The combined effects of the different components can easily be expressed by taking the conservation of electric charge into account. This is formalized in Kirchhoff's law,

$$c_{\mathrm{m}} \frac{\mathrm{d}V_{\mathrm{m}}(t)}{dt} = -I, \tag{4.2}$$

where c_m is the capacitance of the dendritic compartment and the minus sign on the right-hand side is a convention in neuroscience where currents are measured as flowing from outside the cell to inside the cell.

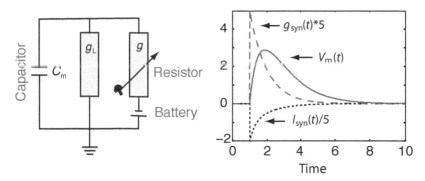

A. Electric circuit of basic synapse

B. Time course of variables

Fig. 4.4 (A) Electric circuit of a simple dendritic compartment to simulate a PSP with capacitance c_m, conductance g_L of the leakage channel, time dependent conductance g of the transmitter–gated ion channel and battery describing the equilibrium potential of the transmitter-gated ion channel. There is no battery for the leakage channel as the resting potential of circuit is set to zero. (B) Results for the numerical integration of the dendritic compartment model. Shown are time courses of the conductance $g(t)$, the synaptic current $I_{syn}(t)$, and the membrane potential $V(t)$. The conductance and current are scaled for better visibility, and the units correspond to the numerical values used in the simulations discussed below.

Eqn 4.2 is a linear differential equation. A differential equation describes the infinitesimal change of a quantity (the voltage in this example) with time, and this change is give by a function on the right-hand side. Solving a differential means to derive the time course of this quantity,

$$\frac{dx(t)}{dt} = f(x, t, ...) \quad \Rightarrow \quad x(t) = ? \tag{4.3}$$

We will mainly solve these equations numerically with simulation programs. Numerical integration in this circumstance simply means to sum all the changes, as given by the function on the right-hand side, from an initial state. Models are often formulated with differential equations, and is therefore recommended to study the brief introduction to differential equations given in Chapter 3.4 in case the reader is not so familiar with these concepts.

In the synaptic model, the current I is produced by two channels, a leakage channel with conductance (inverse of resistance) g_L and a reversal potential of zero (the resting potential of this compartment as we measure everything relative to this voltage), and the neurotransmitter-gated synaptic ion channel with time-varying conductance $g_{syn}(t)$ and reversal potential E_{syn}. The relation between the electric potential, the current, and the conductance is given by Ohm's law $(I = gV)$,

$$I(t) = g_L V(t) - g_{syn}(t)(V_m(t) - E_{syn}). \tag{4.4}$$

The time course of the time-varying synaptic conductance is modelled further with a simple model of the average channel dynamics. In this model we assume that many channels open immediately after binding neurotransmitters, but close stochastically like radioactively decaying material. This open-and-decay process is modelled as

$$\tau_{\mathrm{syn}}\frac{\mathrm{d}g_{\mathrm{syn}}(t)}{\mathrm{d}t} = -g_{\mathrm{syn}}(t) + \delta(t - t_{\mathrm{pre}} - t_{\mathrm{delay}}), \qquad (4.5)$$

where the delta function $\delta()$ is a convenient way to express a term that has an infinitely large contribution in an infinitely small time interval, when its argument is zero. The contribution to the sum (or integral) is finite (see Chapter 3.3). In the case above, a contribution is made at time t_{delay} after a presynaptic spike that occurred at t_{pre}. At other times, this equation results simply in an exponential decay with time constant τ_{syn} (see Chapter 3.4).

Below we discuss a Python program that implements the equations in this section and solves them numerically. The result of this numerical integration after a neurotransmitter binding at time $t = 1$ is shown in Fig. 4.4B. The time evolution of $g(t)$ is shown with a dashed line and is precisely an exponential decay. The opening of the channel produces a synaptic current I_{syn} through the neurotransmitter-gated ion channel (dotted line), where the amount does not only depend on the conductance of the ion channel, but also on the voltage of the membrane relative to the reversal potential of this channel. Thus, if the synaptic channel stays open, then the system comes to an equilibrium where the synaptic current matches the leakage current, and the voltage stabilizes at an intermediate value between zero and the reversal potential. However, the neurotransmitter-gated channels also close rapidly so that the synaptic compartment eventually decays to its resting state.

Simulation

We are now ready to discuss in some detail our first major simulation program. To some extend this is how complicated it gets. The program is an important example in neuroscience and is a simulation of a synapse by implementing the numerical integrating a the coupled differential equations explained before. Most of our simulations takes this form of numerical integrations of differential equations. Indeed, later programs might only appear more difficult as they might incorporate some more abstracts concepts. We also need first to get used to the Python programming language and how this is used in this context.

Programs/EPSP.py

```
1  # Synaptic conductance model to simulate an EPSP
2  import matplotlib.pyplot as plt
3
4  # Setting some constants and initial values
5  c_m=1; V_l=0; V_s=10; tau=1; dt=0.1;
6  g_l=1; g_s=[0];
7  I_l=[0]; I_s=[0];
8  v_m=[0]; t=[0];
9
10 # Numerical integration using Euler scheme
11 for step in range(1,int(10/dt)):
```

```
12    # record the time (in ms) in slot step of vector t
13    t.append(t[step-1]+dt)
14    # simulate opening synaptic chanels around t=1ms
15    if abs(t[step]-1) < 0.0001: g_s[step-1] = 1;
16    # calculate the currents at this time
17    I_l.append(g_l * (v_m[step-1]-V_l))
18    I_s.append(g_s[step-1] * (v_m[step-1]-V_s))
19    # update conductance and membrane potential
20    g_s.append(g_s[step-1]-dt/tau * g_s[step-1])
21    v_m.append(v_m[step-1]-dt/c_m*(I_l[step]+I_s[step]))
22
23 plt.plot(t,v_m,'k');
```

The basic conductance-based synaptic simulation programs to generate Fig. 4.4B is called EPSP.py. This program is not only a demonstration of a basic conductance-based model, but is also the first example of a simulation program based on numerical integration. The principle algorithm implemented in this program is to solve an ordinary differential equation of the form eqn 4.3 with a discrete iterative process,

$$x(t + \Delta t) = x(t) + \Delta t f(x, t, ...), \tag{4.6}$$

which calculates the value of the variable at the next time index (after one time step) from the value at the current time index plus the time step multiplied by the change as specified in the function f. Since it is the first major simulation program in this book, we describe this program line by line in the following.

In Python, every text that follows the hashtag sign, #, is a comment and will not be interpreted by the Python interpreter. We sometimes start the program with a comment that briefly states the purpose of the program in Line 1. We then import necessary libraries for specific function such as the plotting function in this program. Constants are then typically set at the next block of code so that they can easily be found to vary for different experiments. This includes the capacitance of the membrane, c_m, the conductance of the leakage channel, g_L, the time constant which sets the time scale of the opening (or better closing) of the synaptic ion channel, tau_syn, the reversal potential of the synaptic ion channel, E_syn. The last parameter is the integration time step, delta_t, which sets the (time) resolution of the simulation. Note that all the parameters are numbers and do not have units. A numerical simulation program cannot handle physical units and we have to make sure that the values are in the appropriate units. For example, we can interpret the time scale in terms of milliseconds (ms), so that the integration time step is $\Delta t = 0.01$ ms. The conductance of the leakage channel could be 1 Siemens (S), which is the inverse of the resistance measured in Ohms. A more typical value would be that the combined leakage channels in a square centimeter (cm^2) of membrane would be around some milliSiemens (mS). The conductance of other channels have then to be specified in the same units, and the other quantities have to be chosen consistently. We also include initial values for variables that will change with time. These quantities include the conductance of the synaptic ion channel, g_syn[0], which is set to zero so that it is closed at the beginning of the simulation. Consequently, the corresponding current, I_syn[0], is also zero. While we calculate the current from the conductance and membrane potential later, we include the value explicitly here for the first time index, i=0, since we start the iteration below at time index i=1 (the index after one time step). We also start with a zero membrane potential at the first time index, v_m[0]=0, and set the clock for the first time index to zero, t[0]=0.

The numerical integration of the differential equations, which specify the model, start at Line 11. The numerical integration is done using the Euler method (see Chapter 3.4), which simply adds the changes to the initial states for each integration step. The counter for the time step (index) is given by the variable i. The loop specifies that it starts with the value of 1 and is incremented by 1 until the index is equal to 10/0.01=1000. This time corresponds to 10 ms, or more precisely to 9.99 ms since we set the time for the first time index to zero. The actual time is updated in each step in Line 13 and kept in the vector t.

The next lines implement eqn 4.5. Line 15 simulates the opening of the synaptic ion channel after binding of neurotransmitters at time $t = 1$ ms by stetting the conductance at the previous time step to one, which is represented mathematically as the delta function in eqn 4.5. We override the value of the previous time step because this value is used in the next line to calculate the actual value at this current time step. The if statement might have an unexpected form. One might have suspected a statement like if t[i] == 1: .... The problem with this statement is that the left-hand side and the right-hand side have to be exactly the same, bit for bit. For example, 1.000000000001 is not equal to 1. To make sure that the if statement catches the time in the right vicinity, we ask instead that the absolute difference between t[i] and 1 should be less than a small value.

Line 17 and following lines is the simulation of the dynamics of the ion channel without the delta function part in eqn 4.5. The initial value of this conductance is zero, and it will stay like this until we force it to open at $t = 1$ ms in Line 15. After this it will decay since the code specifies that the new value of the conductance will be 'one minus a little bit' of the value at the previous time. The reduction of this value is proportional to the value itself, which is the characteristics of an exponential decay. This can be seen in the solution, the dashed line in Fig. 4.4B. As argued above, we can think of this dynamics as the average number of open channels when the channels close randomly like in a radioactive decay. This simulation does thus not include the precise dynamics of individual ion channels, although we could build such models.

4.2.4 Different levels of modelling

It is good to pause for a moment and realize that we have made two important models that describes the time course of membrane potential in a synapse after neurotransmitter triggered this response. The first model, that of eqn 4.1, is purely heuristic. By this we mean that we merely describe experimental observations by coming up with a mathematical function that mimics this time course to some extent. Such models can be very useful in many circumstances. For example, we can use this function as an input when modelling the further propagation of this signal in the dendrites.

This purely descriptive model is however not so useful when it is necessary to describe the process that causes this behaviour. Our second model was based on more fundamental mechanisms at work during the synaptic process. This model, described by equations 4.2, 4.4, and 4.5, uses the physical descriptions of electric currents in response of a changing conductance to calculate the time course of the membrane potential. The crucial input in this model is that the change in the synaptic conductance due to the opening of an ion channel is described by eqn 4.5. As already mentioned, this basically just describes an exponential decay of the conductance after the instantaneous opening at $t_{\text{pre}} + t_{\text{delay}}$. This in itself is only a macroscopic description of the underlying biophysical processes. Further research has shown that individual ion channels close stochastically after being opened, resulting in an exponential decay of their averaged effect on the synaptic conductance. Of course, we could build models which describe these behaviours in more detail.

The above model and its interpretation is a crude approximation of the synaptic processes. In reality, there is a complicated interplay between different ion channels and even subunits of receptors. The parameters $c_m, g_0, E_{\text{syn}}, \tau_{\text{syn}}$ have therefore no direct relations to specific ion channels and can be chosen arbitrarily to fit experimental data. Dendritic processing is further enriched by several other mechanisms, such as interdendritic calcium waves and BAPs related to active spiking mechanisms, as discussed in the next section. Glial cells can also influence synapses, for example by regulating vesicle release through calcium signalling. The above generic synaptic model does not attempt to explain the detailed workings of synapses, but rather, should be seen as a phenomenological model intended to parameterize experimental findings for convenience.

Electrical potentials have the physical property that they superimpose as the sum of the individual potentials. Many of the models discussed in the literature incorporate linear superposition of synaptic input, meaning that inputs are simply summed up in neuronal models. However, it is important to keep in mind that the membrane potential of a neuron depends on several other factors, such as the physical shape of the dendrites, the voltage dependence of some channels, and other interactions between synaptic ion channels. Also, there is some research that shows complex intercellular calcium signalling and interactions of synapses with genetic information. Most of the current computational models on a network level mostly assume much more stereotyped spiking mechanisms that we describe next. However, the large possibility of sophisticated dendritic computation has led some people, like Carver Mead, to speculate that dendritic computation might lead to the building of truly intelligent systems.

Non-linear interactions between synaptic inputs can add greatly to the information-processing capabilities of neural networks. We will discuss some examples in this book, although this area is still largely unexplored. The basic synaptic models introduced in this chapter are, however, already sufficient to explore many features of spiking neurons and networks. This model is sufficient for most of the discussions in this book and much of the network level computational literature. If necessary, more details of the underlying biochemical and physical mechanisms can be incorporated into the model, but, as we have stressed in Chapter 1, our aim here is not to recreate all details of the brain, but rather to extract essential mechanisms that explain brain functions.

4.3   The generation of action potentials: Hodgkin–Huxley

As discussed in the previous section, the dendritic membrane potential of a neuron can be altered by the release of neurotransmitters from a presynaptic neuron that opens specific synaptic ion channels and allows ions to leave or enter the neuron. This happens at the receiving end of neurons in the denditric tree. We now switch to membrane currents in axons, the sending end of the neurons at the other side of the nucleus. This type of membrane is able to trigger sharp and substantial changes in voltage, so-called action potentials, often simply called a spike. An important ingredient of axonal compartments are voltage-sensitive ion channels. So in contrast to synaptic ion cannels that are mainly triggered by neurotransmitters, these ion channels change their conductance with a change of membrane potential itself. Note that while these mechanisms are traditionally implicated in axonal processing, there are also mechanisms in the dendrites that can generate so-called back-propagating action potentials. However, our focus here is on the classical minimal model as proposed by Alan Hodgkin and Andrew Huxley. These two researchers proposed this model with parameters measured from the giant axon of a squid, although it turns out that their models with comparable parameters describe also the action potentials in vertebrate pyramidal cells. A trace of their original recording of an action potential is shown by Fig. 4.5. It is characterized by a sharp increase (depolarization) of the membrane potential to positive values, followed by a sharp decrease in the membrane potential, undershooting (hyperpolarizing) the resting potential of the neuron before returning to resting potential.

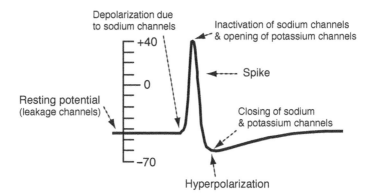

Fig. 4.5 Typical form of an action potential; redrawn from an oscilloscope picture from Hodgkin and Huxley (1939).

It was a major scientific accomplishment by Hodgkin and Huxley when they quantitatively described the form of action potentials with equations summarized in this section. It is not only the beauty of the description that made them famous, but also the fact that they quantified the process leading to the generation of action potentials with mathematical terms that were later identified with ion channels. Their model made specific predictions that could be verified experimentally and by so doing guided further research and many discoveries. Their original paper in the *Journal of Physiology* from 1952 is still worth reading and an excellent example of quantitative work in computational neuroscience.

4.3.1 The minimal mechanisms

A least two types of voltage-dependent ion channels and one type of static ion channel are necessary for the generation of a spike, as illustrated in Fig. 4.6. In contrast to the neurotransmitter-gated ion channels discussed in the previous section, voltage-dependent ion channels open and close as a function of the voltage of the membrane, as symbolized in Fig. 4.2B. A voltage-dependent sodium channel is responsible for the rising phase of action potentials. When neurotransmitter-gated ion channels depolarize neurons sufficiently, voltage-dependent sodium (Na^+) channels open, leading to an influx of Na^+ due to the negative potentials and the lower concentration of Na^+ within the cell. The domination of the sodium channel shifts the membrane potential close to the sodium resting potential, which is around $V_m = +65$ mV.

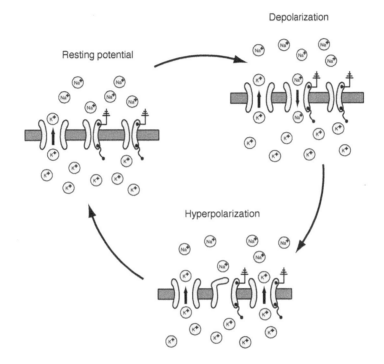

Fig. 4.6 Schematic illustration of the minimal mechanisms necessary for the generation of a spike. The resting potential of a cell is maintained by leakage channels through which potassium ions can flow as a result of concentration differences between the inside of the cell and the surrounding fluid. Voltage-gated sodium channels allow the influx of positively charged sodium ions and thereby the depolarization of the cell. After a short time sodium channels are blocked and voltage-gated potassium channels open. This results in hyperpolarization of the cell. Finally, the hyperpolarization causes the inactivation of voltage-gated channels and a return to the resting potential.

Two contributing processes cause the subsequent falling phase. First, sodium channels inactivate due to blockade of the channels by a part of the protein making up the channels, around 1 ms after the opening of the channels. Second, another type of voltage-dependent channels, potassium (K^+) channels, open, leading to an efflux of K^+. In contrast to voltage-dependent sodium channels, which open nearly instantaneously after crossing the threshold, voltage-dependent potassium channels open about 1 ms after the initial depolarization of the action potential. The dominance of potassium channels drives the membrane potential close to the potassium equilibrium of around $V_m = -80$ mV, undershooting the normal resting potential of the neuron. This hyperpolarization of neurons relative to the resting potential, V_{rest}, of neurons causes the voltage-dependent potassium channels to close and the voltage-dependent sodium channels to deactivate, so that the normal resting potential, V_{rest}, of neurons is eventually recovered.

4.3.2 Ion pumps

Repeated generation of action potentials results in a repeated efflux of K^+ and influx of Na^+. If a neuron repeated the process, as described so far, many times, it would decrease the potassium concentration and increase the sodium concentration within the cell repeatedly, eventually leading to the failure to generate action potentials. Another type of ion channel, not included in Fig. 4.6, is therefore vital for a cell. These specific ion channels are called ion pumps and are illustrated schematically in Fig. 4.2C. Ion pumps can transfer specific ions against their concentration level between the inside and outside of neurons. The price to pay is the large amount of energy necessary for this process. Ion pumps are estimated to account for about 70% of the total metabolic consumption of neurons, or about 15% of the total energy consumption in humans, while the brain accounts for one-fifth of our total energy consumption.

4.3.3 Hodgkin–Huxley equations

Hodgkin and Huxley quantified the process of spike generation with a set of four coupled differential equations, formalizing their measured findings of the giant axon of a squid. The net movement of ions across the membrane is a current that we label with the symbol I_{ion}. The number and permeability of open ion channels determine the electric conductance (the inverse of the resistance), which we label with $\bar{g}_{ion}$. The bar over the g is used here to indicate that this value can change and is therefore a function of possibly several factors. In the following we express the membrane potential relative to the resting potential V_{ion} of each channel and label it with V. The relation between this electric potential, the current, and the conductance is given by Ohm's law,

$$I_{ion} = \bar{g}_{ion}(V - V_{ion}), \tag{4.7}$$

The equilibrium potential for the channel where V_{ion} is the voltage when the force for ion movements due to the concentrations between the inside and the outside of the cell is in equilibrium with the electrical force. This corresponds to a channel-specific battery, as shown in the electric diagram representation of the Hodgkin-Huxley model in Fig. 4.7. The equilibrium potential in the above formula is thereby measured relative to the resting potential of the neuron.

As discussed above, a major component of the general framework for generating an action potential is the fact that the K^+ and Na^+ channels are voltage dependent. Hodgkin and Huxley introduced empirically three dynamic variables, n, m, and h, to describe this voltage dependence and the dynamics of the channels. The variable n describes the activation of the (then unknown) potassium channels, m describes

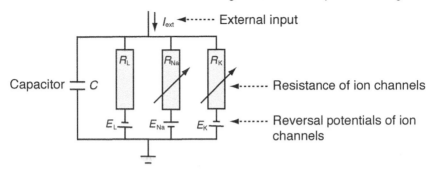

Fig. 4.7 A circuit representation of the Hodgkin–Huxley model. This circuit includes a capacitor on which the membrane potential can be measured and three resistors with their own batteries, modelling the ion channels; two are voltage-dependent and one is static.

the activation of the sodium channels, and h describes the inactivation of the sodium channels. The voltage and time dependence of the conductances is then described in the model by modulating constant conductance values, g_{ion} (without bar), with the voltage and time dependent variables $n(V, t)$, $m(V, t)$, and $h(V, t)$,

$$\bar{g}_K(V, t) = g_K n^4 \tag{4.8}$$

$$\bar{g}_{Na}(V, t) = g_{Na} m^3 h. \tag{4.9}$$

Hodgkin and Huxley chose the dynamics and voltage dependence of the variables so that the experimental data could be approximated reasonably well. They formulated this dynamic with an elegant set of three first-order differential equations, one for each variable,

$$\frac{dx}{dt} = \alpha_x(1 - x) + \beta_x x, \tag{4.10}$$

with $x \in \{n, m, h\}$.

The particular dynamics of the variables and their functional dependence on the membrane potential were chosen by Hodgkin and Huxley to reflect their experimental measurements. These are

$$\alpha_n = 0.01(V + 10)/(\exp(\frac{V + 10}{10}) - 1) \tag{4.11}$$

$$\alpha_m = 0.1(V + 25)/(\exp(\frac{V + 25}{10}) - 1) \tag{4.12}$$

$$\alpha_h = 0.07 \exp(V/20) \tag{4.13}$$

$$\beta_n = 0.125 \exp(V/80) \tag{4.14}$$

$$\beta_m = 4 \exp(V/18) \tag{4.15}$$

$$\beta_h = 1/(\exp(\frac{V + 30}{10}) + 1)) \tag{4.16}$$

These are lengthy-looking functions, but they are just descriptive or phenomenological models to fit the experimental data. They do not provide further insight into the mechanisms of these voltage dependencies. Ultimately this is due to the physical properties of the ion channels. However, we are here mainly interested to simulate the

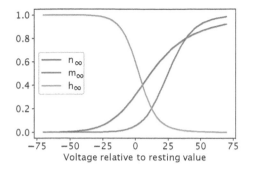

Fig. 4.8 (A) The equilibrium functions for the three variables n, m, and h in the Hodgkin–Huxley model with parameters used to model the giant axon of the squid.

spike dynamics and not the biophysical properties of individual ion channels. So these variables basically describe the opening dynamics of the channels.

To get some more insight that will be useful later, we can make a little mathematical exercise. For this, let us define the variables

$$x_\infty = 1/(\alpha_x + \beta_x) \tag{4.17}$$

$$\tau_x = \alpha_x x_\infty. \tag{4.18}$$

We can then write the above differential equations for the variables $x \in \{n, m, h\}$ in the familiar form

$$\tau_x(V)\frac{\mathrm{d}x}{\mathrm{d}t} = [x - x_\infty(V)]. \tag{4.19}$$

In this way we know how we can interpret functions. The function $x_\infty(V)$ corresponds to an voltage-dependent equilibrium value that is exponentially approached with the voltage dependent time constant $\tau_x(V)$. The voltage-dependence of these asymptotic equilibrium values are shown in Fig. 4.8. It shows that two of the functions have a similar form, and the other is somewhat the inverse of the others. This will give us some hint later how we can further simplify some spiking models. Meanwhile, let us go back to the Hodgkin-Huxley model.

The rest of the implementation of the electric circuit model (Fig. 4.7) is now straight forward and similar to the treatment on the synaptic side. The capacitor with capacitance, C is in parallel with three resistors, each supplied with their own battery setting their reversal potential. One of the resistors is constant, while the other two can change depending on the state of the system. The combined effects of the different components can be expressed by considering the conservation of electric charge due to Kirchhoff's law of the conservation of electric currents,

$$C\frac{\mathrm{d}V}{\mathrm{d}t} = -\sum_{\text{ion}} I_{\text{ion}} + I(t). \tag{4.20}$$

We can now put all pieces together by inserting the three ionic currents discussed above into eqn 4.20 and adding the three differential equations of the form 4.10, resulting in the standard four differential equations of the Hodgkin–Huxley model,

$$C\frac{\mathrm{d}V}{\mathrm{d}t} = -g_\text{K}n^4(V - E_\text{K}) - g_\text{Na}m^3h(V - E_\text{Na}) - g_\text{L}(V - E_\text{L}) + I(t) \tag{4.21}$$

$$\frac{dn}{dt} = \alpha_n(1-n) + \beta_n n \tag{4.22}$$

$$\frac{dm}{dt} = \alpha_m(1-m) + \beta_m m \tag{4.23}$$

$$\frac{dh}{dt} = \alpha_h(1-h) + \beta_h h \tag{4.24}$$

To summarize, the Hodgkin-Huxley equations describe the generation of action potentials by sodium, potassium, and leakage channels. It should be clear that this mechanism is a result of the simultaneous working of many such ion channels. The conductances in the Hodgkin–Huxley equations are hence the net result of individual ion channels in the membrane. The Hodgkin–Huxley model makes thereby the assumption that individual ion channels work independently of each other, an assumption that was recently called into question. Also, note that he densities of the ion channels have to exceed a certain threshold in order to be able to generate an action potential. These conditions normally occur in the axonal membrane, although active action potentials have now been observed in dendrites. The axon can typically be excited at any location when the axon is not myelinated as this blocks the ion channels.

The densities of the ion channels have to exceed a certain threshold in order to be able to generate an action potential. These conditions normally occur in the axonal membrane, although active action potentials have now been observed in dendrites. The axon can typically be excited at any location when the axon is not myelinated as this blocks the ion channels. However, in vivo (which is Latin for 'within the living'), neurons typically initiate action potentials in the axon-hillock. A small change of the membrane potential at the axon-hillock can then generate a large electric signal at this location. The spike generation is hence like an amplifier. At this time we only discussed this amplifier model, and we have still to discuss how this signal is transported down the axon further below.

The Hodgkin–Huxley equations can be easily integrated numerically, and a Python program to accomplish this is given in hh.py with the parameters used originally by Hodgkin and Huxley to model the axon of the giant squid. We first defined some parameters, the maximal conductances and battery voltages as used by Hodgkin and Huxley. We placed them into vectors (Numpy arrays), which makes it possible to write the later equations in compressed form using matrix notation. After the initialization of some more variables we enter a big loop over the time steps over which we want to integrate the Hodgkin–Huxley equations. In this simulation we actually perform an experiment where we switch on an external current between t=30 and t=89, and set it to zero otherwise.

Programs/hh.py

```
1  # Hogdkin-Huxley model
2  import numpy as np
3  import matplotlib.pyplot as plt
4  # Max conductances (in units of mS/cm^2); 0=K,1=Na,2=R
5  g = np.array([36,120,0.3])
6  # Battery voltage ( in mV); 0=n, 1=m, 2=h
7  V = np.array([-12,115,10.613])
8  # Initialization of some variables
9  v=0; x = np.array([0,0,1]); t=0; dt=0.01
10 t_rec=[]; v_rec=[]; x_0_rec=[]
```

```
11  # Integration  with  Euler  method
12  for  step  in  range(1,int(100/dt)):
13       t=t+dt
14       if  t>30  and  t<89:  I_ext=10
15       else:  I_ext=0
16   # alpha  functions  used  by  Hodgkin–and  Huxley
17       Alpha  =  np.array(
18            [0.01*(−v+10)/(np.exp((−v+10)/10)−1),
19             0.1*(−v+25)/(np.exp((−v+25)/10)−1),
20             0.07*np.exp(−v/20)])
21   # beta  functions  used  by  Hodgkin–and  Huxley
22       Beta  =  np.array([0.125*np.exp(−v/80),
23                          4*np.exp(−v/18),
24                          1/(np.exp((−v+30)/10)+1)])
25   # update  x  =  {n,m,h}  variables
26       x  =  x+dt*(Alpha*(1−x)−Beta*x)
27   # calculate  actual  conductances  g  with  given  n,  m,  h
28       gx=np.array([g[0]*x[0]**4,g[1]*x[1]**3*x[2],g[2]])
29  # Ohm's  law
30       I  =  gx*(v−V);
31   # update  voltage  of  membrane
32       v  =  v+dt*(I_ext−sum(I))
33   # record  some  variables  for  plotting  after  equil.
34       t_rec.append(t)
35       v_rec.append(v)
36
37  # Plotting  results
38  plt.plot(t_rec,v_rec);
39  plt.xlabel('Time');  plt.ylabel('Voltage')
40  plt.rcParams.update({'font.size':  15})
41  plt.legend(loc="center  left")
```

For each time step, the voltage of the membrane potential may have changed and we have first to calculate the parameters α and β of eqn 4.10 for each of the parameters m, n, and h. These are the functions that were chosen by Hodgkin and Huxley. With these new values we can update the values for all three parameter in line 25. This corresponds to the integration of the differential equations 4.10 using a simple Euler method (see Chapter 3.4) by replacing this continuous equation with the discrete version

$$x(t + \Delta t) = x(t) + \Delta t(\alpha_x(1 - x(t)) + \beta_x x(t)) \qquad (4.25)$$

The final steps are to use Ohm's law to calculate the corresponding synaptic currents and to update the membrane potential from the synaptic currents and the external current that flow within the small time step Δt for which all of these calculations are done.

The results of this simulation is shown in Fig. 4.9A. Interestingly, there seams to be a spike even before we apply some external current. This is unrealistic and a consequence of our simulation technique. We have started the integration with somewhat arbitrary initial values for the parameters. Hence, we need to first wait until these values converge to realistic values before we include such data in our analysis. This is called equilibration. In the simulation it seem that the voltage approximately reaches an equilibrium value around time $t = 20$. The voltage stays then constant until the external current is switched on at $t = 30$. This generates a spike and also several

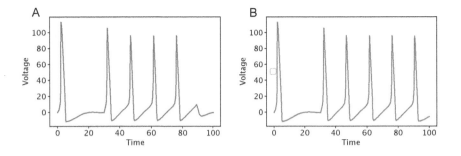

Fig. 4.9 A Hodgkin–Huxley neuron responds with constant firing to a constant external current of $I_\text{ext} = 10 \text{ mA/cm}^2$ between (A) t=30 and t=89 and (B) t=30 and t=90.

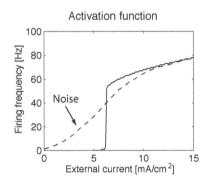

Fig. 4.10 The dependence of the firing rate on the strength of the external current shows a sharp onset of firing around $I_\text{ext}^c = 6 \text{ mA/cm}^2$ (solid line). High-frequency noise in the current has the tendency to 'linearize' these response characteristics (dashed line).

other spikes. Note that the first spike is a bit different than the consecutive spikes as the initial condition for this spike is different to the others. After removing the external current at $t = 89$, the membrane potential will go back to the resting potential.

Interestingly, if we just leave the external current on a little bit longer, until $t = 90$, then there is another spike generated. This is shown in Fig. 4.9B. Thus, there seems to be a kind of threshold when the spike is generated. While is it good to think about such a firing threshold, it is good to point out that this is not a fixed value as it depends on the history of buildup until a point of no return. However, this small detail is usually not a major confound for most of the discussions in this book and in the literature.

These simulations demonstrate that a constant external current with sufficient strength (here $I_\text{ext} = 10 \text{ mA/cm}^2$ leads to a constant firing of the neuron with a stereotyped waveform, as shown in Fig. 4.9. It is remarkable how the form of this simulated action potential captures the essential details of action potentials in real neurons, such as the one shown in Fig. 4.5. Also, when increasing external current, the number of spikes in a fixed interval, also called rate, increases. The function that describes the rate in dependence of input will be called the activation function or the gain function. Simulation results for the activation function of a Hodgkin–Huxley neuron are plotted in Fig. 4.10. The result reveals two more characteristics of the basic Hodgkin–Huxley neuron. First, in the basic model, shown with the solid line in the graph, onset of firing follows a sharp threshold around $I_{ext} = 6 \text{ mA/cm}^2$. Second, there is a fairly limited range of frequencies when the axon fires, starting at about 53 Hz and increasing only slightly with increasing external current. This is interesting because it shows that not all neuronal frequencies are equally likely.

Of course, there is a maximum firing rate with which any neuron can respond not explicitly included in these simulations. The reason for this is that the inactivation of the sodium channels makes it impossible to initiate another action potential for about 1 ms. This time is called the absolute refractory period, which limits the firing rates of neurons to a maximum of about 1000 Hz because then only a maximum of 1 spike in a millisecond, or 1000 spikes in a second, can be generated. Due to the hyperpolarizing action potential it is also relatively difficult to initiate another spike during this time period. This relative refractory period reduces the firing frequency of neurons even further. Of course, most neurons don't even fire close to such high rates, although very fast spiking frequencies have been measured in brainstem neurons, with frequencies sometimes exceeding 600 Hz. In contrast, cortical neurons typically respond with much lower frequencies, sometimes with only a few spikes per second. This cannot be explained by the refractory periods alone.

It is not obvious why cortical neurons fire with such low frequencies and with such irregularly. However, many circumstances influence the firing times of neurons. Among them are the details of charge transmission within dendrites, interactions between PSPs, other types of ion channels, and additional mechanisms not included in the Hodgkin–Huxley equations. Also, very importantly, we have to consider interactions within a network, specifically with inhibitory interneurons. Furthermore, a constant external current is physiologically unrealistic in the working brain, so one has to consider more realistic driving currents to get a better feel for typical response characteristics of a neuron.

To demonstrate how simple alterations in the basic mechanisms can alter the response characteristics of a Hodgkin–Huxley neuron, some results of further simulation are added in Fig. 4.10 with a dashed line. These simulations included some high frequency (1000 Hz) white (Gaussian distributed) noise. Such high-frequency noise could, for example, simulate low-frequency inputs from many presynaptic neurons. This noise was added to the main input current which was constant as in the previous simulations. The results indicate that such noise has the tendency to 'linearize' the f_I curve, resulting in the sigmoid-shaped function plotted as a dashed line in Fig. 4.10. Such response curves are important to model the information transmission in networks, and we will discuss such response curves further at the end of the next chapter when we can compare such curves to population responses.

4.3.4 Propagation of action potentials

Once an action potential is initiated, it will rapidly increase the membrane potential of neighbouring axon sites and thus travel along the axon with a low speed of around 10 m/s. This form of signal transportation within an active membrane is loss-free; the signal is regenerated at each point of the axon membrane and the signal will not deteriorate with distance. This is of major importance since axons can sometimes be very long, on the order of metres. On the other hand, this form of loss-free signal transportation is much slower than simple current transportation within a conductor, such as in an electrical wire or cable, and also consumes a lot of energy, as we mentioned above. It seems that nature responded to these problems by covering axons with a sheath of myelin. This sheath is created by a special type of glial cells, oligodendrocytes in the central nervous system and Schwann cells in the peripheral nervous system. Myelin sheaths change the electrical properties of axons to allow fast, but lossy, signal transfer within axons. However, myelin sheets are regularly interrupted by so-called Ranvier nodes, at which points the action potential can regenerate though the active membrane mechanism. It seems that nature combines, in this way, the advantages of fast and 'cheaper' signal transmission with regenerative amplifiers. It is interesting to note that a large part of the myelination happens after an initial organizational phase of the nervous system, which occurs in humans around their second year of age.

4.3.5 Above and beyond the Hodgkin–Huxley neuron: the Wilson model ◇

The Hodgkin–Huxley equations have taught us the basic concepts of the generation of action potentials. However, mammalian neurons have additional types of ion channels that enable more complex neuronal responses. At least a dozen types of ion channels can be involved in the spike generation of human neocortical neurons. It is fairly straightforward to include other ion channels in models to describe more specifically the electrical properties of specific neurons. Some modelling papers include therefore many coupled differential equations to model many different channels in one compartment. Such models are important to investigate detailed response characteristics of neurons and to investigate the interactions between the different channels. On the other hand, simplifications are also common when studying networks of neurons. Simplifications are often necessary to enable large-scale investigations, and, as discussed in Chapter 1, our scientific strategy is to keep models as simple as possible. Here we illustrate that the original Hodgkin–Huxley equations can be modified in several ways, to simplify the systems for large-scale studies, or to include more of the details of real neurons.

Models that reduce the dimensionality of Hodgkin–Huxley systems have been advanced for many years. For example, we can simplify the Hodgkin–Huxley model by using the results shown in Fig. 4.8. From this figure we see that the rate of inactivation of Na^+ channels is approximately reciprocal to the opening of K^+ channels. We can thus reduce the dimensionality of the model by setting $h = 1 - n$. Furthermore, one can show that the time constant τ_m for the dynamic variables m is small for all values of V. The dynamic for this variable is thus fast and can be approximated with the corresponding equilibrium values, $m_0(V)$. These simplifications reduce the Hodgkin–Huxley model to a two-dimensional system with an action potential very similar to that of the original Hodgkin–Huxley neurons. The model can be further simplified for neocortical neurons. Neocortical neurons often show no inactivation of the fast Na^+ channel, so h can be set to $h = 1$ (or, equivalently, $n = 0$ within our approximations). Following these approximations Hugh Wilson showed that a simplified model with only two differential equations,

$$C\frac{dV}{dt} = -g_K R(V - E_K) - g_{Na}(V)(V - E_{Na}) + I(t) \tag{4.26}$$

$$\tau_R \frac{dR}{dt} = -[R - R_0(V)], \tag{4.27}$$

still behaves similarly to Hodgkin and Huxley's system of four differential equations. The Wilson model described by eqns 4.26 and 4.27 combined the Na^+ and leakage channels into a new single Na^+ channel by including a linear term in the description of the voltage dependence of the new channel. The symbol of the only remaining dynamic modulation variable, R, describes the recovery of the membrane potential.

So far, we have only approximated the principal mechanisms that have already been described by Hodgkin and Huxley. In the following we include two more types of ion channels that seem essential for the more diverse firing properties of mammalian neocortical neurons. The first channel is a cation influx channel with more graded influx characteristics described by a dynamic gating variable T. Such channels, in particular Ca^{2+} channels, are a major ingredient of mammalian nervous systems. The more graded Ca^{2+} influx is mainly responsible for the more graded response characteristics of neocortical neurons compared to those of the giant axon of the squid. The second channel describes a slow hyperpolarizing current, such as that of a common Ca^{2+}-mediated K^+ channel, with a dynamic gating variable H. We will see that this type of channel is essential for the generation of a more complex firing pattern based on spike frequency adaptation. The complete Wilson model of mammalian neocortical neurons includes these types of channels, and is given by

$$C\frac{dV}{dt} = -g_K R(V - E_K) - g_{Na}(V)(V - E_{Na}) \tag{4.28}$$
$$-g_T T(V - E_T) - g_H H(V - E_H) + I(t)$$

$$\tau_R \frac{dR}{dt} = -[R - R_0(V)] \tag{4.29}$$

$$\tau_T \frac{dT}{dt} = -[T - T_0(V)] \tag{4.30}$$

$$\tau_H \frac{dH}{dt} = -[H - 3T(V)], \tag{4.31}$$

with polynomial parametrizations of the voltage dependence of the effective conductances,

$$g_{Na}(V) = 17.8 + 47.6V + 33.8V^2 \tag{4.32}$$

$$R_0(V) = 1.24 + 3.7V + 3.2V^2 \tag{4.33}$$

$$T_0(V) = 4.205 + 11.6V + 8V^2. \tag{4.34}$$

Despite drastic simplifications, such as neglecting the typical inactivation of the Ca^{2+} channels, this model is able to approximate mammalian spike characteristics in great detail. This includes the shape of single spikes, as well as all major classes of spike characteristics, such as regular spiking neurons (RS), fast spiking neurons (FS), continuously spiking neurons (CS), and intrinsic bursting neurons (IB), by choosing appropriate values of the remaining constants. This is shown next.

Programs/Wilson.py

```
 1  # Wilson neuron
 2  import numpy as np
 3  import matplotlib.pyplot as plt
 4  from scipy.integrate import odeint
 5
 6  def ydot(y,t,Iext,g,E,tau):
 7
 8    V=y[0]; R=y[1]; T=y[2]; H=y[3]
 9
10    gNa = 17.8 + 47.6*V + 33.8*V**2
11    R0 = 1.24 +    3.7*V + 3.2*V**2
12    T0 = 4.205 + 11.6*V + 8  *V**2
13    X = np.array([R,gNa,T,H])
14
15    Vdot = -1/tau[0]*(g*X@(V-E)-Iext)
16    Rdot = -1/tau[1]*(R-R0)
17    Tdot = -1/tau[2]*(T-T0)
18    Hdot = -1/tau[3]*(H-3*T)
19
20    return np.array([Vdot,Rdot,Tdot,Hdot])
21
22  # parameters of the model: 0=K  1=Na  2=T  3=H
23  g = np.array([26,1,2.25,9.5])
24  E = np.array([-0.95,0.50,1.20,-0.95])
25  tau = np.array([1,4.2,14,45])
26
27  #1: Equilibration: no external input
28  Iext=0; y0=np.zeros(4); y0[0]=-1
29  t=np.arange(0,100,0.1)
30  y = odeint(ydot, y0, t, args=(Iext,g,E,tau))
31  #2: Integration with external input
32  Iext=1; y0=y[-1,:];
33  t=np.arange(0,200,0.1)
34  y = odeint(ydot, y0, t, args=(Iext,g,E,tau))
35  plt.plot(t,y[:,0])
36  plt.xlabel('Time'); plt.ylabel('Membrane potential')
```

Simulations of the Wilson model can be done with the programs `Wilson.py`. The following simulations were done with fixed values of the constants as suggested by Wilson, namely $E_{Na} = 50$ mV, $E_K = -95$ mV, $E_T = 120$ mV, $E_R = E_K$, $C = 100$ μF/cm, $g_{Na} = 1$, $g_K = 26$, $\tau_T = 14$ ms, $\tau_R = 45$ ms. The simulations also use a constant external driving current, $I_{ext} = 1$ nA. Ignoring the slow, calcium-mediated potassium channel ($g_H = 0$) and setting $\tau_R = 1.5$ ms, $g_T = 0.25$ results in constant rapid spiking, as shown Fig. 4.11A. Such spike trains are typical for inhibitory interneurons in the mammalian neocortex when stimulated with a constant current.

Excitatory neurons typically have more complex behaviour, with slower spike rates and elongated spikes. In the following simulations, we therefore use a time constant of $\tau_R = 4.2$ ms. The inclusion of a slow, calcium-mediated potassium channel ($g_H = 5$), with a slightly smaller calcium conductance ($g_T = 0.1$), results in the spike train shown in Fig. 4.11B. The slow hyperpolarizing channel has the important effect of reducing the firing rate after initial stimulation of the neuron. This spike rate adaptation is sometimes called fatigue. The firing rates of such regularly spiking neurons are often reduced to about half of their initial value in about 50 ms, and some neurons even cease

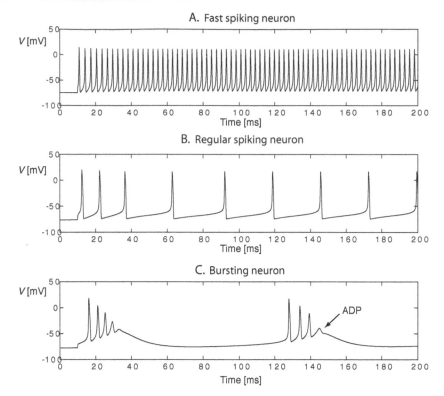

Fig. 4.11 Simulated spike trains of the Wilson model. (A) Simulates fast spiking neuron (FS) typical of inhibitory neurons in the mammalian neocortex $(\tau_R = 1.5$ ms, $g_T = 0.25$, $g_H = 0)$. (B) Simulated regular spiking neuron (RS) with longer interspike time intervalls $(\tau_R = 4.2$ ms, $g_T = 0.1)$. The slow, calcium-mediated potassium channel $(g_H = 5)$ is responsible for the slow adaptation in the spike frequency. (C) This graph demonstrates that even more complex behaviour, typical of mammalian neocortical neurons, can be incorporated in the Wilson model. The parameters $(\tau_R = 4.2$ ms, $g_T = 2.25$, $g_H = 9.5)$ result in a typical bursting behaviour, including a typical after-depolarizing potential (ADP) [see also Wilson, *Journal of Theorretical Biology* 200: 375–88 (1999)].

firing altogether.

Another important class of neurons, showing short bursts interleaved with silent phases, can be simulated by increasing the slow hyperpolarizing conductance ($g_H = 9.5$) as well as the calcium conductance ($g_T = 2.25$). The firing response of such a neuron is shown in Fig. 4.11C. Such bursting neurons typically show a long-lasting after-depolarizing potential (ADP), which is also present in the Wilson model.

4.4 FitzHugh-Nagumo model

The final spiking model we discuss tin this section has been very influential in neuroscience. It emerged shortly after the introduction of the Hodgkin-Huxley model and has been very useful in comprehending many of the dynamical features of neuron-like dynamical systems like the Hodgkin-Huxley model. The FitzHugh-Nagumo model was specifically introduced to simplify Hodgkin-Huxley equations while being able to preserve and analyze more rigorously the dynamical features of such systems. Richard FitzHugh proposed the model in 1961 as a generalization of the van der Pol oscillator, while Jin-ichi Nagumo and colleagues realized this model with a proposed circuit diagram as shown in Fig. 4.12. As we outlined before, the Hodgkin-Huxley equations has been so important as they specifically parameterized the dynamic equations along identifiable synapses, while the model discussed here is more focused on qualifying the dynamic properties as a whole. Due to its simplicitym, it is also a useful model of a spiking neuron in itself when we are not studying specific aspects of individual ion channels. So while these models are somewhat more abstract, similar models such as the ones discussed in the next chapter have been shown to simulate even more dynamical features that are presumably created by details in the neurons that are not captured by the Hodgkin-Huxley model.

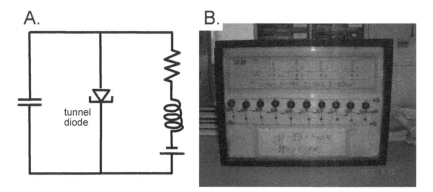

Fig. 4.12 (A) The circuit diagram of the FitzHugh-Nagumo neuron as suggested by Naguno (1962). (B) The physical implementation by Naguno (photograph courtesy of Kazuyuki Aihara).

The model equations of the FitzHugh-Nagumo model are much simpler than the Hodgkin-Huxley model and are two-dimensional similar to the basic Wilson model that we discussed before. A two-dimensional model is useful as it allows the illustration of its phase space that has highly motivated the theoretical understanding of their dynamical properties within dynamical systems theory. This two variables are the voltage-like variable v and a recovery variable w that drives the reset of the voltage after buildup:

$$\frac{dv(t)}{dt} = v - v^3/3 - w + I_{\text{ext}} \tag{4.35}$$

$$\tau \frac{dw(t)}{dt} = 0.08(v + 0.7 - 0.8w) \tag{4.36}$$

Numerically integrating these equation should be familiar now and is give in the program FN.py. The spike train of this neuron is shown in Fig. 4.13A. While the individual spikes do not seem to fit exactly the time-course of the spike in the giant axon of the squid, the emphasis of this model is the understanding of the dynamical systems aspects of neurons. The phase diagram, which is a plot of the two variables

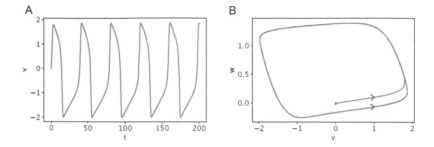

Fig. 4.13 (A) The regular firing of the FitzHugh-Nagumo neuron. (B) The phase diagram of the FitzHugh-Nagumo neuron.

Programs/FN.py

```
1  #FitzHugh−Nagumo model
2  import matplotlib.pyplot as plt
3
4  # Parameters and initialization
5  Iext=0.5; v=[0]; w=[0]; t=[0]; dt=0.1
6
7  for step in range(1,int(200/dt)):
8      # record time steps
9      t.append(t[step−1]+dt)
10     # numerical integration and recording
11     v.append(v[step−1]+dt*(v[step−1]−v[step−1]**3/3−w[step−1]+Iext))
12     w.append(w[step−1]+dt*0.08*(v[step−1]+0.7−0.8*w[step−1]))
13
14 plt.plot(t,v); plt.xlabel('t'); plt.ylabel('v')
```

against each other, is shown in Fig. 4.13B. We started the system with arbitrary initial conditions that might not be biologically realistic. This is illustrated with the red circle at the beginning of the trajectory. Also, we indicated the time evaluation of this trajectory with two black arrowheads. The important part here is that the system quickly approaches a limit cycle that is characteristic for the oscillatory behaviour of the voltage and reset parameter for that matter. Many more characterizations of a dynamical system can be made with dynamical systems theory, but at this time we will move on to finalize this chapter to outline how the synaptic mechanisms can be integrated with the morphology of a neuron.

4.5 Neuronal morphologies: compartmental models

We have discussed the effects of neurotransmitter-gated ion channels, leakage channels, and voltage-dependent ion channels on the membrane potential of a neuron. To get a comprehensive view of the state of a neuron we must also include the conductance properties and the physical shape of the neuron. In contrast to axons with active membranes able to generate action potentials, dendrites have been seen historically more like passive conductors, analogous to long cables. Note that dendrites also have active ion channels generating BAPs. Non-linear effects in dendrites are also important. However, many general features of dendrites in a subthreshold regime can be studied using passive cable equations, so this approximation is used to outline the principal idea behind compartmental modelling. The physics of conducting cables was worked out in the mid-nineteenth century by William Thomson (Lord Kelvin), enabling the first transatlantic communication cables. Many researchers have since applied this theory to neural transmission such as Wilfrid Rall, who has contributed much to the theory and its applications. Taking these missing links into account, we will only outline the basic idea behind compartmental models in this section. Such modelling alone is an active and important part of computational neuroscience. Indeed, modern tools in this area will include mechanisms to include many details of neurons and enable sophisticated network simulations.

4.5.1 Cable theory

To get a feeling for some equations involved in compartmental modelling, we will briefly outline the cable equation. This equation describes the spatio-temporal variation of an electric potential along a cable-like conductor driven by an injected current I_{inj}. For an idealized one-dimensional linear cable, the equation is given by

$$\lambda^2 \frac{\partial^2 V_m(x,t)}{\partial x^2} - \tau_m \frac{\partial V_m(x,t)}{\partial t} - V_m(x,t) + V_0 = R_m \, I_{inj}(x,t). \qquad (4.37)$$

This is a partial differential equation, second-order in space and first-order in time. Partial derivatives are symbolized by ∂ instead of total derivatives symbolized by d. Partial derivatives only consider explicit dependencies on the parameters and ignore implicit dependence on other parameters. This differential equation is formally a hyperbolic differential equation in case you want to look it up in mathematics books. The solution of this equation, $V_m(x,t)$, describes the potential of the cable at each location of the cable and how it varies at each location with time. The constant λ describes the physical properties of the cable and has the dimensions of Ω cm. For example, a cylindrical cable of diameter d, in an equipotential surrounding, has a lambda parameter of

$$\lambda = \sqrt{\frac{dR_m}{2R_i}}, \qquad (4.38)$$

where R_m is the specific resistance of the membrane and R_i is the specific intracellular resistance of the cable. A specific resistance is the resistance of a piece of material with constant cross-section, divided by the volume of the resistor. Membrane resistance is, of course, much larger than the intracellular resistance, which explains why most of the current flows within the dendritic tree. Note that the lambda parameter changes with the diameter of the cable. The time constant τ_m also depends on the physical properties of the cable and is given by

$$\tau_m = R_m C_m, \qquad (4.39)$$

where R_m is the specific resistance of the membrane, or the inverse of the leakage conductivity, and C_m is the specific capacitance, the capacitance per unit area.

The solutions of eqn 4.37 also depend on the form of the injected current $I_{inj}(x, t)$, and analytical solutions can only be given for some simple examples which are nevertheless instructive. Note that the equation can be integrated numerically in more general situations as discussed later. It is clear that the cable potential should reach a stable configuration (distribution within the cable) if the injected current is not time dependent. For example, if we consider a semi-infinite cable that starts at $x = 0$ with a fixed potential $V_0 = R_m I_0$ and extends to infinity thereafter, then the potential decays exponentially with

$$V_m = V_0 e^{-\frac{x}{\lambda}}. \tag{4.40}$$

This exponential decay is, of course, a problem for information transmission and the signal in a long cable has to be amplified periodically in order for it to be transmitted over large distances. Note that in the case of signal transmission we have to solve the cable equation in the presence of a time-varying current. However, the general features of a decaying signal also hold in this case.

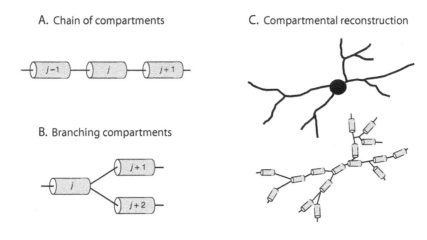

Fig. 4.14 Short cylindrical compartments describing small equipotential pieces of a passive dendrite or small pieces of an active dendrite or axon when including the necessary ion channels. (A) Chains and (B) branches determine the boundary conditions of each compartment. (C) The topology of single neurons can be reconstructed with compartments, and such models can be simulated using numerical integration techniques.

If we include voltage-dependent ion channels as in the Hodgkin–Huxley equations, we have a voltage-dependent injected current. In this case we have to solve the nonlinear cable equation where $I_{inj}(x, t)$ in eqn 4.37 is replaced with $I_{inj}(V_m(x, t), t)$ which depends explicitly on V_m, which in turn varies spatially and temporally. No general analytical solution can be given for this equation, but we can use numerical integration techniques to solve the equation for particular cases.

4.5.2 Physical shape of neurons

The cable equations depend on the physical properties of the cable through the parameter λ, and it is time to take the physical shape of neurons into account. The first step in solving the cable equations for cables with structures other than a simple homogeneous linear cable is to divide the cable into small pieces (for example, small cylindrical cables), where each piece has to be small enough so that the potential within each unit is approximately constant. We call this unit a compartment (see Fig. 4.14A). Each compartment is governed by a cable equation for a finite cable, which is a first-order differential equation in time, as we have seen above. For small compartments we can assume a constant potential within the compartment. However, we also have to take the boundary conditions into account. This can be done by replacing the continuous space x with discrete spatial locations labelled with indices, such as x_j, and replace the spatial differentials with differences,

$$\frac{\partial^2 V(x,t)}{\partial x^2} \to \frac{V_{j+1} - 2V_j(t) + V_{j-1}(t)}{(x_{j-1} - x_j)^2}. \tag{4.41}$$

With similar formulas we can take branching cables (as illustrated in Fig. 4.14B) into account. A neuron is therefore simulated with a discrete model of small cylinder-like cables as illustrated in Fig. 4.14C. This compartmental model is governed by a set of first-order differential equations in time, since we have replaced the spatial differentials with difference equations. The number of compartments should be large enough to accurately represent a neuron. In practice, the number of compartments needed to get good approximations of the real neuron depends on the complexity of the neuron. Models with a few hundred to several thousand compartments have been used in the literature to represent single neurons very accurately.

4.5.3 Neuron simulators

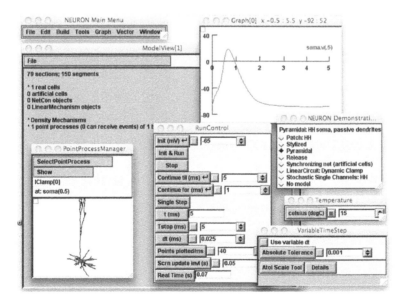

Fig. 4.15 Example of the NEURON simulation environment. The example shows a simulation with a reconstructed pyramidal cell, in which a short current pulse was injected.

The set of coupled differential equations defining a compartmental model can be solved numerically. While numerically solving differential equations is, in principle, straightforward, as discussed in Chapter 3.4, there are many details to be considered for efficient numerical integration. These include the stability of solutions and efficient use of computational resources. It is therefore useful to employ special-purpose software that implements appropriate numerical techniques so that computational neuroscientists can concentrate on the biological questions. Compartmental models have often been analysed numerically by replacing their equations with equivalent representations of electrical components and using circuit simulation programs such as SPICE to solve the systems.

The most popular simulator today called NEURON https://neuron.yale.edu/neuron) that was developed by M. L. Hines, J. W. Moore, and N. T. Carnevale from Duke and Yale Universities. Its distribution package includes an example of a three-dimensional reconstruction of a pyramidal cell, as shown in Fig. 4.15. In the shown example, we injected a 20 nA current at $t = 1$ ms for 0.5 ms at the location on the dendrite indicated by the blob and cursor in the graphical outline of the cell. We then measured the response at the soma, which can be seen in the graph window. The passive dendrite passed the current on to the soma with some delay and a more gradual response. The new versions of such simulation programs also include many specific cellular mechanisms and some support for network simulations. All of these simulation packages include tutorials that are highly recommended for further studies. Also, the Allen Institute now has an extensive list of models for many neuron types from the mouse and human cortex together with the data from which these models were constructed.

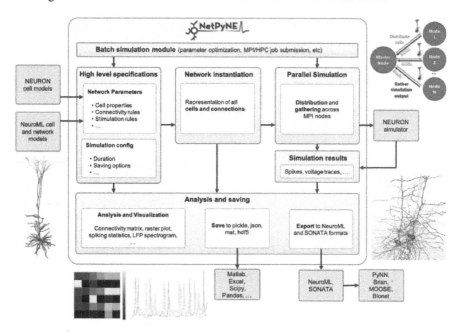

Fig. 4.16 Outline of the NetPyNe tool for simulating and analysing neurons and networks [from Dura-Bernal et al., NetPyNE, a tool for data-driven multiscale modelling of brain circuits, *eLife* 2019.

While Neuron is a sophisticated tools, there have been many developments since its introduction. The power of this and related tools is that there is now a large database of models as well as integrations to analysis tools. An exciting recent tool call NetPyNe for 'Networks using Python and NEURON'. This tool allows the import and definition of neuron models and networks and to simulate an analyse such models. An outline is shown in Fig. 4.16.

5 Integrate-and-fire neurons and population models

In keeping with the minimalist approach to modelling, this chapter introduces a variety of further abstractions of neurons. We start with discussing the all important leaky integrate-and-fire (LIF) neuron together. While this model is complex as a whole, the simplicity of the subthreshold dynamics allows for some interesting calculations. We also introduce more recent generalizations of this basic model to allow again to incorporate more realistic feature of specific neuronal groups. In the middle section of this chapter, we discuss some general aspects information processing with spiking neurons that will set the stage for our final abstraction of neural systems. That is, we make another important leap to describe the collective behaviour of groups of neurons, also known as population models or rate models. Population nodes are the basis for many system-level investigations in cognitive neuroscience and are used frequently in later sections of this book. This chapter is an important start of abstractions that are necessary to tackle more system-level information-processing principles.

5.1 The leaky integrate-and-fire models

Many computational studies in the literature are based on strongly simplified versions of the mechanisms present in real neurons or even that of conductance-based models. The are several reasons for such simplifications. Often, simplifications are necessary to make computations with large numbers of neurons tractable. Simplifications are also useful scientifically to highlight the minimal features necessary to enable certain emergent properties in the networks. It is, of course, an important part of every serious study to verify that the simplifying assumptions are appropriate in the context of specific question to be analyzed via a model. Also, a strong motivation for the following models is that the form of spikes generated by neurons is very stereotyped and it is therefore unlikely that the precise details of spike shape are crucial for information transmission in a nervous system on the level discussed in this book. In contrast, spike timing certainly has some influence on the processing of spiking elements in networks that we will explore further below. Thus, for the questions we are going to ask, it is not important to describe the precise form of a spike, only the integration of synaptic input leading to a generation and the following recovery process of a spike. We therefore neglect the detailed ion-channel dynamics and concentrate instead on approximating the dynamic integration of synaptic input, spike timing, and resetting after spikes.

The main effects of sodium and leakage channels, which are important in the rising phase of a spike, is that they drive the neuron to higher voltages with input and let the voltage decay to its resting potential otherwise. Neglecting the non-linearities captured

Fundamentals of Computational Neuroscience. Third edition. Thomas P. Trappenberg,
Oxford University Press. © Oxford University Press 2023. DOI: 10.1093/oso/9780192869364.003.0005

by the non-linear voltage dependence of sodium channels, we can approximate the subthreshold dynamics of the membrane potential with a simple linear differential equation according to Kirchoff's law (see eqns 4.20 and 4.2),

$$\tau_{\mathrm{m}}\frac{\mathrm{d}v(t)}{\mathrm{d}t} = -(v(t) - E_L) + RI(t), \tag{5.1}$$

where E_L is the resting potential. Such a system is also called a leaky integrator. We have introduced a time constant τ_{m} determined mainly by the capacitance of a one-compartment model and the average conductances of the sodium and leakage channels. The input current $I(t)$ can have different sources, such as artificially applied current in experimental settings or synaptic input. We will specify this later for specific models.

While the subthreshold buildup of the membrane potential is modelled in some detail, a major simplification is made once the membrane potential is large enough to trigger an action potential. At this point we used the full set of Hodgkin–Huxley equations to model the form of the spike in Chapter 4. However, we are now only interested in the fact that a spike was generated at time t^{f} when the threshold θ was reached. Mathematically we can write this as

$$v(t^{\mathrm{f}}) = \theta. \tag{5.2}$$

Assuming that there is a fixed threshold is only a crude approximation of real spike generation. The Hodgkin–Huxley equations already show that the value of no return, which is the amount of buildup from which spiking cannot be prevented by turning off the stimulus, depends on the form (or curvature) of current buildup. Also, some cortical neurons in vivo display a strong variability of this threshold as well as other variabilities that are ignored here.

To complete the model we also have to reset the membrane potential after a neuron has fired. Several mechanisms can be considered here which will be explored further below. A particularly simple choice is to reset the membrane potential to a fixed value v_{res} immediately after a spike, for example,

$$v(t^{\mathrm{f}} + \delta) = v_{\mathrm{res}}, \tag{5.3}$$

where δ is an infinitesimally small time step in the continuous formulation, or a finite time step in discrete versions, as used in numerical simulations. We can incorporate an absolute refractory time by holding the membrane potential constant, $v = v_{\mathrm{res}}$ for a certain period of time after the spike. A more graded refractoriness can be simulated with a smoother functional description instead of the sudden reset of the membrane potential, but most of the simulations discussed in this book will not depend crucially on these details. Equations 5.1–5.3 define the (leaky) integrate-and-fire neuron, although a better name would probably be a leaky integrate-and-fire-and-reset neuron. It is also often abbreviated as LIF neuron or IF neuron. Such a model neuron is illustrated schematically in Fig. 5.1.

While the form of the IF neuron as presented here is rather general, this neuron model is commonly used in conjunction with specific input currents for specific modelling studies. For example, we can think of this current as supplied externally in experiments or we could describe the current which is produced from specialized

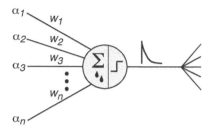

Fig. 5.1 Schematic illustration of a leaky integrate-and-fire neuron. This neuron model integrates (sums) the external input, with each channel weighted with corresponding synaptic weighting factors w_i, and produces an output spike if the membrane potential reaches a firing threshold.

processes of sensory cells. In many network simulations, we are mainly concerned with the sum of synaptic currents generated by firings of presynaptic cells. This sum of synaptic currents depends on the efficacy of individual synapses, which are described by a synaptic strength value, w_j, for each synapse, labelled by an index j representing each presynaptic neuron. We also call this value the connection strength, synaptic efficacy, or simply weight value. In the following, we assume that there are no interactions between synapses so that we can write the total input current to the neuron under consideration as the sum of the individual synaptic currents where each postsynaptic response to a presynaptic event, written as an α-function that we discussed in Section 4.2.3, is multiplied by a weight value (synaptic efficiency)

$$I(t) = \sum_j \sum_{t_j^f} w_j \alpha(t - t_j^f). \tag{5.4}$$

The variable t_j^f denotes the firing time of the presynaptic neuron of synapse j, in contrast to the firing time of the postsynaptic neuron above, which has no index. Thus, we parameterized the time course of synaptic response with the function $\alpha(t)$ such as used in eqn 4.1. Alternatively, we could use a conductance-based model of synapses as in eqns 4.4–4.5. The major simplification of IF neurons is the spike generation that is simply replaced by a note that a spike occurred and a reset of the potential.

5.1.1 Response of IF neurons to very short and constant input currents

The importance and illustrative simplicity of the LIF model allows for some more detailed derivation of some of its behaviour. The whole set of equations describing an IF neuron are non-linear due to the reset of the membrane potential after each spike, and typically have to be integrated numerically. However, the dynamic equation for the subthreshold membrane potential leading up to a spike, eqn 5.1, is mathematically an inhomogeneous linear differential equation that can be solved analytically. To simplify the following equations we will set $E_L = 0$ so that the membrane potential v is measured relative to this resting potential. We discuss the solutions in this section for some instructive case.

We start with the case of an IF neuron that is driven by a very short input pulse, a very short input current $I(t)$ which is not sufficient to elicit a spike. Mathematically we write this short input pulse as a delta function $I(t) = \delta(t)$ as mentioned in Chapter 3.3. It is hard to imagine that this form can be realized in nature; it would mean having an input pulse that is infinitely strong but has zero duration. However, it is possible to define the delta function properly as a limiting process of a finite pulse, for example, as a Gaussian bell curve, and making the duration smaller while keeping the integral over this function constant. With this limiting process, we can solve the differential equation 5.1.. Say we start at a situation where the initial potential shortly before time $t = 0$ is equal to zero. We then apply a very short input pulse that drives the potential at time $t = 0$ to $v(t = 0) = 1$. After this, there is no remaining input current, so that eqn 5.1 becomes a simple homogeneous differential equation for all times $t > 0$, given by

$$\tau_\mathrm{m} \frac{\mathrm{d}v(t)}{\mathrm{d}t} + v(t) = 0. \tag{5.5}$$

The solution of this differential equation is an exponential function that can easily be verified by inserting the result into the differential equation. The membrane potential decays exponentially after a short external current is applied,

$$v(t) = \mathrm{e}^{-t/\tau_\mathrm{m}}. \tag{5.6}$$

The time scale of this decay is given by the time constant τ_m.

Another example where we can integrate the subthreshold dynamic equations is an IF neuron driven by a constant input current that is low enough to prevent firing. This will lead, after some transient time, to a stationary state where the membrane potential will not change any further because the input current no longer changes. When the membrane potential does not change we have

$$\frac{\mathrm{d}v}{\mathrm{d}t} = 0. \tag{5.7}$$

Inserting this into eqn 5.1 yields the equilibrium potential for large times given by

$$v = RI. \tag{5.8}$$

We chose the condition where the input current is small enough to not elicit a spike. This condition can now be specified further as $RI < \theta$. We only calculated the equilibrium solution of the membrane potential after a constant current had been applied for a long time. The differential equation for constant input can also be solved for all times after the constant current $I_\mathrm{ext} = \mathrm{const}$ is applied, as in

$$v(t) = RI(1 - \mathrm{e}^{-t/\tau_\mathrm{m}} + \frac{v(t = 0)}{RI}\mathrm{e}^{-t/\tau_\mathrm{m}}), \tag{5.9}$$

which can be verified by inserting this solution into the differential equation. This solution has two parts: the last term describes the exponential decay of potential at $v(t = 0)$, as before, and the first term describes the increase of the membrane potential due to the input current. This solution is illustrated in Fig. 5.2A. The neuron does not fire in this case because we have used a relatively small input current, relative to the firing threshold of the neuron, $RI < \theta$. In contrast, if the mean external current is larger than the threshold, $RI > \theta$, then the neuron fires regularly with a constant time between spikes, the interspike interval. This is shown in Fig. 5.2B from simulations with the simulation program LIF.py.

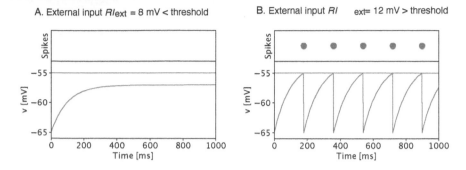

Fig. 5.2 Simulated spike trains and membrane potential of a leaky integrate-and-fire neuron. The threshold is set at $\theta = 10$ mV and is indicated as a dashed line. (A) Constant input with strength $RI_{ext} = 8$ mV, which is too small to elicit a spike. (B) Constant input of strength $RI_{ext} = 12$ mV, strong enough to elicit spikes in regular intervals. Note that we did not include the form of the spike itself in the figure but simply reset the membrane potential while indicating that a spike occurred by plotting a dot in the upper figure.

Programs/LIF.py

```
1  # Simulation of (leaky) integrate-and-fire neuron
2  import numpy as np
3  import matplotlib.pyplot as plt
4
5  # parameters of the model
6  dt=0.1          # integration time step [ms]
7  tau=10          # time constant [ms]
8  E_L=-65         # resting potential [mV]
9  theta=-55       # firing threshold [mV]
10 RI_ext=8    # constant external input [mA/Ohm]
11
12 # Integration with Euler method
13 v_rec=np.array([])
14 t_rec=np.array([])
15 s_rec=np.array([])
16 t_step=0; v=E_L
17 for t in range(int(100/dt)):
18     s=v>theta
19     v=s*E_L+(1-s)*(v-dt/tau*((v-E_L)-RI_ext))
20     v_rec=np.append(v_rec,v)
21     t_rec=np.append(t_rec,t)
22     s_rec=np.append(s_rec,s)
23
24 # Plotting results
25 ax1 = plt.axes([0.2, 0.7, 0.7, 0.2])
26 ax1.plot(t_rec,s_rec,'.',markersize=20)
27 ax1.axis([0, 100/dt, 0.5, 1.5])
28 plt.xticks([], []); plt.yticks([], [])
29 plt.ylabel('Spikes')
30
31 ax2 = plt.axes([0.2, 0.2, 0.7, 0.5])
32 ax2.plot(t_rec,v_rec)
33 ax2.plot([0, 100/dt],[-55, -55],'--');
34 ax2.axis([0, 100/dt, -66, -53])
35 plt.xlabel('Time [ms]'); plt.ylabel('v [mV]')
```

5.1.2 Rate gain function

We can calculate the time an IF neuron needs for a constant input current to reach threshold, called the first passage time, from the solution in eqn 5.9. We can choose the time scale so that the last spike occurs at $t = 0$, which is also the time at which the membrane potential is reset, $v(t = 0) = v_{res}$. The first passage time, t^f, is then given by the time when the membrane potential reaches the firing threshold, $v(t^f) = \theta$. This is calculated from eqn 5.9 to be

$$t^f = -\tau_m \ln \frac{\theta - RI}{v_{res} - RI}, \tag{5.10}$$

where ln is the natural logarithm (logaritmus naturalis), which is the inverse of the exponential function. The inverse of the first passage time defines the firing rate,

$$\bar{r} = (t^{ref} - \tau_m \ln \frac{\theta - RI}{v_{res} - RI})^{-1}, \tag{5.11}$$

where we included an absolute refractory time t^{ref}. This function is the activation function of an IF neuron which is illustrated in Fig. 5.3 for several values of the reset potential, v_{res}, and absolute refractory time, t^{ref}. This function quickly reaches asymptotic linear behaviour after a quick onset with external currents exceeding the threshold value. A threshold-linear function is often used to approximate the activation function of IF neurons.

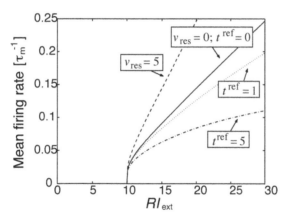

Fig. 5.3 Activation function of a leaky integrate-and-fire neuron for several values of the reset potential v_{res} and refractory time t^{ref}. The firing rate is given in units of the inverse time constant. The neuron fires only when the input is strong enough for the membrane potential to reach threshold ($RI_{ext} = 10$ in this case). The mean firing rate increases for larger reset potentials and shorter refractory times.

The activation function of a neuron can be measured experimentally, similar to the simulations by applying constant external currents of different magnitude to an isolated neuron in a Petri dish. Such in vitro recordings can be used to examine the principal neuronal parameters that we need to understand for biologically faithful simulations. However, we have already seen that such activation functions also depend on noise in the system, as was illustrated for a Hodgkin–Huxley neuron in Fig. 4.10. We will now discuss some noise models that can be used to revise this activation function.

5.1.3 The spike-response model ◇

In the previous section we integrated the equation describing simple IF neurons with constant currents driving the neurons, and we calculated the responses of the neurons to very short current pulses. When thinking about information transmission in neurons we are much more interested in time-varying input currents, such as those generated by presynaptic spike trains. We can formally integrate the dynamic differential equation 5.1 for any time-dependent inputs. To show this, we use our previous results showing the response of neurons to very short external current pulses. The idea of the solution is to express an arbitrary external current stream $I(t)$ as a collection of many very short pulses modulated by the strength of the input signal at the particular time. The response to each current pulse is an exponential function, as we have seen before. The general solution can thus be expressed as a sum over all the exponential responses to very short current pulses. The sum is actually an integral because we have a term for each infinitesimal time step. The time course of an IF neuron in response to an arbitrary input current $I(t)$ can be written as an integral equation,

$$v(t) = R \int_0^\infty \mathrm{e}^{-s/\tau_\mathrm{m}} I(t-s)\mathrm{d}s. \tag{5.12}$$

The integration variable s stands for all the times that precede the time t, and current pulses at such times influence the membrane potential at time t by an amount that depends exponentially on the time distance s. This means that more recent spikes have a larger influence on the membrane potential than more distant spikes.

The input current $I(t)$ can be generated with electrodes penetrating a neuron, and we could apply different forms of this current to study the responses of neurons. The following is an outline of the equations specifically for the interesting case of synaptic inputs generated by presynaptic firing. We need to take into account the resetting mechanisms in the IF neurons, which we ignored in eqn 5.12. We will account for the response in the membrane potential following a presynaptic spike and the change in the membrane potential following a postsynaptic spike by using two separate terms, labelled with ϵ and η, respectively. Hence, the membrane potential of the leaky integrate-and-fire model can be expressed as the sum of the individual potentials η and ϵ due to the linearity of the differential equation 5.1. The description of the membrane potential is therefore split into the following components

$$v(t) = \sum_j \sum_{t_j^\mathrm{f}} w_j \epsilon(t - t^\mathrm{f}, t - t_j^\mathrm{f}) + \sum_{t^\mathrm{f}} \eta(t - t^\mathrm{f}). \tag{5.13}$$

This equation includes a sum over several ϵ terms, one for each synapse multiplied by the corresponding weight value. The changes in membrane potential described by the ϵ terms can depend, in general, on the last postsynaptic spike at time t^f if the ion channels are voltage-dependent. The main feature encoded in this ϵ term is the influence of the postsynaptic membrane potential on the firing history of the individual presynaptic spikes t_j^f, as determined by eqn 5.12. We can include in this term the specific form of the input current generated by a synaptic event that we parametrized by the α-function in Chapter 4. This can be written as

$$\epsilon(t - t_j^{\mathrm{f}}) = R \int_0^\infty \mathrm{e}^{-s/\tau_{\mathrm{m}}} \alpha(t - t_j^{\mathrm{f}} - s)\mathrm{d}s, \tag{5.14}$$

for a synaptic input at synapse j.

The second term in eqn 5.13 (the η term) describes the reset of the membrane potential after a postsynaptic spike has occurred. We can write this in a form similar to that of the expression for the synaptic response, by including a short negative delta current with the strength of the threshold

$$RI_{\mathrm{res}} = -\theta\delta(t - t^{\mathrm{f}}). \tag{5.15}$$

The integral 5.12 for this special reset current is given by

$$\eta(t - t^{\mathrm{f}}) = -\theta\mathrm{e}^{-(t-t^{\mathrm{f}})/\tau_{\mathrm{m}}}. \tag{5.16}$$

The firing time t^{f}, written without an index, is the firing time of the postsynaptic neuron, given by solving the equation

$$v(t^{\mathrm{f}}) = \theta, \tag{5.17}$$

in contrast to the presynaptic neuron firing times that have an index, t_j^{f}. Note that the functions η and ϵ can often be solved analytically for particular choices of reset mechanisms and α-functions, respectively. Some examples are summarized in Table 5.1. The integrated form of the IF neurons, defined by eqns 5.17 and 5.13, is called the spike-response model. We will use this model to derive descriptions of the average behaviour of populations of neurons later in this chapter.

5.1.4   The Generalized LIF model

The leaky integrate-and-fire (LIF) neuron captures some of the essential components of a firing neuron, namely a subthreshold integration of currents, the firing of a neuron with sufficient buildup of the membrane potential, and the reset of the membrane potential after a spike. As already pointed out, several details of this model are oversimplified, and more biological details might be important to include depending on the specific investigative questions. For example, it was already mentioned that there is strictly speaking no fixed firing threshold, and also that the reset and refractoriness after the spike are more refined. An important step for computational modellers has been made at the Allen Institute for Brain Science. Researchers there have defined a systematic series of generalized LIF (GLIF) models with added details.

Defining generalized leaky integrate-and-fire models was thereby part of a large undertaking to characterize many types of neurons from the mouse and the human cortex, and that included detailed conductance-based models as already mentioned in Chapter 4.5.3. From all these cell types, they have derived a series of five models with increasing complexity to include systematically specific types of features of various neurons. These additions are outlined here.

Table 5.1 Examples of spike response functions (right column) describing the membrane potential in response to the corresponding forms of postsynaptic potentials (left column) used in simulations and analytical models. The firing time of the presynaptic neuron is t^f, and t^d is the duration of the α-pulse in the second example. τ^m and τ^s are time constants

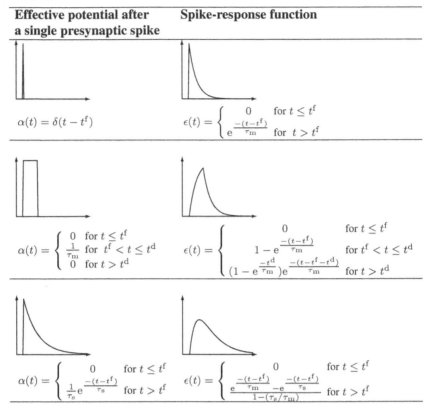

Effective potential after a single presynaptic spike	Spike-response function
$\alpha(t) = \delta(t - t^f)$	$\epsilon(t) = \begin{cases} 0 & \text{for } t \le t^f \\ e^{\frac{-(t-t^f)}{\tau_m}} & \text{for } t > t^f \end{cases}$
$\alpha(t) = \begin{cases} 0 & \text{for } t \le t^f \\ \frac{1}{\tau_m} & \text{for } t^f < t \le t^d \\ 0 & \text{for } t > t^d \end{cases}$	$\epsilon(t) = \begin{cases} 0 & \text{for } t \le t^f \\ 1 - e^{\frac{-(t-t^f)}{\tau_m}} & \text{for } t^f < t \le t^d \\ (1 - e^{\frac{-t^d}{\tau_m}})e^{\frac{-(t-t^f-t^d)}{\tau_m}} & \text{for } t > t^d \end{cases}$
$\alpha(t) = \begin{cases} 0 & \text{for } t \le t^f \\ \frac{1}{\tau_s}e^{\frac{-(t-t^f)}{\tau_s}} & \text{for } t > t^f \end{cases}$	$\epsilon(t) = \begin{cases} 0 & \text{for } t \le t^f \\ \dfrac{e^{\frac{-(t-t^f)}{\tau_m}} - e^{\frac{-(t-t^f)}{\tau_s}}}{1 - (\tau_s/\tau_m)} & \text{for } t > t^f \end{cases}$

The base model is called LIF$_1$ which corresponds to the model we discussed in Chapter 5.1. We summarize this here again with replacing the time constant with $\tau_m = RC$ to conform with their notation:

$$\frac{dv(t)}{dt} = \frac{1}{C}(I(t) - \frac{1}{R}(v(t) - E_L)) \tag{5.18}$$

$$v(t^f) = \theta \tag{5.19}$$

$$v(t^f + \delta) = v_{\text{res}}. \tag{5.20}$$

The first equations describes the subthreshold dynamics, the second the firing when a firing-threshold is crossed, and the third the reset of the potential after the spike.

The second model, LIF$_2$, includes the effect that the firing threshold depends on previous firings which is termed a biologically defined threshold model. This model does include a decaying additional threshold value θ_s that triggers an increase of $\Delta\theta_s$ with each spike and then decays exponentially with decay constant b_s,

$$\frac{d\theta_s(t)}{dt} = -b_s\theta_s + \Delta\delta(t - t_f)\delta\delta\theta_s \tag{5.21}$$

$$v(t^f) = \theta + \theta_s(t) \tag{5.22}$$

$$v(t^f + \delta) = E_L + f_v(v(t) - E_L) + \Delta V. \tag{5.23}$$

The reset potential has thereby two more parameters, f_v and Δv.

The third model, LIF_3, takes the base model LIF_1 and adds after-spike currents. This addition is meant to simulate the effects of different ion channels such as the rapidly changing sodium and potassium channels. These currents are added with their own time scale k_j, a multiplicative constant R_j and an additive constant A_j,

$$\frac{dI_j(t)}{dt} = -k_j I_j(t) \tag{5.24}$$

$$\frac{dv(t)}{dt} = \frac{1}{C}(I(t) + \sum_j I_j(t) - \frac{1}{R}(v(t) - E_L)) \tag{5.25}$$

$$I(t^f + \delta) = R_j I_j(t) + A_j \tag{5.26}$$

The fourth models, LTF_3, combines the biologically defined threshold with the after-spike currents. The last model, LIF_5, adds then to this another effect of the threshold, that of a voltage dependence,

$$\frac{d\theta_v(t)}{dt} = a(v(t) - E_L) - b_v(\theta_v(t) - \theta) \tag{5.27}$$

$$v(t^f) = \theta + \theta_s(t) + \theta_v(t) \tag{5.28}$$

$$v(t^f + \delta) = E_L + f_v(v(t) - E_L) + \Delta V. \tag{5.29}$$

This model introduces two more constants, namely a and f_v.

Defining these models is not the only contribution of the Alan institute. What makes these models very valuable for future investigations is that the inventors also developed a procedure to fit these models to recording of specific neurons. In this way, the investigators have established parameters of the models for specific neuron types which will be useful for direct comparisons of models with recording data.

5.1.5 The McCulloch–Pitts neuron

Before leaving the section which introduces spiking neurons, we should finally mention one of the oldest and simplest neuron models, which was introduced by Warren McCulloch and Walter Pitts in 1943. This model has the form of a logical unit, which sums input values, x_i^{in}, to determine the net input,

$$h = \sum_i x_i^{\mathrm{in}}. \tag{5.30}$$

The unit becomes active if the net input is larger than a threshold value, θ,

$$x^{\mathrm{out}} = \begin{cases} 1 & \text{if } h > \theta \\ 0 & \text{otherwise} \end{cases}. \tag{5.31}$$

Many information-processing capabilities of neural networks can be discussed and demonstrated with McCulloch–Pitts units. Before using this model in later chapters we should therefore say a few words about the interpretation of this model. While McCulloch and Pitts certainly had neurons in mind, it is clear that this model does not capture the precise time course of a membrane potential. Rather, this model should be seen as a model for operations in discrete time steps. While this time step could, in principle, be very small to capture rapidly changing signals, it is also clear that McCulloch and Pitts considered computational tasks of neurons rather than the description of physical properties of neurons. A better view of the relevant scale of the time step is therefore several tens of milliseconds, and we could interpret activity during this time step as the occurrence of one or more spikes during this interval. If we want to take different numbers of spikes in such a time step into account, then we might want to change the activation function (eqn 5.31) to allow a more graded output. The output would then represent a temporal average of spike counts.

The use of temporal averaging by the brain has been questioned, since responses would then be much longer than observed experimentally. However, we could go a step further in our abstraction and consider the logical unit of McCulloch and Pitts as a reflection of a population of functional connected neurons which will become active in response to a specific input. Activation of this population does then reflect the presence of certain input patterns, and we can imagine that individual neurons can contribute to a number of populations, as envisioned by Donald Hebb for his cell assemblies. The population approach is an important contribution to brain modelling. Such models are formally introduced in Section 5.5, and the computational abilities of such logical units are explored in Chapter 7. While the interpretation of the McCulloch–Pitts neuron is not always clear, this should not distract from the importance of this model to illuminate computational principles in brain processing, including spike processing in a discrete time model.

5.2 Spike-time variability ◇

5.2.1 Biological irregularities

Neurons in the brain do not fire regularly, rather, they seem extremely noisy. Neurons that are relatively inactive emit spikes with low frequencies that are very irregular. Also, high-frequency responses to relevant stimuli are often not very regular. Single-cell recordings transmitted to a speaker sound very much like the irregular ticking of a Geiger counter when exposed to radioactive material. A histogram of the interspike intervals of one cortical cell is shown in Fig. 5.4A. This prefrontal cell fired around 15 spikes/s without a noticeably task-relevant pattern. The interspike interval distribution shows great variability. The firing pattern of this cortical cell is therefore not well described with the constant interspike intervals generated by the simple IF neurons studied in Section 3.1. A convenient measure of the variability of spike trains is the coefficient of variation, which is defined by the ratio of the standard deviation σ and the mean μ,

$$C_V = \frac{\sigma}{\mu}. \tag{5.32}$$

This value is $C_V \approx 1.09$ for the cell data shown in Fig. 5.4A. Recordings in the brain often show a high value of variability such as $C_V \approx 0.5\text{--}1$ for regularly spiking neurons

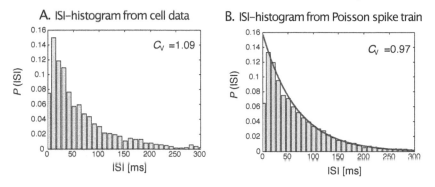

Fig. 5.4 Normalized histograms of interspike intervals (ISIs). (A) Data from recordings of one cortical cell (Brodmann's area 46) that fired without task-relevant characteristics with an average firing rate of about 15 spikes/s. The coefficient of variation of the spike train is $C_V \approx 1.09$ [data courtesy of Stefan Everling]. (B) Simulated data from a Poisson-distributed spike train in which a Gaussian refractory time has been included. The solid line represents the probability density function of the exponential distribution when scaled to fit the normalized histogram of the spike train. Note that the discrepancy for small interspike intervals is due to the inclusion of a refractory time.

in the primary visual cortex (V1) and the medial temporal lobe (MT), as pointed out by Softky and Koch (1993). Regular firing of an IF neuron has an inconsistent value of $C_V = 0$.

The distribution of the interspike intervals shown in Fig. 5.4A shows an exponentially decaying tail after a rapid onset determined by the refractory period. The exponential distribution, or more formally the probability density function of this distribution, given by

$$\text{pdf}^{\text{exponential}}(x; \lambda)(x) = \lambda e^{-\lambda x}, \tag{5.33}$$

has only one parameter, $\lambda = 1/b$, where b is equal to the mean, and, at the same time, the standard deviation of an exponential distributed random variable. The coefficient of variation for the exponential distribution is therefore $C_V = 1$. The number of events, when the time between events is exponentially distributed, is given by the Poisson distribution,

$$\text{pdf}^{\text{Poisson}}(x; \lambda)(x) = \sum_{i=1}^{x} \lambda^i \frac{e^{-\lambda}}{i!}, \tag{5.34}$$

and spike trains in computational studies are often generated with a Poisson process. A Poisson process is a process that results in a variable being Poisson distributed. An important characteristic of a Poisson process is that there is no memory of past events. That is, at any given time there is an equal likelihood that the next spike occurs. This is, of course, not the case in the refractory time, which accounts for reductions in the number of small interspike intervals. The exponential distribution is shown in Fig. 5.4B, together with a corresponding simulation of a modified Poisson process which is described in more detail below.

The heuristic modelling of spike trains discussed so far does not describe the processes producing the noise. Also, there are several further factors that we need to take into account, including inhibition in the network and other contributing factors from irregularities in the biological system. To begin with, the input to the system, such as sensory input from the environment, is not constant as is assumed in the simulations above. Moreover, on a single-cell level we expect many structural irregularities to contribute to the irregular behaviour of neurons. These include the diffuse propagation of neurotransmitters across the synaptic cleft, the opening and closing of ion channels, the propagation of the membrane potential along dendrites with varying geometries, the nature of biochemical processes, and the probabilistic nature of transmitter releases by axonal spikes. It is beyond the scope of this book, and beyond the scope of most models in computational neuroscience, to try to describe the nature of these irregularities in detail. Instead, we often incorporate the sum of all these irregularities into our models by including noise in the simulations.

5.2.2 Noise models for IF neurons

How can we include noise in the neuron models to describe some of the stochastic processes within neuronal responses? For simplicity, we will discuss this for the IF model, although similar procedures can be applied to other models. We want to determine the stochastic firing times of neurons. In order to do so we can use three principal methods to include a stochastic component in the IF model. These are illustrated in Fig. 5.5.

The noise models commonly used for IF neurons can be summarized as:

1. **Stochastic threshold**: We can replace the threshold, which the membrane potential has to pass in order to generate a spike, with a noisy threshold

$$\theta \rightarrow \theta + \eta^{(1)}(t). \tag{5.35}$$

2. **Random reset**: We can reset the membrane potential to a random reset potential

$$v^{\text{res}} \rightarrow u^{\text{res}} + \eta^{(2)}(t). \tag{5.36}$$

3. **Noisy integration**: The integration mechanisms in neurons can be noisy such that the leaky integrator of the IF neurons may be better described by a stochastic differential equation (which is equivalent to saying that the integrator is not noisy but it integrates noisy inputs)

$$\tau_{\text{m}} \frac{dv}{dt} = -v + RI_{\text{ext}} + \eta^{(3)}(t). \tag{5.37}$$

With appropriate choices for the distribution function of the random variables $\eta^{(1)}, \eta^{(2)}$, and $\eta^{(3)}$ we can produce equivalent results for the stochastic processes of a neuron, although the same probability distribution for each random variable can produce different results for each noise model. In practice, we want to choose distributions that are appropriate for capturing experimental data, so which noise model to choose is more a question of convenience. For analytical treatments it is often most convenient to use a random threshold model. Although there is little evidence that the firing thresholds of real neurons change over time, this noise model is equivalent to the other noise models, so modelling of stochastic processes in neurons can be done in

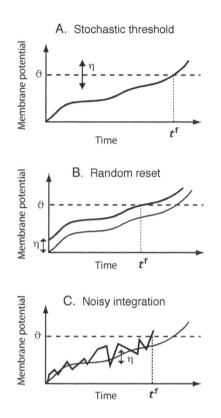

Fig. 5.5 Three different noise models of integrate-and-fire neurons. (A) Stochastic threshold, (B) random reset, and (C) noisy integration. t^f is the time of firing, θ the firing threshold, and η is a random variable [adapted from W. Gerstner, in *Pulsed neural networks*, Maass and Bishop (eds), MIT Press (1998)].

this way. Numerical studies frequently use noisy input to model stochastic processes in the brain. This model has the simple interpretation of noisy synaptic transmission that can be observed in real neuronal systems. Analytical treatments of this model are difficult, although it is straightforward to integrate noise in this fashion in numerical studies, as shown below.

5.2.3 Simulating the variability of real neurons

While the choice of the noise model depends primarily on convenience, an important remaining question is the appropriate choice of the random process, including the probability distribution, and the time scale on which those fluctuations are relevant. We cannot give general answers to these questions as the particular choice depends strongly on the nature of the question and the particular neural system under investigation. Appropriate choices have to be made to fit experimental data whenever the precise form of fluctuations is relevant. In the following, we only give a flavour of the effects of including noise in the IF model by considering noisy input (noise model 3). In the

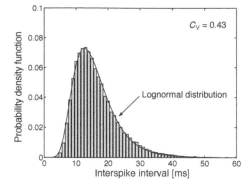

Fig. 5.6 Simulated interspike interval (ISI) distribution of a leaky IF neuron with threshold $\theta = 10$ mV and time constant $\tau_m = 10$ ms. The underlying spike train was generated with noisy input around the mean value $RI = 12$. The fluctuations were therefore distributed with a standard normal distribution. The resulting ISI histogram is well approximated by a lognormal distribution (solid line). The coefficient of variation of the simulated spike train is $C_V \approx 0.43$.

following example we use a normally distributed input current produced by adding white noise to a constant input current,

$$I_{\text{ext}} = \bar{I}_{\text{ext}} + \eta \quad \text{with} \quad \eta \in N(0,1). \tag{5.38}$$

Normally distributed input signals are a good approximation when we consider independent synaptic input from many equally distributed neurons as stated by the central limit theorem (see Chapter 3.5). The interspike interval (ISI) distribution of an IF neuron with mean input $R\bar{I}_{\text{ext}} = 12$ mV and threshold $\theta = 10$ mV is shown in Fig. 5.6.

This distribution is approximated well by a lognormal distribution,

$$\text{pdf}^{\text{lognormal}}(x; \mu, \sigma) = \frac{1}{x\sigma\sqrt{2\pi}} e^{-\frac{(\log(x)-\mu)^2}{2\sigma^2}}. \tag{5.39}$$

A fit of the data to this distribution is shown as a solid line in Fig. 5.6. The coefficient of variation of these data is $C_V \approx 0.43$, approaching the lower end of cortical variability of interspike intervals. This is remarkable since we considered only one source of noise. We can, for example, assume this noise results from the noisy internal mechanisms of integration within the neuron, and we could then consider, in addition, noisy input from the variability in the input spike trains themselves. There are several other ways to increase the variability of spikes in simple IF neurons, such as using partial and noisy reset after a spike has occurred. This effectively increases the gain in the relation between input current and output spike frequency and has been argued to describe the variability seen in experiments very well.

The last example we want to discuss is an IF neuron that is driven by independent presynaptic spike trains with exponential interspike intervals (Poisson spike trains). Results from such simulations are shown in Fig. 5.7. There, we have taken as input 500 Poisson-distributed spike trains with refractory corrections as discussed above. The mean firing rate of the input neurons was set to 20 Hz, which was lowered slightly to

19.3 Hz due to the Gaussian refractory time with a 2 ms time constant. We took only 500 independent presynaptic spike trains into account as they should represent the fraction of presynaptic neurons that are active in a particular task (for example, 10% of the inputs to a neuron with 5000 presynaptic neurons). Each presynaptic spike was set to elicit an EPSP in the form of an α-function (eqn 4.1) with amplitude $w = 0.5$ and time constant of 2 ms for all synapses. The synaptic input of all the input spike trains was then large enough to keep the average incoming current, that is, the sum over all EPSPs, larger than the firing threshold of the neuron.

The sum of the EPSPs for the first 1000 ms in this experiment is illustrated by the upper curve in Fig. 5.7A, and the firing threshold is indicated as a dashed line. The average exceeds the firing threshold of the IF neuron, and this, in turn, results in a regular firing pattern with a high firing rate of around 118 Hz. This result is similar to the response of an IF neuron to a constant input as discussed in Section 5.1.1. The ISI distribution, plotted in Fig. 5.7B, has low variance, and the coefficient of variation of this model neuron is only $C_V = 0.12$. Note that these simulations did not include any noise in the neuron model itself; they only included noise in the driving input currents. Noise in the neuron model would further increase the coefficient of variation.

If we lower the effect of each incoming spike by lowering the amplitude of the α-function to $w = 0.25$, then we get an average postsynaptic current, which is shown for the first 1000 ms of the simulation in the lower curve of Fig. 5.7A. The average sum of EPSPs was $R\bar{I}_{ext} = 9.7$ mV in this simulation, which is just below the firing threshold of the neuron. The fluctuations due to the random processes of the incoming spike trains are then crucial, and the neuron shows an irregular firing pattern with an average firing rate of 16 Hz. The corresponding ISI histogram is shown in Fig. 5.7C. The coefficient of variation is $C_V = 0.58$, exceeding the lower boundary found in experiments. The question is, of course, how a neuron can adjust the combined strength of incoming spikes to function in this balanced, more biologically realistic, regime. It is rather difficult to achieve the right level of input strength, as it seems to require a fine-tuning of the strength parameter by hand. The question of synaptic scaling must be investigated further, and possible factors that need to be considered include inhibition in networks, synaptic plasticity, as well as explicit scaling mechanisms.

5.2.4 The activation function depends on input

A final, important, point is that the activation or gain function of a neuron depends on variations in the input spike train. This can be shown analytically for an IF neuron that is driven by a noisy current with normally distributed values. The IF dynamics of eqn 5.1 is then a stochastic differential equation as we have argued before in connection with noise model 3. The stochastic differential equations of the leaky IF neuron can still be solved formally. The first passage time as given in eqn 5.10 is then a random variable for which we can calculate the mean first passage time. These calculations were carried out by Tuckwell who showed that the average firing rate for a stochastic IF neuron is given by

$$\bar{r} = (t^{ref} + \tau_m \int_{(v^{res} - R\bar{I}_{ext})/\sigma}^{(\theta - R\bar{I}_{ext})/\sigma} \sqrt{\pi} e^{v^2} [1 + \mathrm{erf}(v)] \mathrm{d}v)^{-1}, \tag{5.40}$$

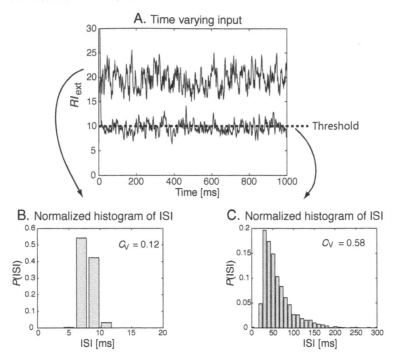

Fig. 5.7 Simulations of an IF neuron that has no internal noise but is driven by 500 independent incoming spike trains with a corrected Poisson distribution. (A) The sums of the EPSPs, simulated by an α-function for each incoming spike with amplitude $w = 0.5$ for the upper curve and $w = 0.25$ for the lower curve. The firing threshold for the neuron is indicated by the dashed line. The ISI histograms from the corresponding simulations are plotted in (B) for the neuron with EPSP amplitude of $w = 0.5$ and in (C) for the neuron with EPSP amplitude of $w = 0.25$.

where σ is the variance of the Gaussian signal and erf is the error function as described in Chapter 3.5, eqn 3.54. The firing rate is not only a function of the mean input current, but also depends on higher moments (for example, variance, skewness, etc.) of the distribution describing the input signal. The important result to keep in mind is that the mean firing time of an IF neuron depends on the precise form of the input spike train, not only on the mean firing rate of the inputs,

$$\bar{r} = \bar{r}(\mu, \sigma, ...). \tag{5.41}$$

Some examples of the mean firing rates of an IF neuron as a function of the mean firing rates, μ, of presynaptic spike trains, as specified by eqn 5.40, are illustrated in Fig. 5.8. This figure shows the response curves for three different values of the standard deviation $sigma$ of presynaptic firings. The activation function for a low-variance input spike train has a sharp transition, as we have seen before in Fig. 5.3, and the firing rate of the neuron will soon approach its maximal firing rate, as determined by the inverse of the absolute refractory time for means of the input current exceeding the firing threshold. Also note that the effective threshold, the point where the strong increase of the firing rate with external input starts, is lower than the hard threshold imposed on the IF neuron model. With increasing variance, the strong non-linear response is

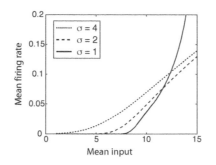

Fig. 5.8 The activation function of an IF neuron driven by an external current that is given a normal distribution with mean $\mu = R\bar{I}$ and variance σ^2. The reset potential was set to $v_{\mathrm{res}} = 5\mathrm{mV}$ and the firing threshold of the IF neuron was set to $\theta = 10\mathrm{mV}$. The three curves correspond to three different variance parameters.

'linearized', similarly to the linearization by noise in the Hodgkin–Huxley model (see Fig. 4.10). In the population models introduced below, we can take the structure of the driving signals into account with activation functions that depend on the mean input current as well as the higher moments of the distribution of the input signals. This is, unfortunately, often neglected in the application of such models in the literature.

5.3 Advanced integrate-and-fire models

5.3.1 The Izhikevich neuron

The subthreshold dynamic of leaky IF neurons, eqn 5.1, is linear in v and is therefore beneficial for analytic calculations and is also somewhat efficient in numerical implementations. The drawbacks of the basic IF model are that it might not sufficiently approximate the subthreshold dynamic of a neuronal membrane potential and that it does not include the variety of response patterns seen in real neurons. Whether it is sufficient or not depends on the scientific question under investigation. While there are, of course, more detailed models, as we discussed in Chapter 4, their computational demand is often prohibitive for use in large-scale network simulations.

However, Eugene Izhikevich has proposed an intermediate model which is computationally efficient while still being able to capture a large variety of response properties of real neurons.

This model neuron is described by two coupled differential equations, one for the membrane potential v, and one for a recovery variable u,

$$\frac{dv(t)}{dt} = 0.04v^2(t) + 5v(t) + 140 - u + I(t) \tag{5.42}$$

$$\frac{du(t)}{dt} = a(bv - u), \tag{5.43}$$

along with the corresponding reset conditions,

$$v(v > 30) = c \ \text{ and } \ u(v > 30) = u + d. \tag{5.44}$$

The equations describe the membrane potential v in mV for a given external current I in mA, and the time scale corresponds to ms, and includes four parameters a, b, c, and d. In contrast to the IF neuron, and more consistent with real neurons and Hodgkin–Huxley type models, this model does not have a constant firing threshold. The reset voltage of $v = 30$ is far above the regime where spike generation could be stopped by the removal of external current. The model does, therefore, better incorporate the critical regime of spike initiation. Furthermore, through the inclusion of a recovery variable that models the inactivation of sodium channels and hyperpolarizing potassium channels, typical spike patterns of biological neurons can be simulated. The constant values in eqn 5.42 are chosen so that the model can fit a large variety of neural behaviour.

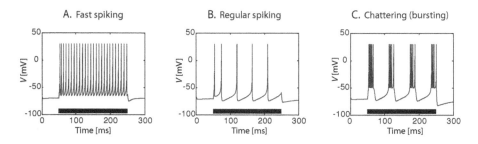

Fig. 5.9 Different spike pattern of a Izhikevich neuron by varying some parameters around their base values $a = 0.02, b = 0.2, c = -65$ and $d = 2$. The bar on the bottom of the graphs indicates the times at which a constant current of 10 mA was applied. (A) Fast spiking results from a fast recovery constant, $a = 0.1$. (B) Regular spiking with a large reset value of the recovery variable, $d = 8$. (C) Bursting behaviour simulated with $d = 2$ and a high value for the voltage reset, $c = -50$.

The four parameters a, b, c, and d can be set to simulate different type of neurons. Fig. 5.9 shows examples with the recommended base values of $a = 0.02, b = 0.2, c = -65$ and $d = 2$, unless stated otherwise. The parameter a sets the time scale of the recovery variable with low values corresponding to slow recoveries. For example, a value of $a = 0.1$ results in the fast spiking shown in Fig. 5.9A, where the bar at the bottom indicates the interval when a current of $I = 10$ was applied. Such fast spiking with little spike-time adaptation is similar to the basic IF neuron with a small time constant and is common in some types of inhibitory neurons. More common for excitatory neurons in the cortex is a spike rate with fatigue to constant input, like that shown in Fig. 5.9B. To simulate this neuron, the base parameters were used except for the parameter describing the reset of the recovery variable, d, which was set to $d = 8$. An interesting bursting behaviour (Fig. 5.9C) can be seen when using a high value for the voltage reset parameter, $c = -50$, and moderate recovery variable reset of $d = 2$. The parameter b, not varied in these simulations, describes the sensitivity of the recovery variable to fluctuations of the membrane potential. This model is implemented in the program `Izhikevich.py`.

Programs/Izhikevich.py

```
1  #Izhikevich model
2  import matplotlib.pyplot as plt
3
```

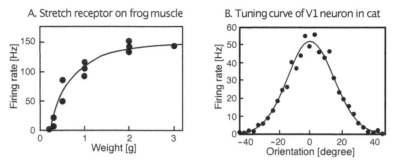

Fig. 5.10 (A) Data from Adrian's original work showing the firing rate of a frog's stretch receptor on a muscle as a function of the weight load applied to the muscle [redrawn from Adrian, *Journal of Physiology (Lond.)* 61: 49–72 (1926)]. (B) Response (tuning curve) of a neuron in the primary visual cortex of the cat as a function of the orientation of a light stimulus in the form of a moving bar [data from Henry, Dreher, and Bishop, *Journal of Neurophysiology* 37: 1394–1409 (1974)].

```
4  # Parameters and initialization
5  a=0.02; b=0.2; c=−65; d=2
6  Iext=10.; v=[−65]; u=[−65*b]; t=[0]; dt=0.5
7
8  for step in range(1,int(200/dt)):
9      # record time steps
10     t.append(t[step−1]+dt)
11     #numerical integration and recording of Izhikevich equations
12     v.append(v[step−1] +
13       dt*(0.04*v[step−1]**2+5*v[step−1]+140−u[step−1]+Iext))
14     u.append(u[step−1]+dt*a*(b*v[step−1]−u[step−1]))
15     if v[step]>30:
16         v[step−1]=30; v[step]=c
17         u[step]=u[step]+d
18
19 # Plotting results
20 plt.plot(t,v); plt.xlabel('t'); plt.ylabel('v')
```

5.4 The neural code and the firing rate hypothesis

Neuroscientists try to decipher the neural code by searching for reliable correlations between firing patterns and behavioural consequences, or correlations, between sensory stimuli and neural activity patterns. The most robust findings typically show modulations of the firing rate of neurons with sensory stimuli. For example, one of the first scientists to use microelectrode recordings in the 1920s, after sufficient amplification of the small electrical signals became available through vacuum tubes, was the English physiologist Edgar Douglas Adrian. One of the first effects he recognized was that the number of spikes of a neuron often increases when increasing the strength of a stimulus. An increasing firing rate is easily detectable and still dominates the neurophysiological search for stimuli that 'drive' a neuron.

An example of a rate code that was explored by Adrian is that of the stretch receptor on the frog muscle which increases with increasing weights on the muscle, as shown in Fig. 5.10A. In general, firing rates of sensory neurons increase considerably in a short time interval following the presentation of an effective stimulus to the recorded neuron. The response of a neuron to various stimuli is sometimes captured in response curves. For example, the response curve of a sensory neuron in the primary visual cortex, also called the tuning curve of the neuron, is shown in Fig. 5.10B. Simple cells in this visual area respond to orientations of bars moved through the receptive field of the neuron, which is the area in the physical world for which this neuron is responsive. While firing rates dominate physiological descriptions of neuronal responses, and much of the further discussions in this book, we should not overlook the fact that other parts of spike patterns can convey information. We therefore take a short side tour into this topic.

5.4.1 Correlation codes and coincidence detectors

Information processing in the brain usually includes modulations of firing rates. This is not very surprising as we expect a variation in the number of spikes with varying input currents. However, we want to ask if only the firing rate is used in the brain to convey information. A rare example where the firing rate does not show the relevant information is shown in Fig. 5.11. The figure displays the response of two neurons in the primary auditory cortex to a 4 kHz tone with an amplitude envelope shown at the top. Fig. 5.11B shows the average firing rate at 5 ms intervals over many trials for each neuron. No significant variation of the firing rate can be seen in either of the neurons. However, some stimulus-locked variation in the relative spiking of the two neurons can be seen when plotting the rate of spikes from one neuron that occurred within a short fixed interval of the spiking of the other reference neuron (Fig. 5.11C). This rate indicates the probability of co-occurrence of the spikes of the two neurons, which is a nice example where behavioural correlates can only be seen in the correlation between the firing patterns of two neurons.

In contrast, for a receiving leaky IF neurons, the close temporal proximity of spikes is relevant. A perfect integrator, which sums the input of synaptic input without leakage, is illustrated for the case of two driving inputs in Fig. 5.12A. The membrane potential accumulates the synaptic currents triggered by the presynaptic spikes and therefore counts the number of presynaptic spikes since the last reset of the membrane potential. In the case of a leaky integrator, illustrated in Fig. 5.12B, the membrane potential decays after an increase caused by presynaptic spikes, and the neuron becomes sensitive to the relative timing of spikes of different presynaptic neurons. Such a leaky integrator with a small time constant can be used as a coincidence detector.

A neuron generates a spike after the membrane potential reaches a threshold, at which time the membrane potential must be reset (not included in Fig. 5.12). With the thresholds indicated by dashed lines in Fig. 5.12, both neurons, the integrator and the coincidence detector, would fire at the same time. However, the reason for the firing would be very different in the two cases. In the first case, that of a perfect integrator, the neuron fires because four presynaptic spikes occurred since the last firing of the neuron. This neuron would also fire at this time if one of the two last simultaneous spikes occurred at an earlier time. In contrast, the spike of the leaky integrator only occurs because of the occurrence of two simultaneous presynaptic spikes. With a higher firing threshold, larger than the effect of the sum of two simultaneous EPSPs, it is also possible to employ such a leaky integrator neuron to detect the coincidence of

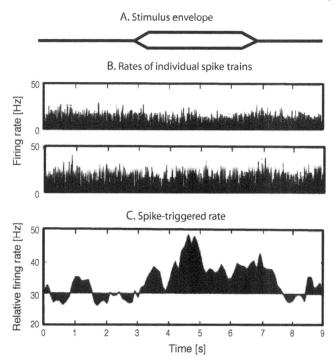

Fig. 5.11 An example of the response of some neurons in the primary auditory cortex that do not show significant variations in response to the onset of a 4 kHz tone with the amplitude envelope shown in (A). (B) Average firing rates in 5 ms bins of two different neurons. (C) Spike-triggered average rate that indicates some correlation between the firing of the two neurons that is significantly correlated to the presentation of the stimulus [from DeCharms and Merzenich, *Science* 381: 610–13 (1996)].

more than two spikes. The time window of coincidence depends on the decay constant and the time course of the EPSPs. Thus, temporal proximities of spikes can make a difference in the information processing of the brain.

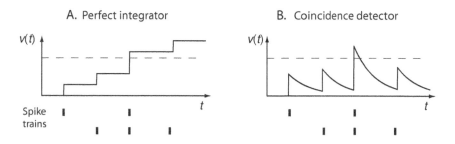

Fig. 5.12 Schematic illustration of (A) a perfect integrator and (B) a leaky integrator that can be utilized as coincidence detector. In this example the membrane potential $v(t)$ integrates short current pulses of the two spike trains shown at the bottom.

5.4.2 How accurate is spike timing?

It is a widely held belief that neural spiking is not very reliable, and that there is a lot of variability in neuronal responses. Another demonstration of spike-time variability, from experiments by Buračas and colleagues, is shown in Fig. 5.13 for responses of a cell in the middle temporal area (MT) that responds to the movement of visual stimuli. The top graph of Fig. 5.13A shows the response of the neuron in several trials to a stimulus with constant velocity, as indicated at the bottom. The middle graph shows the trial average. The data indicate a reliable initial neuronal response. After this initial response the neuron still fires rapidly; however, the times of these spikes are different in each trial. Some people search for a neural code in the firing pattern of neurons in response to a constant pattern. The data in Fig. 5.13A indicate that there might not be much information in the continuing firing pattern of the neuron due to the enormous variability.

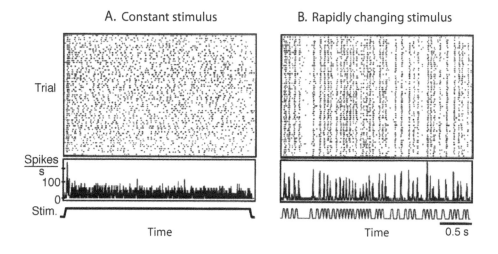

Fig. 5.13 Spike trains (top) and average response over trials (middle) of an MT neuron to a visual stimulus with either constant velocity (A) or altering velocity (B) as indicated in the bottom graph [adapted from Buračas et al., *Neuron* 20: 959–69 (1998)].

Data like those shown in Fig. 5.13A lead to the impression that neuronal spike times are very variable and imprecise. However, this has to be viewed in relation to the experimental situation. Fig. 5.13B shows the response of the same neuron to a rapidly varying stimulus. The response of the neuron follows the variations in the stimulus rapidly with little jitters. Each neuron does not always respond with a spike to the changing velocity of the stimulus, and some spikes still occur in between the stimulus changes. However, the majority of spikes follow the changing stimulus rapidly. Thus, sensory events can elicit a rapid cascade of neuronal activity through a neuronal network which, in turn, can lead to rapid recruitment of neurons along processing pathways. In other words, populations of neurons can rapidly convey information in a neural network.

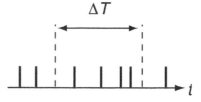

Fig. 5.14 Temporal average of a single spike train with a time window ΔT that has to be large compared to the average interspike interval.

5.5 Population dynamics: modelling the average behaviour of neurons

Simulation of networks of many thousands of spiking neurons has become tractable on recent computer systems. However, even with the increasing power of digital computers, we are barely able to simulate neural systems with spiking neurons on the scale of functional units in the brain, not to mention models on a scale comparable to that of the central nervous system. Furthermore, as discussed in Chapter 1, our aim is not so much to reconstruct the brain in all its detail, but rather to extract the principles of its organization and functionality. Many of the models in computational neuroscience, in particular on a cognitive level, are therefore based on descriptions that do not take the individual spikes of neurons into account, but instead describe the average activity of neurons or neural populations.

In this section we introduce population models and discuss their relationship to populations of spiking neurons. The aim is to highlight under what conditions these common approximations are useful and faithful descriptions of neuronal characteristics. It is clear that rate models cannot incorporate all aspects of networks of spiking neurons. However, many of the principles behind information processing in the brain can be illuminated on the level of population models, and many of the features of population models have been confirmed with spiking neurons.

5.5.1 Firing rates and population averages

It is important to recognize that neurophysiological recordings of single cells have been very successful in correlating the firing rates of single neurons with the behavioural perceptions, or responses, of a subject. It is common in physiological studies to derive an instantaneous firing rate with the help of a sliding window in the spike train. For example, as illustrated in Fig. 5.14, we can estimate the average temporal spike rate of a neuron with a fixed window of size ΔT,

$$\nu(t) = \frac{\text{number of spikes in } \Delta T}{\Delta T}$$

$$= \frac{1}{\Delta T} \int_{t-\Delta T/2}^{t+\Delta T/2} \delta(t' - t^{\text{f}}) \mathrm{d}t', \tag{5.45}$$

where t^{f} is the firing time of the neuron. This defines, for small time windows, the instantaneous firing rate. It is also possible to calculate a weighted average with different kernel functions which often give smoother results. For example, it is common in physiological studies to use a Gaussian window that does not have the sharp boundaries of the rectangular time window above. The firing rate of a neuron at time t is then defined by

$$\nu(t) = \frac{1}{\sqrt{2\pi}\sigma} \int_{-\infty}^{+\infty} \delta(t' - t^{\mathrm{f}}) e^{(t'-t)^2/2\sigma^2} \, \mathrm{d}t'. \tag{5.46}$$

The physiological estimates of the firing rates of single neurons often include an average over several trials under equal experimental conditions. Such averages over repetitions are necessary because the firing of a neuron in a single trial is very noisy. This is a valid experimental estimation procedure as it has been found that such averages correlate well with behavioural responses. However, it is also clear that averaging over several trials is not an option for the brain, where responses to a single stimulus must be possible. Also, the temporal averaging explained above can only be employed by the brain in a limited way since the time windows of averaging have to be much smaller than the typical response time of the organism, which can be on the order of 100 ms. Thus, mainly population activity is relevant for information processing in the brain.

The brain does not rely on the information of a single spike train. Indeed, such reliance would make the brain very vulnerable to damage or reorganization. We therefore conjecture that there must be a subpopulation, or pool of neurons, with similar response properties, as illustrated in Fig. 5.15. The neurons in these subpopulations of a cortical module may act in a statistically similar way. This would explain why single-neuron recordings have been so successful in correlating single-neuron measurements to behavioural findings. Thus, we conjecture that the temporal average of single neurons measured in repeated physiological experiments approximates the neuro-computationally relevant average population activity $A(t)$ of neurons,

$$A(t) = \lim_{\Delta T \to 0} \frac{1}{\Delta T} \frac{\text{number of spikes in population of size N}}{N}$$

$$= \lim_{\Delta T \to 0} \frac{1}{\Delta T} \int_{t-\Delta T/2}^{t+\Delta T/2} \frac{1}{N} \sum_{i=1}^{N} \delta(t' - t_i^{\mathrm{f}}) \mathrm{d}t'. \tag{5.47}$$

Since this average employs a sum over many neurons (in contrast to eqn 5.45), it is possible to use much smaller time windows. In the limit of very small time windows, we can also write the last equation in differential form,

$$A(t)\mathrm{d}t = \frac{1}{N} \sum_{i=1}^{N} \delta(t' - t_i^{\mathrm{f}}), \tag{5.48}$$

which we will use later to derive formulas for population dynamics.

It is difficult to verify this conjecture directly with experiments, as this would demand the simultaneous recording of many thousands of neurons. Recording with multiple electrodes is, to a large extent, beyond a current experimental feasibility, and brain imaging currently averages over too many neurons to be able to verify our conjecture. Local field potentials may come closest to such population recordings, when the populations are spatially localized. The conjecture is, however, supported indirectly by several known experimental facts, such as the existence of cortical columns

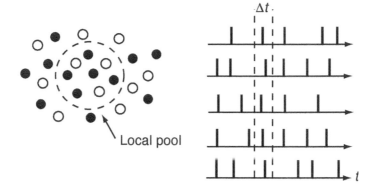

Fig. 5.15 Pool or local population of neurons with similar response characteristics. The pool average is defined as the average firing rate over the neurons in the pool within a relatively small time window [adapted from W. Gerstner, in *Pulsed neural networks*, Maass and Bishop (eds), MIT Press (1998)].

where neurons with very similar responses are found. The remainder of this chapter is dedicated to the introduction of dynamic models for such populations.

5.5.2 Population dynamics for slow varying input

To describe the average behaviour of a pool of neurons, we divide the population into subpopulations of neurons of the same type, with similar response properties. For simplicity, we assume further that the neurons in this pool have the same membrane time constant τ_m, the same mean numbers and synaptic efficiencies of afferents, receive the same input current I^{ext}, and do not interact. We now guess that the dynamics of such a neuronal pool can be described by a leaky integrator similar to the subthreshold dynamics of the individual IF neurons,

$$\tau \frac{dA(t)}{dt} = -A(t) + g(RI^{ext}(t)). \tag{5.49}$$

The function g is a population activation function, that describes the influence of the external current on the activation of the pool. We will discuss several activation functions in the next section. For now, it is sufficient to have a linear function $g(x) = x$ in mind. It is clear that the dynamic eqn 5.49 can only be an approximation of the pool dynamics. The motivation for this description is that, when at any instance in time only a small number of neurons in the pool is firing, we expect that the population dynamics are mainly characterized by the subthreshold dynamics to slowly varying input currents. The time constant in eqn 5.49 for slowly varying input currents should then be close to the average membrane time constants of the neurons in the pool.

The description given in eqn 5.49 is particularly appropriate when we analyse asymptotic stationary states of neuronal networks. Stationary states are states that do not change under the dynamics of the system, and by asymptotic we mean that these are the states after the initial transient behaviour has levelled off. Saying that the states do not change under the dynamics of the system can be expressed mathematically as $dA/dt = 0$. Including this in eqn 5.49 yields

$$A(t) = g(RI^{\text{ext}}(t)). \tag{5.50}$$

This is, of course, only true for constant input because the state cannot be stationary with varying input. However, the formula should also hold, to a good approximation, with slowly varying input. Many information-processing capabilities of neural networks have been studied in this limit, as shown in later chapters.

5.5.3 Motivations for population dynamics ◇

The population dynamic given by eqn 5.49 is the basis for many studies in cognitive neuroscience, and much research has gone into its justification. A lot of such studies use techniques developed in statistical physics, since the task has some similarity to deriving thermodynamic descriptions from the underlying physical movement of molecules. The principle is to start with a large number of coupled differential equations (spiking neurons in our case) and to find methods and approximations so that the large set of coupled equations can be replaced by a dynamic equation of the mean. Wilson and Cowan (1972) were among the first to argue in this way, and Brunel and Wang (2001) derived more advanced mean field models for neurons with different ion channels. We will not look at these derivations in detail, but we will outline briefly such arguments, as advanced by Wulfram Gerstner and Leo van Hemmen, which are generalizations of the Wilson–Cowan integral equations.

Recall from Section 5.1.3 that the membrane potential in the spike response model is given by

$$v_i(t) = \sum_{t^{\text{f}}} \eta(t - t^{\text{f}}) + \sum_j \sum_{t_j^{\text{f}}} w_{ij}\epsilon(t - t_j^{\text{f}}), \tag{5.51}$$

where we have ignored the possible dependence of the ϵ term on the postsynaptic firing, but included new indices i for the postsynaptic neurons, as we are now interested in a population of such neurons. We will again assume a specific kind of population of N neurons in which each neuron reacts in a similar way to input and has, on average, a synaptic efficiency specified by the constant w_0,

$$w_{ij} = \frac{w_0}{N}. \tag{5.52}$$

We also assume that there is no spike-time adaptation in the neurons, that the total number of neurons in the population stays constant, and that we, formally, have an infinitely large population of neurons in which only the means of the random variables matter. Using the definition of the population average (eqn 5.48) we can thus express the mean influence of the postsynaptic potential using the rate of the population as

$$v_\epsilon(t) = w_0 \int_0^\infty \epsilon(t')A(t - t')\mathrm{d}t'. \tag{5.53}$$

Finally, we have to take noise into account, which can be done with either of the noise models mentioned in Section 5.2.2. In general, we can define a probability density $P_v(t|t^{\text{f}})$ with which a neuron fires at time t when it has a membrane potential v and has fired previously at times t^{f}. The membrane potential does depend on the population rate, as specified in eqn 5.53. The population rate at time t can thus be expressed as the sum (or integral) of all the population rates at previous times, multiplied by the probabilities of firing at the corresponding times (see Gerstner in *Neural Computation* 12:43–89, 2000, and references therein, for details)

$$A(t) = \int_{-\infty}^{t} P_v(t|t^f) A(t^f) dt^f. \tag{5.54}$$

This dynamic is exact in the limit of an infinite pool of neurons, and the equation can be solved for particular probability densities, $P_v(t|t^f)$, derived from the noise models. It is possible to use such descriptions directly in simulations, although it requires the calculation of large sums, which is computationally demanding. It is therefore still desirable to derive approximations of population dynamics in differential form, and the derivation from the integral equations makes it possible to precisely specify the assumptions that have to be made. Wulfram Gerstner has discussed this issue in great detail (see 'Further reading'). He has shown that, in the adiabatic limit, in which the cell assembly responds only slowly to slowly varying inputs that do not cause specific collective phenomena of the neurons in the cell assembly (such as synchronization or phase locking), the population dynamics can be approximated with differential equations in the form of eqn 5.49 with an activation function of the form

$$g(x) = \frac{1}{t^{\text{ref}} - \tau \log(1 - \frac{1}{\tau x})}, \tag{5.55}$$

where t^{ref} is an absolute refractory time. This result tells us that the average activation function of the population is similar to the activation function of a single IF neuron (compare to eqn 5.11), although only in the adiabatic limit. This activation function, eqn 5.55, is plotted in Fig. 5.16A with an absolute refractory time of $t^{\text{ref}} = 1$ ms and a time constant of $\tau = 5$ ms.

Some activation functions of single neurons that have been measured electrophysiologically have shown similar response characteristics. An example of an activation function measured from a hippocampal pyramidal cell is shown in Fig. 5.16B. The figure shows the instantaneous firing rate (discharge frequency) of such a neuron in response to a 1.5 s rectangular current stimulus, with different amplitudes measured in nanoamperes (nA). The instantaneous firing rate was derived from the inverse of the first interspike interval. The neuron quickly adapted to the stimulus (not shown in the figure) so that instantaneous firing based on subsequent spikes would be much smaller. Keep in mind that we are comparing two different definitions of activation functions in Fig. 5.16, a population response in Fig. 5.16A to an averaged single neuron response in Fig. 5.16B. The similarity of the forms could be the result of the particular way in which the measurements are performed. Activation functions are typically measured in experiments with isolated neurons, which could account for the similarity of this response to the average response of a population to slowly varying inputs. Such experimental measurements neglect possible interactions in vivo that could alter the effective gain function considerably. It is important to keep in mind the different interpretations of activation functions used in the following models. Most often we will consider population models with slowly varying inputs.

We described in this section the line of thought for deriving population models from averaging over populations. While these bottom-up arguments are of great importance

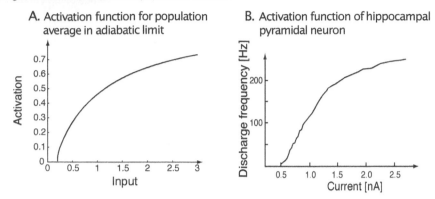

Fig. 5.16 (A) The activation function of eqn 5.55 that can be used to approximate the dynamics of a population response to slowly varying inputs (adiabatic limit). (B) Examples of physiological activation functions from a hippocampal pyramidal cell. The discharge frequency is based on the inverse of the first interspike interval after the cell started to respond to rectangular current pulses with different strength [redrawn from Lanthorn, Storm, and Anderson, *Experimental Brain Research* 53: 431–43 (1984)].

and have resulted in many advancements in the field, it is clear that many approximations and assumptions have to be made in order to allow an analytical treatments of such systems. However, we should not forget that many simulation studies have shown that findings of population models can be reproduced with models of spiking neurons. Furthermore, many examples in the remainder of this book demonstrate that population, or rate, models can capture behavioural data and characteristics of neural processing in the brain. The top-down motivation of such models, the ability of the models to capture a wide variety of neuronal data, should also be taken into account for such models.

5.5.4 Rapid response of populations

We stressed several times that the population dynamics of eqn 5.49 should only hold for slowly varying inputs, and can indeed break down under several circumstances. To demonstrate this, we consider a pool of equivalent IF neurons all with the same time constant $\tau_m = 10$ ms, and all receiving the same noisy input $I^{\text{ext}} = \bar{I}^{\text{ext}} + \eta$ with $\eta = N(0, 1)$. A simulation of such a 'network' of independent model neurons (no connections between the neurons) is shown in Fig. 5.17. In this simulation, we have switched the external input, at time $t = 100$ ms, from a low magnitude $R\bar{I}^{\text{ext}} = 11$ mV to a higher magnitude $R\bar{I}^{\text{ext}} = 16$ mV. The spike count follows the jump in the input almost instantaneously. The reason for this is that at each instant of time there is a subset of neurons that are close to threshold. These neurons can respond quickly to the input, and the other neurons have time to follow quickly. The population rate calculated with the population dynamics in eqn 5.49 follows only slowly this change of input when the time constant is set to $\tau = \tau_m$. The simulation demonstrates that very short time constants, much shorter than typical membrane time constants, have to be considered when using this model to approximate the dynamics of population responses to rapidly varying inputs.

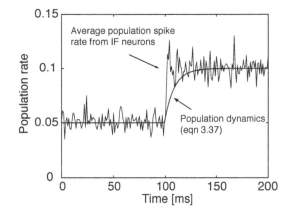

Fig. 5.17 Simulation of a population of 1000 independent integrate-and-fire neurons with a membrane time constant $\tau_m = 10$ ms and threshold $\theta = 10$ mV. Each neuron receives an input with white noise around a mean $R\bar{I}^{\text{ext}}$. This mean is switched from $R\bar{I}^{\text{ext}} = 11$ mV to $R\bar{I}^{\text{ext}} = 16$ mV at $t = 100$ ms. The spike count of the population almost instantaneously follows this jump in the input, whereas the average population rate, calculated from eqn 5.49 with a linear activation function, follows this change of input only slowly when the time constant is set to $\tau = \tau_m$.

We have used noise in the models of spiking neurons while leaving any noise out of the model for the population average. The reason for this is that the noise is essential for the argument with spiking neurons. We have not included noise in the population dynamics so as to outline the average response of the node. Adding noise introduces fluctuations into this curve that seem to resemble fluctuations in the average of spiking nodes. However, analysis of the mean response would certainly bring the difference to light. Adding noise to the population node just to make it look more realistic would only obscure the general argument. In contrast, the noise in a population of spiking neurons might be essential for information processing in the brain.

While the simulation demonstrates that the simplest population model fails to describe the rapid onset of neuronal responses in populations of spiking neurons, we should also stress that the asymptotic increase of the population response is well captured by the population node. For many models in cognitive neuroscience it is this fact which is modelled and thus sufficient for many explanations of system-level processes. Also, faster responses can be modelled by input-dependent time constants τ or by input that is explicitly dependent on fluctuations in the input as, for example, captured by the mean field analysis of Brunel and Wang.

5.5.5 Common activation functions

While we have already discussed the population activation function in the limit studied by Wulfram Gerstner, it should be clear that more complicated interactions in the neuronal population can, in principle, lead to other such functions g. We also call this function the activation function, which is often termed transfer function in neural network studies. This function describes the net effect of various processes within a neuronal group that transforms a given input into the specific output of the neuron assembly. As the neural population itself can implement various response characteristics, it is possible that this function can have various forms beyond the monotone activation functions of single neurons discussed before. Some frequently used functions are illustrated in Table 5.2.

The first example is the linear function, g^{lin}, which relates the sum of inputs directly to the output. Linear units can often be treated analytically and can provide us with many insights into the working of networks. Many other activation functions can also be approximated by piecewise linear functions. A simple example of such a non-linear function is the step function, g^{step}. This function only returns two values and therefore produces binary responses. This activation function was used by McCulloch and Pitts (1943), and a node with this activation function is therefore called a McCulloch–Pitts node.

The third example, the threshold-linear function g^{theta}, is similar to the linear functions, except that it is bounded from below. Limiting the node activities from below is sensible as negative activity has no biological equivalent. This activation function is a good approximation of the population activation functions derived in the spike response model. Besides the lower limit on the firing rate, it is also biologically sensible to limit the maximal response of the node. This is because the rate of neuronal groups is limited by the refractory times of neurons, and limited number of neurons can be active at any given time. A simple realization of such an activation function is a combination of the threshold-linear function and the step function. However, a more frequently used activation function in this class is the sigmoid function g^{sig}, illustrated as the fourth example in Table 5.2. This function bounds the minimal and maximal responses of a node, while interpolating smoothly between these two extremes. This type of activation function is most frequently used in neural network and connectionist models, for reasons that will become apparent in Chapter 7. It also approximates the activation function of noisy IF neurons well, as we saw in Chapter 4. The last function in the table is very different to the former in the sense that it is a non-monotonic function. The example shown is a radial-basis function, one of a group of general functions that are symmetrical around a base value. The particular example g^{gauss} is the famous Gaussian bell curve.

Suffice it to say that these are only a few examples of possible activation functions. We have only outlined the general shape of these functions, and it should be clear that these shapes can be modified. The functions often include parameters with which some characteristics of the functions can be changed, such as the slope and offset of a function. For example, we can generalize the sigmoid function in the table with

$$g^{\text{sig}} = \frac{1}{1 + \exp(-\beta(x - x_0))}, \tag{5.56}$$

where increasing the value of the parameter β increases the steepness of the curve, and x_0 shifts the curve along the abscissa. Keep in mind that these are not the only possible forms of activation functions. Networks of nodes with different activation functions have different characteristics and it is worth exploring the dependence of network characteristics on the specific activation functions. However, it is also interesting to note that many of the information-processing capabilities of networks of such nodes do not depend critically on the precise form of the activation function. Several types of activation function lead to similar network abilities in the sense that we do not have to fine-tune the functions in order to demonstrate network abilities.

Table 5.2 Examples of frequently used activation functions and their basic implementation in MATLAB

Type of function	Graphical represent.	Mathematical formula	MATLAB implementation
Linear		$g^{\mathrm{lin}}(x) = x$	X
Step		$g^{\mathrm{step}}(x) = \begin{cases} 1 & \text{if } x > 0 \\ 0 & \text{elsewhere} \end{cases}$	floor(0.5*(1+sign(x)))
Threshold-linear		$g^{\mathrm{theta}}(x) = x\,\Theta(x)$	x.*floor(0.5*(1+sign(x)))
Sigmoid		$g^{\mathrm{sig}}(x) = \dfrac{1}{1+\exp(-x)}$	1./(1+exp(-x))
Radial-basis		$g^{\mathrm{gauss}}(x) = \exp(-x^2)$	exp(-x.^2)

5.6 Networks with non-classical synapses

We introduced population nodes in the last section by assuming an assembly of neurons that behave with similar response profiles. We also assumed that such nodes are summing all weighted inputs, reflecting the additive characteristics of currents. However, we already mentioned in Chapter 4 that single neurons show also non-linear interactions between different input channels; for example, in the case of shunting inhibition. It is therefore likely that population nodes can interact in a non-linear way. This chapter introduces briefly a basic non-linear (multiplicative) interaction between population nodes as this will be used in some of the models described later in this book.

5.6.1 Logical AND and sigma–pi nodes

An example of a strong non-linear interaction between two ion channels is a spiking neuron with a firing threshold that requires at least two spikes in some temporal proximity to each other. A single spike alone, in this case, cannot initiate a spike. Only if two spikes are present within the time interval, on the order of the decay time of EPSPs, can a postsynaptic spike be generated. This corresponds to a logical AND function. We can represent such an AND function with a multiplicative term of two binary presynaptic terms, r_1 and r_2, with values one, indicating that a presynaptic spike at a particular synapse is present, or zero, indicating that no presynaptic spike is present. Thus, the dependence of the activation of such a node from two inputs is described by a multiplicative term such as $h = r_1 r_2$.

We can generalize this idea for population models. Let us consider two independent presynaptic spike trains with average firing rates r_j^{in} and r_k^{in}, respectively. The average firing rate determines the probability of having a spike in a small interval. The probability of having two spikes of the two different presynaptic neurons in the same interval is then proportional to the product of the two individual probabilities. This forms the basis of a simple model of non-linear interactions between synapses in a rate model that includes non-linear interactions between synapses. The activation of a node i in this model is given by

$$h_i = \sum_{jk} w_{ijk} r_j^{\text{in}} r_k^{\text{in}}, \qquad (5.57)$$

where the weight factor w_{ijk} describes now the overall strength of two combined synaptic inputs. The activation of postsynaptic neurons in this model depends on the sum (mathematically depicted by the Greek letter $\sum$) of multiplicative terms (mathematically depicted by the Greek letter $\prod$), and such a node is therefore called a sigma–pi node. Notes that the product of four terms $x_1 x_2 x_3 x_4$ can be written with this shorthand notation as $\prod_{i=1}^{4} x_i$, although we have not used this notation here as we have only two factors in the product and the notation would actually make the formula look more cluttered. The model can be generalized to other forms of non-linear interactions between synaptic channels by replacing the product of the presynaptic firing rates with some function of presynaptic firing rates, for example, $r_j^{\text{in}} r_k^{\text{in}} \rightarrow g(r_j^{\text{in}} r_k^{\text{in}})$, but the simple multiplicative model already incorporates essential features of non-linear ion channel interactions that are sufficient for most of the models discussed in this book. Note that we can also view such interactions as modulatory effects of one synaptic input on the other synaptic input.

5.6.2   Divisive inhibition

Equation 5.57 is an example of two non-linear interacting excitatory channels. An analogous model of an interaction between an excitatory synapse and an inhibitory synapse can be written as

$$h_i = \sum_{jk} w_{ijk} r_j^{\text{excitatory}} / r_k^{\text{inhibitory}}. \qquad (5.58)$$

This is an example of divisive inhibition which models the effects of shunting inhibition as mentioned in Chapter 4. Inhibitory synapses on the cell body often have such shunting effects (see Fig. 5.18A), whereas inhibitory synapses on remote parts of the dendrites are better described by subtractive inhibition. It is possible that synapses in between have effects that interpolate between these two extremes.

5.6.3   Further sources of modulatory effects between synaptic inputs

Interactions between synapses can result from a variety of other sources in biological neurons. An obvious source is voltage-dependent synapses that are in physical proximity to each other as illustrated in Fig. 5.18B. A good example are NMDA receptors that are blocked for low membrane potentials. If the membrane potential is raised by

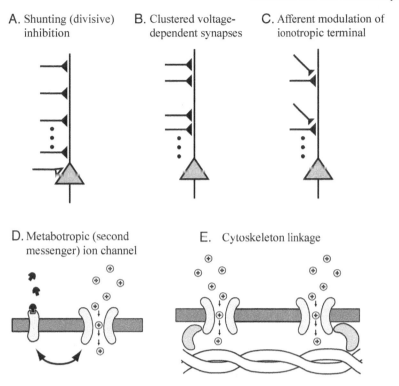

Fig. 5.18 Some sources of non-linear (modulatory) effects between synapses as modelled by sigma–pi nodes. (A) Shunting (divisive) inhibition, which is often recorded as the effect of inhibitory synapses on the cell body. (B) The effect of simultaneously activated voltage-gated excitatory synapses that are in close physical proximity to each other (synaptic clusters) can be larger than the sum of the effect of each individual synapse. Examples are clusters of AMPA and NMDA type synapses. (C) Some cortical synaptic terminals have nicotinic acetylcholine (ACh) receptors. An ACh release of cholinergic afferents can thus produce a larger efflux of neurotransmitter and thereby increase EPSPs in the postsynaptic neuron of this synaptic terminal. D. Metabotropic receptors can trigger intracellular messengers that can influence the gain of ion channels. (E) Ion channels can be linked to the underlying cytoskeleton with adapter proteins and can thus influence other ion channels through this link.

an EPSP from another non-NMDA synapse in its proximity, then it is possible that the blockade is removed so that the combined effect of a non-NMDA synapse together with the NMDA synapse is much larger than the sum of the activation through each synapse alone. The physical proximity is necessary as the EPSP in a passive dendrite decays with distance, so that the non-linear effects are largest for nearby synapses. The non-linear effects can also reach larger distances between synapses with local active dendrites that can activate more remote dendrites through active spike propagation.

Examples of a direct influence of specific afferents on the release of neurotransmitters by presynaptic terminals are also known. This is illustrated schematically in Fig. 5.18C. An example is cholinergic afferents that emit acetylcholine (ACh). This can bind to ACh receptors at a presynaptic terminal that opens calcium channels. The excess of calcium in the presynaptic terminal then triggers an enhanced release of neurotransmitters by a presynaptic action potential. This is an example of the modulation of an ionotropic synapse. A more diffuse modulation can be achieved with metabotropic receptors (see Fig. 5.18D). Such receptors initiate intracellular chemical reactions leading to second messengers that can influence the efficiency or gain of different ion channels. A more direct linkage between ion channels is possible through adapter proteins that link ion channels to the underlying cytoskeleton in a neuron (Fig. 5.18E). More research is necessary to understand all the details of such mechanisms. We are mainly concerned here with the principal potentials of such modulatory effects between presynaptic neuron activities, and we will employ such mechanisms in some models discussed in later chapters.

6   Associators and synaptic plasticity

So far, we have neglected some of the most exciting and central mechanisms of brain processing, those of synaptic plasticity and learning in networks. Neurons are connected to form networks, and a neural network is not only characterized by the topology of the network, but also by the connection strength, w_{ij}, between two neurons or two population nodes. In this chapter we discuss how connection strengths can be changed in a usage-dependent way through a biological phenomena called synaptic plasticity. Synaptic plasticity is the physical basis of learning in neural systems which we will discuss later. Here, we start with a general discussion of associators, which summarize the essence of plasticity mechanisms and their importance for cognitive brain processing. We then present the neurophysiological basis of plasticity and some specific models of plasticity. The final part of this chapter discusses some consequences of plasticity rules, in particular weight distributions, and explains some strategies for weight scaling and weight decay. The chapter ends with an application of a basic Hebbian rule with weight decay to principal component analysis.

6.1   Associative memory and Hebbian learning

Neural networks are characterized by a collection of connection strengths, w_{ij}, between neurons or population nodes. We can code the network architecture with a large matrix that specifies all the weights between all the nodes in the network. A weight of zero indicates that there is no functioning connection between two neurons. We can loosely differentiate two forms of plasticity:

- **Structural plasticity** is the mechanism describing the generation of new connections and thereby redefining the topology of the network.
- **Functional plasticity** is the mechanism of changing strength values of existing connections.

Also, it is sometimes useful to distinguish developmental mechanisms from adaptations in mature organisms. The formation and maintenance of neuronal networks in the brain must be, to a large extent, genetically coded. However, not all the details can be coded with the fairly small number of genes in the human genome, estimated to be around 20,000–25,000, not to mention the current view that only a small percentage of these genes are thought to be used to construct particular proteins that guide the functionality of the organisms. Genes can, however, influence attractor substances that guide the growth of neurites during brain development and the maintenance of synapses, as discussed later. Brain development can also be influenced by environmental circumstances. Adaptive mechanisms are thus thought to be very important for brain functions, at least for the fine tuning of parameters in brain networks.

Fundamentals of Computational Neuroscience. Third edition. Thomas P. Trappenberg,
Oxford University Press. © Oxford University Press 2023. DOI: 10.1093/oso/9780192869364.003.0006

During neural development of mammalian organisms, it is thought that brains start highly connected and that during infancy many of the connections get pruned. Also, it has been found that there are critical periods during which normal development of specific neuronal organizations can be easily disturbed. Providing new synaptic contacts does not only require that axons grow close to dendrites, but that axons develop release sites, that dendrites incorporate synaptic ion channels, and that glial cells provide supporting functionality. While brain development and structural plasticity are important areas of research, many of our discussions in later chapters focus on the ability of adaptive networks in general, without distinguishing between different forms of plasticity that are certainly present in biological organisms. Most of the following discussion is concerned with learning rules that are widely attributed to functional plasticity.

6.1.1 Hebbian learning

The idea that the brain can change and adapt by building associations had already appeared by the end of the 19th century. For example, Sigmund Freud proposed the law of association by simultaneity in 1888 which very much resembles the general principles explained in this section. However, the central role of associative learning as an organizing principle in the brain became popular only later with an influential book by the Canadian psychologist Donald O. Hebb. In his book, *The organization of behaviour*, which was published in 1949, he even speculates on the functional implementation of learning:

> When an axon of a cell A is near enough to excite cell B or repeatedly or persistently takes part in firing it, some growth or metabolic change takes place in both cells such that A's efficiency, as one of the cells firing B, is increased.

Hebb had no means of observing synapses directly, which makes this hypothesis a wild guess by our standards. But his book had a great influence on many researchers as it was one of the first concrete proposals about how the brain organizes itself to implement the cognitive functions underlying behaviour. In particular, Hebb proposed that cell assemblies, formed dynamically in response to external stimuli, carry out much of the information processing in the brain. The basic physical mechanisms that support these plastic changes in the brain, he argued, are some synaptic changes which he speculated to be 'some growth or metabolic change'. Likely the most important component of his hypothesis for us is the functional basis for this change, that of a functional meaningful correlation between presynaptic and postsynaptic activity. This important insight is summarized as 'what fires together, wires together'. While this phrase could be interpreted more towards structural plasticity, it should be understood here in terms of synaptic plasticity, or in Hebbian's sense, in what fires together should wire together more strongly. It is only much more recently that the physiology of synaptic plasticity has been observed in some detail. This newer research shows that Hebb's qualitative description, as quoted above, is remarkably accurate and captures most of the essential organizational principles in the nervous system. Activity-dependent plasticity that depends on pre- and postsynaptic activity is often called Hebbian plasticity or Hebbian learning in Hebb's honour.

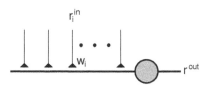

Fig. 6.1 A simplified neuron that receives a large number of inputs r_i^{in}. The synaptic efficiency is denoted by w_i and the output of the node by r^{out}.

6.1.2 Associations

A major hypothesis quantified by computational models is that synaptic plasticity enables memory and learning, as discussed extensively in later chapters. Human memory is very different from that of digital computers. Memory in a digital computer consists of a device where information is stored, similar to a shelf. When recalling information from the computer memory we have to tell the computer internally where to find this memory using a memory address. Failing to specify the memory address precisely results in complete loss of this memory as it cannot then be recalled. Even an error of one bit in the memory address turns out to be fatal for memory recall. Natural systems cannot work with such demanding precision.

The human memory system is different in many respects from conventional computer memory. We are often able to recall vivid memories of events from small details. For example, when visiting some places of your childhood it is likely that the images of the locations, although not exactly the same as years ago, will trigger vivid memories of friends and certain incidents that occurred at these places; a picture with only part of the face of a friend can be sufficient to recognize him and to recall his name, or, if someone mentions the name of a friend, it is possible to remember certain facial features of this person. In contrast to digital computers, we are able to learn associations that can trigger memories based on related information, that is, only partial information can be sufficient to recall memories. It is this type of memory that we think is essential for human cognitive processes. While computer scientists sometimes call this content addressable memory, we will generally call this an associative memory or associator.

Synaptic plasticity is the necessary ingredient behind forming associations, and we will now illustrate the principal idea of Hebbian associative learning using a simplified neuron as illustrated in Fig. 6.1. We will later use these mechanisms extensively in associative networks, illustrated in Fig. 6.2. Such associative architectures were proposed around 1960 independently by Bernd Widrow (Madaline) and Karl Steinbuch (Lernmatrix). While we now use the language of neurons, the same arguments apply for associative learning in networks of population nodes, as primarily used in the later chapters of this book. We showed only a few presynaptic axons which synapse on the model node in Fig. 6.1. However, it is important to keep in mind in the following discussion that neurons receive input from a large number of sources, as mentioned before. A cortical neuron receives on the order of 5000–10,000 synapses from other neurons, although only a small subset, fewer than 1%, of active synaptic channels can be sufficient to elicit a presynaptic spike if the synaptic efficiencies are sufficient and synaptic events fall within certain temporal windows.

Let us discuss the example illustrated in Fig. 6.3. There, a certain event, such

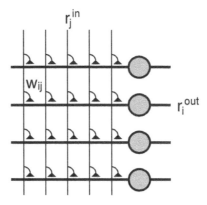

Fig. 6.2 A network of associative nodes. Each component of the input vector, r_i^{in}, is distributed to each neuron in the network. However, the effect of the input can be different for each neuron as each individual synapses can have different efficiency values w_{ij}, where j labels the neuron in the network.

as the presence of particular smell, is reflected in the firing of a subset of the input channels to the neuron (Fig. 6.3A). We have used only a small subset of presynaptic neurons to represent the input stimulus in accordance with distributed, yet sparse, coding discussed further below. In Fig. 6.3A we represent the odour stimulus, say the smell from a BBQ when cooking hamburgers, with an input pattern that represents spikes in input channels 1, 3, and 5. The synaptic efficiencies of these input channels are assumed to be large enough to elicit a postsynaptic spike. For example, we can take the spiking threshold to be $\theta = 1.5$ and assume initially that the synaptic weights of only these input channels have the values $w_i = 1$, as shown on the right site of Fig. 6.3A. The input pattern is then sufficient to elicit a postsynaptic spike. This can easily be verified by comparing the internal activation of the neuron,

$$h = \sum_i w_i r_i^{in} = 3, \tag{6.1}$$

with the firing threshold of the neuron ($\theta = 1.5$). These values of the synaptic weights are also sufficient to enable the neuron to fire in response to partial input. For example, if only channels 1 and 3 are on, then $h = 2 > \theta$ and the neuron still fires. This is very important for brain processes since the input pattern might not always be complete due to noisy processing or partial sensory information. In this way, the brain can achieve pattern completion, the ability to complete the representation of a partial stimulus.

Another stimulus, such as the sight of the hamburger when opening the BBQ, represented in the model as a presynaptic input to the last three incoming channels in Fig. 6.3B, is not able to elicit the response of this neuron with the current values of synaptic weights. In order to associate the visual cue of a hamburger with an odour signalling the smell of a hamburger, we have to modify the synaptic weights. For this we adopt the following strategy:

Increase the strength of the synapses by a value $\Delta w = 0.1$ if a presynaptic firing is paired with a postsynaptic firing.

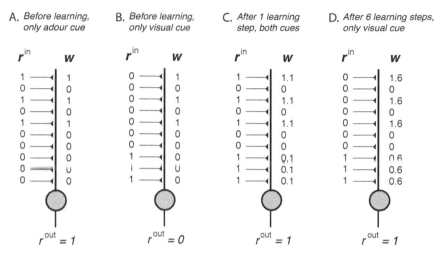

Fig. 6.3 Examples of an associative node that is trained on two feature vectors with a Hebbian-type learning algorithm that increases the synaptic strength by $\Delta w = 0.1$ each time a presynaptic spike occurs in the same temporal window as a postsynaptic spike.

This learning rule modifies the synaptic weights, so that after one simultaneous presentation of both stimuli, the visual cue and the cue representing the odour, the weights have the values illustrated in Fig. 6.3C. After six consecutive learning iterations, we end up with the synaptic weights shown in Fig. 6.3D. How fast we achieve this point depends on a learning rate, which we set to 0.1 in this example.

The visual cue of a hamburger alone is sufficient to elicit the response of the neuron after only 5 or 6 simultaneous presentations of both stimuli. The firing of this neuron is then associated with both the presence of a visual image of a hamburger and the presence of a cue representing the smell of a hamburger. If this neuron, or this neuron in combination with other neurons in a network, elicits a mental image of a hamburger, then the presence of only one cue, the smell or the sight of the hamburger, is sufficient to elicit the mental image of a hamburger. Therefore, the odour and the visual image of a hamburger are associated with its mental image. Such associations are fundamental for many cognitive processes.

6.1.3 Hebbian learning in the conditioning framework

The mechanisms of an associator, as outlined above, rely on the fact that the first stimulus, the odour of the hamburger, was already effective in eliciting a response of the neuron before learning. This is a reasonable assumption since we could start with random networks in which some neurons would be responsive to this stimulus before learning. Thus, we can assume that we have selected such a neuron in our example from a large set of neurons responsive to all kinds of stimuli, based on a random initial weight distribution. Although the synaptic strengths of these input channels change with the learning rule, we call the initial stimulus the unconditioned stimulus (UCS) because the response of the neuron to this stimulus was maintained. The main reason for this labelling is that we want to distinguish this input, which is already effective, from the second stimulus, the visual image of the hamburger. For the second input the response of the neuron changes during learning, and so we call the second stimulus the conditioned stimulus (CS). The input vector to the system is thus a mixture of UCS and CS as illustrated in Fig. 6.4A.

Several variations of this scheme are known to occur in biological nervous systems. One of these is outlined in Fig. 6.4B. We stressed that it is crucial for the UCS in the previous scheme to elicit a postsynaptic neural response, which was incorporated in our example above by using sufficiently strong synapses in the input channels of the UCS. Alternatively, as illustrated in Fig. 6.4B, the fibres carrying the UCS can have many synapses on to the postsynaptic dendrite that can ensure the firing of the node. For example, mossy fibres in the hippocampus are axons that generate very strong contacts with postsynaptic neurons. Another example is climbing fibres in the cerebellum, which have many hundreds of synapses with a single Purkinje cell. The cerebellum has been implicated in motor learning, and it has been suggested that the UCS provides a motor error signal for such learning mechanisms. We will elaborate on this in Chapter 10.

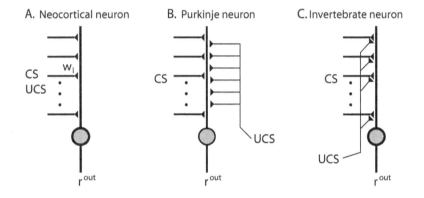

Fig. 6.4 Different models of associative nodes resembling the principal architecture found in biological nervous systems such as (A) cortical neurons in mammalian cortex and (B) Purkinje cells in the cerebellum, which have strong input from climbing fibres through many hundreds or thousands of synapses. In contrast, the model as shown in (C) that utilizes specific input to a presynaptic terminal as is known to exist in invertebrate systems, would have to supply the UCS to all synapses simultaneously in order to achieve the same kind of result as in the previous two models. Such architectures are unlikely to play an important role in cortical processing.

Another model is illustrated in Fig. 6.4C. Here, we have indicated a specific modulatory mechanism using a separate input to presynaptic terminals, which can induce presynaptic changes. Such mechanisms exist in invertebrates, for example, in the sensorimotor system of the sea slug Aplysia. Such mechanisms could be specific for each presynaptic terminal and would thus be non-Hebbian by definition. To achieve the same results as in the other two models, which depend globally on the firing of the postsynaptic neuron, we would have to supply the UCS signal to all synaptic inputs simultaneously. Such an architecture is much more elaborate to realize in larger nervous systems and seems to be absent in vertebrate nervous systems. This demonstrates that different synaptic mechanisms and information-processing principles may be present in vertebrate and invertebrate nervous systems.

The example of Fig. 6.3 illustrates that it is possible to store information with associative learning; after imprinting an event–response pattern, the response can be recalled from partial information about the event. This is the primary reason that synaptic plasticity is thought to be the underlying principle behind associative memory and other important information-processing abilities in the brain. Of course, the basic learning rule used above has to be extended to incorporate important details not captured in the example. For example, the learning rule outlined in the example increased all the relevant synaptic weights. This synaptic potentiation results in an increase of the complete weight vector after some time if the presentation of many different input vectors is coupled with random firing of the postsynaptic node. The synaptic weights would then become extremely large and so the response of the node becomes unspecific to input patterns since it would respond to noisy input. Some form of synaptic weakening, called synaptic depression, including some competitive depression between synapses, is therefore important. Also, the temporal structure of the firing pattern can be relevant in the learning rule, as suggested by Hebb. We will review recent experimental findings that verify this hypothesis in the following section.

6.1.4 Features of associators and Hebbian learning

Associations, together with some form of distributed representation discussed further in Chapters 7, lead to important characteristics of networks of associative nodes. These characteristics are essential for brain-style information processing and the modelling of cognitive processes. The following is a brief summary of such characteristics which we will study further in different parts of this book.

Pattern completion and generalization

We have seen that a stimulus capturing only part of a pattern associated with an object can still trigger a memory of that object. This means that networks support recall of details of an object which were not part of the stimulus. This ability to recall from partial input is also termed pattern completion. It relies on a distributed representation of an object stimulus so that some missing components of a feature vector can be added. Pattern completion is based on the calculation of some form of overlap, or similarity, of an input vector with a weight vector that represents the pattern on which the node was trained. An example of such a similarity measure is the dot product between the pattern input vector and the vector of the synaptic efficiencies. We also need non-linearity in the output function, such as a firing threshold, which is characteristic of neurons and neural populations. Then, as long as the overlap between the input pattern and the trained pattern is large enough, an output is generated that is equivalent to the output of the trained pattern. Thus, the output node responds to all patterns with a certain similarity to the trained pattern, an ability that is called generalization.

Prototypes and extraction of central tendencies

A closely related ability of associative nodes, or networks, is the ability to extract central tendencies. This occurs when training associative nodes on many similar, but not equivalent, examples. The weight vector then represents an average over these examples, which we can interpret as a prototype. Such training sets are typical in natural environments. For example, each person has an individual face, while there are still many common features in all faces. Another reason for training sets with many, slightly different, patterns, is that the training set is derived from the same object, which is represented over time with fluctuating patterns due to some noisy processes in the encoding procedure. The prototype extraction ability of associators can then be used to achieve noise reduction, an ability that is important in the case of noisy processing systems, such as the brain and technological applications.

Graceful degradation

The loss, or inaccuracy, of some components of a neural system, such as some synaptic connections or even whole neurons, should not markedly affect the system. Associative networks often degrade gracefully in that a large amount of synapses have to be removed before the system produces a large amount of error. Even the loss of nodes can be tolerated if the information feeds into an upstream processing layer with associative abilities that can archive pattern completion from partial information. Such fault tolerance is essential in biological systems.

6.2   The physiology and biophysics of synaptic plasticity

In Chapter 4 we reviewed how a spike elicits the release of neurotransmitters in chemical synapses through which presynaptic spikes can influence the state of postsynaptic neurons. In this section, we briefly review the physiology and biochemical mechanisms which are thought to be involved in changing the response characteristics of neurons, with a focus on activity-dependent functional plasticity. We should keep in mind the possibility that several components of the synaptic machinery can change in plasticity experiments. Possible changes include the number of release sites, the probability of neurotransmitter release, the number of transmitter receptors, and the conductance and kinetics of ion channels.

6.2.1   Typical plasticity experiments

Long-lasting changes of synaptic response characteristics, including the average amplitude and latency of EPSPs, were first demonstrated experimentally in 1973 by Timothy Bliss and Terje Lømo in hippocampus cultures. Some exemplary results of such typical plasticity experiments are shown in Fig. 6.5A. The shown experiments are based on measurement of evoked field potentials (EFPs) in the striatum of mice, a subcortical structure involved in motor control. The graph shows the change in EFP amplitude, compared to average initial measurements (here at times from $t = -10$ min to $t = 0$ min). At time $t = 0$, a high-frequency stimulus was applied. The recording of EFP amplitudes after this plasticity-inducing tetanus shows increased EFP amplitude. While the initial, strong response will often decay somewhat after some minutes, many experiments have shown long-lasting effects over hours, days, or more, which is very long on the scale of brain processing. Such changes in synaptic efficacy are there-

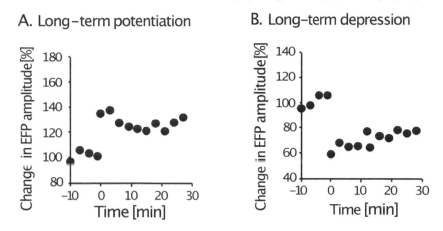

Fig. 6.5 (A) Change in evoked field potential in the striatum after a high-frequency stimulation at time $t = 0$. (B) Demonstration of LTD in similar experiments [adapted from Dang, Yokoi, Yin, Lovinger, Wang, and Li, *Proceedings of the National Academy of Science* 103: 15254–9 (2006)].

fore termed long-term potentiation (LTP) since the average amplitude of the EPSP increased. Other experiments have shown that long-term changes can be of either sign. For example, stimulations with low frequencies at $t = 0$ result in lowering average EFP amplitudes. An example is shown in Fig. 6.5B. Such long-lasting changes are called long-term depression (LTD). Such mechanisms can support the associations discussed in the previous section. In particular, LTP can enforce associative responses to a presynaptic firing pattern that is temporally linked to postsynaptic firing, while LTD can facilitate the unlearning of presynaptic input that is not consistent with postsynaptic firing. It is interesting to note that these experiments by Dang et al. also showed that preventing LTP in the striatum disrupted learning of motor skills in which the striatum is implicated.

Changes in EFP amplitudes are not the only effects that are measured in plasticity experiments. Bliss and Terje Lømo already noted that the latency of evoked postsynaptic spikes responses can be affected. Also, recent experiments by Alan Fine and Ryosuke Enoki in hippocampal slices of rats have shown that the probability of transmitter release can be modulated in plasticity experiments. Some results of their experiments are illustrated in Fig. 6.6. Fig. 6.6A shows time courses of EPSP responses to pairs of presynaptic stimulations. A pair of probe stimuli was used since it is often observed that the second pulse is more effective than the first pulse in eliciting a postsynaptic response. This is a form of short-term plasticity which is called paired-pulse facilitation. After measuring the initial response in the neuron, a high-frequency stimulus was applied, indicated by vertical bars in the figure. The increase in the EPSP amplitude following the high-frequency stimulation is similar to that seen in the experiments discussed earlier. These experiments also show that a further potentiation was achieved with another high-frequency stimulus.

The investigators also imaged single synapses with calcium-sensitive fluorescent dyes. The time course of changes in the fluorescence are plotted in Fig. 6.6B. While these measurements also show the effects of paired-pulse facilitation, the amplitudes

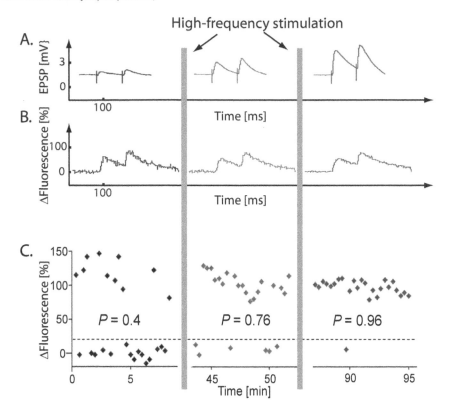

Fig. 6.6 Plasticity experiment in hippocampal slices in which not only EPSPs were measured, but in which, additionally, postsynaptic calcium-dependent fluorescence signals at single synapses were imaged [data courtesy of Alan Fine and Ryosuke Enoki].

are comparable after each LTP tetanus and so do not show a synaptic increase proportional to the increase in EPSPs. However, they do respond faithfully when transmitter has been released from the presynaptic terminal. An important effect of the LTP tetanus can be seen in Fig. 6.6C. This figure shows the change in fluorescence for several trials in the different phases of the experiment. The results show that not every presynaptic stimulus produced a postsynaptic response; the fraction of times that a postsynaptic event was observed can be equated with the probability of transmitter release, as mentioned in Section 4.2. Furthermore, the probability of release increased considerably after each high-frequency stimulus. Other experiments by the group have shown that the probability of release can be altered bidirectionally, increasing the probability with high-frequency stimuli and decreasing the probability when the stimuli are paired in a specific way with postsynaptic spikes as discussed in the next section. The advantage of the imaging technique is that the results in Fig. 6.6B and C can be attributed to a single synapse, while the EPSP measurements are likely to measure effects of several synapses. The increase in EPSP amplitude can thus be a population effect, in which the increased probability of getting a postsynaptic event in each of a number of synapses can increase the summed effect of measuring the EPSP in the soma.

6.2.2 Spike timing dependent plasticity

The classic plasticity experiments discussed above typically use high-frequency presynaptic stimulations to induce LTP and lower-frequency stimulations to induce LTD. These stimulations need to be strong enough to 'drive' the postsynaptic neuron, reflecting Hebb's postulate of a causal relation between postsynaptic and presynaptic spikes. Henry Markram, and others, have further investigated the necessary causal relation between pre- and postsynaptic spiking by varying the time between externally induced pre- and postsynaptic spikes. An exemplary result of such experiments in hippocampal cultures by Guo-chiang Bi and Mu-ming Poo is shown in Fig. 6.7A. The measurements were done in a voltage clamp so that currents are measured here. The data show the relative changes of EPSC amplitudes for different values of the time differences between pre- and postsynaptic spikes, Δt. These results indicate that there is a critical time window for plasticity of around $|\Delta t| \approx 40$ ms. No synaptic plasticity could be detected for differences of pre- and postsynaptic spike times with absolute values much larger than this time window. Changes in excitatory postsynaptic current (EPSC) amplitudes are largest for small positive differences (LTP) or small negative differences (LTD) in the pre- and postsynaptic spike times. The decrease in synaptic plasticity can be fitted reasonably well with an exponential decay of the absolute difference between spike times.

While the data in Fig. 6.7A are obtained from hippocampal cells in vitro, similar relations have also been found in neocortical slices, as well as in vivo, with similar sizes of plasticity windows. However, the asymmetrical form of Hebbian plasticity, shown again schematically on the right in Fig. 6.7A, is not the only possible form for dependence of synaptic plasticity on the relative spike times. Some additional examples are illustrated schematically in Fig. 6.7B–E. Examples are known in which the critical difference window for LTD is much larger compared to that for LTP, as illustrated schematically in Fig. 6.7B. LTP and LTD can also be reversed relative to the difference in pre- and postsynaptic spiking (Fig. 6.7C). For example, positive differences in spike timings induce LTD when synaptic plasticity is triggered in Purkinje cells in the cerebellum. Purkinje cells are known to be inhibitory, and such changes can therefore reduce inhibition in the targets of Purkinje cells. There are also examples of symmetrical Hebbian plasticity illustrated in Fig. 6.7D and E. Such plasticity windows seem more appropriate when considering bursting neurons. It is important for computational neuroscientists to explore the functional roles of the different forms of Hebbian plasticity.

6.2.3 The calcium hypothesis and modelling chemical pathways

The physiological experiments described above illustrate the consequences, in terms of synaptic efficacy, when the synapses are exposed to specific stimulations. While this is most relevant for understanding the functional consequences of synaptic plasticity that we will explore later in this book, it is also important to understand the mechanisms leading to the findings discussed above. Although there are still many unknowns, calcium is an important ingredient. In particular, Artola and Singer, and earlier John Lisman, have advanced the hypothesis that different levels of calcium trigger different biochemical pathways, as illustrated in Fig. 6.8. Calcium triggers the phosphorylation

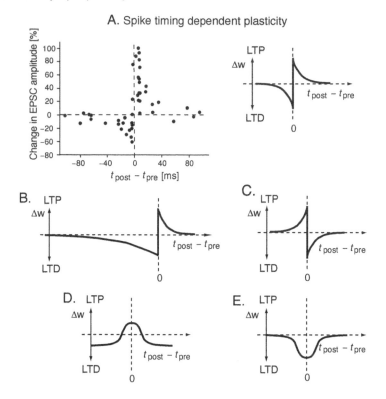

Fig. 6.7 (A) The relative changes in excitatory postsynaptic current (EPSC) amplitudes for various time differences between the time of an induced presynaptic spike and the time of an induced postsynaptic spike [data re-drawn from Bi and Poo, *Journal of Neuroscience* 18: 10464–72 (1998)]. The form of plasticity is stylized on the right. (B–E) Several examples of the schematic dependence of synaptic efficiencies on the temporal relations between pre- and postsynaptic spikes [adapted from Abbott and Nelson, *Nature Neuroscience* 3: 1178–83 (2000)].

of proteins through enzymes such as CaM kinase II, which can alter the efficiency of existing AMPA receptors and can promote the insertion of new AMPA channels in the long term. Specifically, high levels of calcium promote LTP though phosphorylation, whereas moderate levels of calcium lead to dephosphorylation and LTD. This is consistent with findings by Artola and Singer for conditions leading to LTP and LTD, for which we will describe corresponding learning rules in the next section.

To relate this hypothesis to the activity of neurons, we need to think about the mechanisms that influence postsynaptic calcium levels. There are several sources of postsynaptic Ca^{2+}, as schematized in Fig. 6.8. The binding of glutamate can directly influence the postsynaptic calcium level in two ways. First, this occurs through AMPA receptors that gate ion channels with some Ca^{2+} permeability, but the resulting postsynaptic Ca^{2+} level from this source is thought to be moderate. Second, glutamate triggers Ca^{2+} release from internal Ca^{2+} stores. These sources of Ca^{2+} are indirectly triggered by glutamate binding. Glutamate binding also leads to an increase in the membrane potential that can indirectly enable Ca^{2+} entry though voltage-gated Ca^{2+} channels (VGCC). Finally, the largest influx of Ca^{2+} is enabled through NMDAR

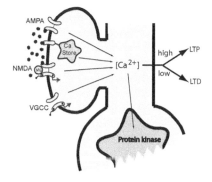

Fig. 6.8 Illustration of the calcium hypothesis which states that high levels of calcium promote LTP, whereas moderate levels lead to LTD. The figure includes common sources of postsynaptic calcium and indicates that calcium drives protein kinases in the nucleus.

channels. However, as discussed before, NMDAR channels are blocked, even after glutamate release, by magnesium ions (Mg^{2+}). Only a strong postsynaptic depolarization removes this blockage, allowing a large increase in postsynaptic Ca^{2+}. The necessary, strong depolarization of the membrane potential is likely provided by back-propagating action potentials (BAPs), as mentioned before. Thus, NMDAR channels provide mechanisms for a Hebbian condition, those of presynaptic activity (indicated by glutamate binding to NMDAR) and postsynaptic activity (indicated by BAPs).

The hypothesis that NMDAR and postsynaptic Ca^{2+} are involved in synaptic plasticity is backed up by demonstrations that the blockade of NMDAR with antagonistic drugs, or prevention of the rise in postsynaptic calcium concentrations, abolishes synaptic plasticity. Note that we have discussed mainly postsynaptic mechanisms of long-lasting plasticity. However, as mentioned before, there is evidence that presynaptic modifications are important for synaptic plasticity and learning. For example, the above-mentioned modulation of transmitter release probabilities can support long-lasting postsynaptic changes or contribute to learning and information processing in its own way. It is also possible that postsynaptic processes influence presynaptic processes through glial cells which wrap around synapses and interact with both the pre- and postsynaptic sides through direct chemical and electrical couplings and other Ca^{2+} channels. A direct presynaptic influence is also possible though retrograde messengers such as nitric oxide. Such mechanisms for conveying information back from the postsynatic terminal to presynaptic boutons are not required in invertebrate systems with specific terminals on presynaptic boutons (Fig. 6.4C). Presynaptic changes in synaptic plasticity seem to be important in such systems through the temporally linked transmitter release of the UCS input and the activation of a specific presynaptic terminal.

It is possible to model the intracellular chemical pathways related to synaptic plasticity directly. An example of chemical pathways in D1 receptors of spiny neurons of the striatum is shown in Fig. 6.9, as summarized by Nakano, Doi, Yoshimoto, and Doya. These synapses are particularly interesting since they are regulated not only by glutamate, but also by dopamine (DA) input from the substantia nigra. Experiments by Jeff Wickens and colleagues have shown that stimulation of cortical input alone

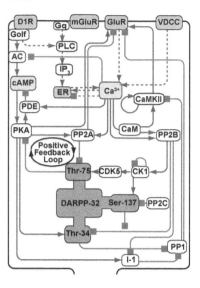

Fig. 6.9 Signalling pathways in the D1 receptors of striatal spiny neurons [adapted from Nakano, Doi, Yoshimoto, and Doya, *Society for Neuroscience* 676.5 (2007)].

results in LTD. Only in combination with DA input could LTP be induced. Nakano et al. modelled the signalling network shown in Fig. 6.9 based on AMPA receptor trafficking, insertion of AMPA receptors when phosphorylated by kinases and removal when dephosphorylated by phosphatases while regulated by DA and Ca^{2+} concentration. The authors found DA- and Ca^{2+}-dependent plasticity, with low levels leading to LTD and high levels to LTP. We will come back to such dependencies in Section 6.3.2.

6.3 Mathematical formulation of Hebbian plasticity

In neural network models, synaptic plasticity is described by a change of weight values, **w**, between nodes. Hence, the weight values are not static but can change over time. Unfortunately, we do not know much about the precise time course of synaptic changes, and most experiments can only explore modifications after certain training intervals. It is thus appropriate to express the variation of weight values only after time steps, Δt, in a discrete fashion as,

$$w_{ij}(t + \Delta t) = w_{ij}(t) + \Delta w_{ij}(t_i^{\mathrm{f}}, t_j^{\mathrm{f}}, \Delta t; w_{ij}). \tag{6.2}$$

We have indicated here the dependence of the weight changes on various factors. For activity-dependent synaptic plasticity it is clear that weight changes should depend on the firing times, t^{f}, of the pre- and postsynaptic neurons. We included in this formula the possibility that the weight changes depend on the current value of the synaptic strength. Weight-dependent plasticity is an important factor, discussed further below, since the strength of biological synapses can certainly only vary within some interval. Different instantiations of the generic rule in eqn 6.2 are discussed in this section.

6.3.1 Spike timing dependent plasticity rules

To explore the consequences of experimental findings of synaptic plasticity in networks of spiking neurons, experimental data are often interpreted with heuristic models that parameterize certain aspects of the experimental findings. For example, spike timing dependent plasticity (STDP) rules are commonly used to describe plasticity with spiking neurons. As argued above, spike timing is essential for plasticity. Unfortunately, the amount of synaptic change depends on many factors when simply viewed as a function of pre- and postsynaptic activity. Bi and Poo used well-isolated pairings of single pre- and postsynaptic spikes to demonstrate STDP curves, as shown in Fig 6.7A. We have already discussed the calcium hypothesis of synaptic plasticity, and it is therefore expected, and seen in experiments, that different spike patterns can result in different plasticity curves. The following rules only apply strictly for isolated spike pairings. Additional specifications have to be included if, for example, multiple spikes or overlapping bursts are considered. The specific theoretical interpretation of the experimental data by Bi and Poo has thus to be applied cautiously. The rule is discussed here mainly because it has gained much influence in computational neuroscience,

In the situation of STDP as explored by Bi and Poo, we can write the rule for the synaptic efficiency change in dependence on the relative timing between a postsynaptic spike at t^{post} and presynaptic spike at t^{pre} as

$$\Delta w_{ij}^{\pm} = \epsilon^{\pm}(w) K^{\pm}(t^{\mathrm{post}} - t^{\mathrm{pre}}). \tag{6.3}$$

This form includes a weight-dependent learning rate, $\epsilon^{\pm}(w)$, and term that depends on the relative spike timings, $K^{\pm}(t^{\mathrm{post}} - t^{\mathrm{pre}})$. Also, we allowed for different functional forms of LTP (labelled with superscript '+') and LTD (labelled with superscript '−'). Following the experimental findings shown in Fig. 6.7A, the kernel function $K^{\pm}(t^{\mathrm{post}} - t^{\mathrm{pre}})$ is commonly taken to have an exponential form,

$$K^{\pm}(t^{\mathrm{post}} - t^{\mathrm{pre}}) = \mathrm{e}^{\mp \frac{t^{\mathrm{post}} - t^{\mathrm{pre}}}{\tau^{\pm}}} \; \Theta(\pm[t^{\mathrm{post}} - t^{\mathrm{pre}}]). \tag{6.4}$$

We also allowed for different decay scale in potentiation and depression with different constants τ^{+} and τ^{-}. $\Theta(x)$ is a threshold function that restricts LTP and LTD to the correct domains of positive and negative differences between pre- and postsynaptic spiking, respectively.

The basic asymmetrical Hebb rule (eqn 6.3 with kernel of eqn 6.4) suggests that when a postsynaptic spike follows a presynaptic spike in a small time window of a few milliseconds, then the synapse is potentiated. The next question, not addressed with the data in Fig 6.7A, is about what happens with repeated spike pairings. It is clear that the process cannot go on forever. Synaptic efficacies must be restricted between a lower value (typically zero) and some upper value. A weight-dependent learning rate, $\epsilon^{\pm}(w)$, was therefore included in the formulation of eqn 6.3. The precise form of the weight-dependence is not yet established experimentally, and discussions of different forms of weight-dependent learning rates has become a major topic in theoretical studies. For example, a learning rule with a constant learning rate, also called an additive learning rule, is often considered. Such a learning rule might be reasonable, at least in some interval of synaptic weights,

$$\epsilon^{\pm} = \begin{cases} a^{\pm} & \text{for } w_{ij}^{\min} \leq w_{ij} \leq w_{ij}^{\max} \\ 0 & \text{otherwise} \end{cases} , \tag{6.5}$$

where $a^{\pm}$ are constants for LTP and LTD. We call this rule an additive rule with absorbing boundaries, since theoretical weight changes outside the plasticity interval are absorbed by the boundaries. An alternative rule is a multiplicative rule, with more graded non-linearity when approaching the boundaries,

$$\epsilon^{+} = a^{+}(w^{\max} - w_{ij}) \tag{6.6}$$

$$\epsilon^{-} = a^{-}(w_{ij} - w^{\min}). \tag{6.7}$$

It is also possible to consider other functional forms of learning rates. Distributions of synaptic weights can depend on the precise form of weight dependence, as discussed further below.

6.3.2 Hebbian learning in population and rate models

In models that describe the average behaviour of single neurons (rate models) or cell assemblies (population models), we cannot incorporate the spike timings. We have therefore to fall back on a description of plasticity that depends only on the activity of pre- and postsynaptic nodes. The essence of Hebbian learning rules is then captured by the observation that the plasticity depends on the correlation of pre- and postsynaptic firing. Of course, these models can then not be used to investigate specific spike timing dependent issues, but as we discussed in the Chapter 1, different models are necessary for different types of questions. However, it is also a good idea to confirm some assumptions of population models with spiking models.

Most Hebbian plasticity rules used in population models have a functional form that can be expressed as

$$\Delta w_{ij} = \epsilon(t, w)[f_{\text{post}}(r_i)f_{\text{pre}}(r_j) - f(r_i, r_j, w)] \tag{6.8}$$

between a postsynaptic node i with a firing rate r_i, and a presynaptic node j with firing rate r_j. We included several parameters (constants or functions) in order to summarize popular rules in population models. The term ϵ represents the overall strength of changes and is often called the learning rate. The learning rate can depend on various factors, such as the weight values themselves, to confine weight values to a prescribed interval. Also, the learning rate is sometimes made explicitly time-dependent to describe, for example, external modulation of synaptic plasticity or developmental plasticity with different plasticity domains.

The functions f_{pre} and f_{post} depend on the firing rates of the pre- and postsynaptic nodes, respectively. For example, Eduardo Renato Caianiello was among the first[1] to specify Hebb's postulate mathematically with linear functions for f_{pre} and f_{post} in what he called the mnemonic equation,

$$\Delta w_{ij} = \epsilon(w)[r_i r_j - f(w)]. \tag{6.9}$$

The term f describes weight decay. We ignore weight decay in the following versions of Hebbian rules and discuss this separately in the next section. Therefore, keep in

---

[1] Stephen Grossberg had already discovered such systems in the late 1950s, but his papers were not published until 10 years later.

Function used in BCM rule

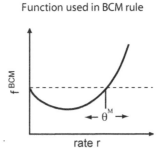

Fig. 6.10 Function as used in BCM theory with a modifiable threshold θ^M. BCM theory was invented by [Bienenstock, Cooper, and Munro [*Journal of Neuroscience* 2:32–48 (1982)].

mind that the rules below have to be augmented with weight scaling in some form to achieve stable learning. For simplicity, we consider constant values for the learning rate in the following. The most basic Hebbian rule has then the form

$$\Delta w_{ij} = \epsilon r_i r_j, \tag{6.10}$$

which captures the correlation between the variables r_i and r_j. However, the functions f_{pre} and f_{post} typically include some plasticity thresholds, as seen in brain experiments. For example, in the generic form of a Hebbian rule introduced by Terrance Sejnowski, these thresholds are set equal to the average firing rates $\langle r_i \rangle$, where the angular brackets are used to denote the average of the quantity enclosed over many trials with different stimuli. The corresponding Hebbian learning rule,

$$\Delta w_{ij} = \epsilon(r_i - \langle r_i \rangle)(r_j - \langle r_j \rangle), \tag{6.11}$$

is called the covariance rule since the average change of the weight value with this rule,

$$\langle \Delta w_{ij} \rangle = \epsilon \langle (r_i - \langle r_i \rangle)(r_j - \langle r_j \rangle) \rangle \tag{6.12}$$
$$= \epsilon(\langle r_i r_j \rangle - \langle r_i \rangle \langle r_j \rangle),$$

is proportional to the covariance between pre- and postsynaptic firing. This is also called a cross-correlation function when ϵ is a proper normalization constant. This learning rule captures the basic suggestion of Hebb in that LTP is induced when the presynaptic firing rate and the postsynaptic firing rate are both systematically below, or above, their average firing rates, and that LTD is induced when one of the firing rates is below average while the other remains above.

We can distinguish the two conditions of LTD even further. When the firing rate of a presynaptic node is above average while the firing rate of the postsynaptic node is below average, then the weight of this specific synapse should be reduced as it cannot be relevant for the functional relevant postsynaptic firing. This only concerns a specific synapse, and this form of plasticity is therefore termed homosynaptic LTD (with Greek prefix homo = same). In contrast, when the postsynaptic node is active above the average firing rate, then all synapses of presynaptic nodes that are firing

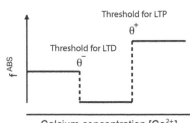

Function used in basic ABS rule

Fig. 6.11 A piecewise linear step function that provides three domains for synaptic plasticity, no change for $x < \theta^-$, LTD for $\theta^- < x < \theta^+$, and LTP for $x > \theta^+$. The dependent variable, x, is assumed to be calcium concentration in the Ca $^{2+}$ hypothesis of Lisman [*Proceeding of the National Academy of Science* 86: 9574–8 (1989)] and Artola and Singer [*Trends in Neuroscience* 16: 480–7 (1993)].

below average should be reduced to make the neuron respond more specifically to relevant input. We call this form of plasticity heterosynaptic LTD (with Greek prefix hetero = other) to stress that this type of plasticity concerns all the synapses of a postsynaptic neuron.

The covariance rule of eqn 6.11 captures the basic Hebbian learning necessary for building associators. It is in this sense a minimal model for Hebbian plasticity, which we will use frequently in later discussions. However, some variations of the basic Hebbian rule are important to notice, specifically rules for synaptic plasticity commonly called BCM theory after their inventors Elie Bienenstock, Leon Cooper, and Paul Munro. The basic plasticity rules in the BCM theory has the form

$$\Delta w_{ij} = \epsilon(f^{\mathrm{BCM}}(r_i; \theta^M)(r_j) - f(w)). \tag{6.13}$$

The function f^{BCM} is outlined in Fig. 6.10. Low rates lead to LTD whereas high rates lead to LTP. Most importantly, the threshold between LTD and LTP, θ^M, is modifiable and can depend on the rate of the postsynaptic neuron. For example, the threshold becomes higher when the postsynaptic neuron becomes more active. Such a sliding threshold has not only been observed experimentally, but is also an important ingredient in keeping the system stable with this learning rule. BCM theory has been applied in particular to developmental plasticity, as in the formation of cortical maps.

A new interpretation of the BCM rule in terms of the calcium hypothesis was provided by Alain Artola and Wolf Singer, based on earlier work by Artola, Bröcher and Singer. The ABS model follows the calcium hypothesis by assuming a lower $[\mathrm{Ca}^{2+}]$ threshold, Θ^-, to induce LTD and a higher $[\mathrm{Ca}^{2+}]$ threshold, Θ^+, to induce LTP. This hypothesis can be written in a form similar to the BCM rule above,

$$\Delta w_{ij} = \epsilon([\mathrm{Ca}^{2+}])(f_{\mathrm{ABS}}([\mathrm{Ca}^{2+}]; \theta^+, \theta^-) - f(w)). \tag{6.14}$$

A simple example of a function f_{ABS} is outlined in Fig. 6.11. This function is constant in the different domains set by the threshold values,

$$f_{\mathrm{ABS}}(x) = \begin{cases} 0 & \text{for } x < \theta^- \\ -1 & \text{for } \theta^- < x < \theta^+ \\ 1 & \text{for } x > \theta^+ \end{cases},$$ (6.15)

although it is possible that there is a concentration dependence within these domains. This formulation in eqn 6.14 is only indirectly dependent on the activities of the pre- and postsynaptic nodes since the calcium concentration $[Ca^{2+}]$ is a function of several processes. For example, as reviewed in Fig. 6.8, postsynaptic calcium concentration is mediated by activation of different voltage-dependent and ligand-gated calcium channels, including NMDA and non-NMDA channels, and internal calcium stores. The calcium concentration depends on postsynaptic depolarization, which in turn depends on activation in the presynaptic cell. The activity dependence of the calcium level can be a complicated function of the presynaptic activities. However, if we assume a monotone, and mainly linear, relation between activity and calcium concentration, then we can write a simplified model such as

$$\Delta w_{ij} = \epsilon(f_{\mathrm{ABS}}(r_i; \theta^-, \theta^+)\mathrm{sign}(r_j - \theta^{\mathrm{pre}})),$$ (6.16)

where θ^{pre} is the minimal presynaptic activation for potentiation. We could consider refined versions of f_{ABS} where the amount of potentiation and depression is varied with activity, but the essence of associative plasticity is already captured in this basic rule.

All the above rules must be augmented with mechanisms to keep weights bounded. For example, we can incorporate weight-dependent learning rates or weight-decay terms, as discussed further in Section 6.4. In the simplest case, we could just restrict the number of learning steps, or confine the weights to a certain interval. However, we can also consider more dynamic mechanisms, such as the activity-dependent threshold in the BCM theory.

Simulation

Here we will briefly show that the basic Hebbian plasticity rule can be implemented compactly in Python. The basic Hebbian rule for rate models, eqn 6.10, states that a term

$$\Delta w = ba$$ (6.17)

is added to the previous weight w, where a is the firing rate of the presynaptic node and b is the firing rate of the postsynaptic node, both for a given training example. We can incorporate all the synapses on a postsynaptic node by collecting the weight values in a vector $\mathbf{w}$, and the rates of the presynaptic nodes in a column vector $\mathbf{a}$. We use a row vector to collect the weights on a single postsynaptic node, but we always write rates of nodes as column vectors. Similarly, we can also consider a column vector, $\mathbf{b}$, of the training rates of all postsynaptic neurons. The learning rule can then be written as

$$\Delta \mathbf{w} = \mathbf{b}\mathbf{a}'.$$ (6.18)

We used thereby the prime symbol to indicates the transpose of a vector which converts a column vector into a row vector. The weights $\mathbf{w}$ are now collected in a matrix since we multiply a column vector with a row vector. For example, let's consider three presynaptic nodes with rates $a = (1, 2, 3)'$ and two postsynaptic nodes with rates $b = (4, 5)'$. The weight matrix is then

$$\mathbf{w} = \begin{pmatrix} 4 \\ 5 \end{pmatrix} (1, 2, 3) = \begin{pmatrix} 4 & 8 & 12 \\ 5 & 10 & 15 \end{pmatrix}. \tag{6.19}$$

That is, the weight matrix has components, w_{ij}, where the first index labels positions in a column (the index of the postsynaptic node) and the second index labels positions in a row (the index of the presynaptic node),

$$\mathbf{w} = \begin{pmatrix} w_{11} & w_{12} & w_{13} & \dots & w_{1n^{\text{in}}} \\ w_{21} & w_{22} & w_{23} & \dots & w_{2n^{\text{in}}} \\ \cdot & \cdot & \cdot & \dots & \cdot \\ \cdot & \cdot & \cdot & \dots & \cdot \\ \cdot & \cdot & \cdot & \dots & \cdot \\ w_{n^{\text{out}}1} & w_{n^{\text{out}}2} & w_{n^{\text{out}}3} & \dots & w_{n^{\text{out}}n^{\text{in}}} \end{pmatrix} \tag{6.20}$$

The number n^{in} is the number of presynaptic neurons, and n^{out} is the number of postsynaptic neurons. A useful trick is to remember that the first label stands for 'to' and the second label for 'from', as in $w_{\text{to from}}$, or $w_{\text{post pre}}$.

If we serially apply all training vectors, then the change in weight values is the sum of all the changes from individual training examples. To write this mathematically, we collect all the column vectors of different training examples into an array, so that we get matrices $\mathbf{a}$ and $\mathbf{b}$ with components $a_{i\mu}$ and $b_{i\mu}$ for training example μ. The Hebbian weight matrix after training all the examples is then given by adding to the initial matrix $\mathbf{a}^0$ the sum over all the training examples, which can be written for the components,

$$w_{ij} = w_{ij}^0 + \sum_{\mu} b_{i\mu} a_{i\mu}. \tag{6.21}$$

The second term on the right-hand side corresponds to a matrix multiplication of the form $\mathbf{ba}'$. Thus, eqn 6.18 corresponds to training all patterns with an initial weight matrix of $\mathbf{a}^0 = 0$. This formula can be written directly into Python. For example, in program `weightDistribution.py`, discussed further in Section 6.4.2, the training is done with

```
w=(rPost-np.mean(rPost))@(rPre-np.mean(rPre)).T/npat
```

where `rPost` and `rPre` are matrices for postsynaptic and presynaptic rates of all training examples and the average is calculated with the Numpy function `mean()`. This rule is therefore an implementation of the covariance rule, eqn 6.11.

6.3.3 Negative weights and crossing synapses

A basic fact that should be observed in learning rules is that synaptic values are always positive, since these values represent weights. However, as discussed in Section 4.2, IPSPs reduce the overall membrane potential. Thus, in neurons or population nodes that sum all the inputs, we can describe inhibitory synapses with negative weights. Of course, the type of synapse depends on the specific receptor type and cannot change. Thus, synaptic learning rules should not change the sign of weight values. While this is obvious for synapses in single neurons, either in spiking neurons or in rate models where the node represents the average frequency of single neurons, the situation for weights in population nodes is not so obvious.

As argued in Section 5.5, a population node represents a collection of neurons, and the 'synapses' of such a node describe the average influence of one population of neurons on another population of neurons. These populations could, in principle, contain excitatory and inhibitory neurons in what we call mixed population nodes. The influence of one mixed population on another could be either excitatory or inhibitory. Moreover, learning in the system, and synaptic plasticity within the mixed populations, could even change the overall effect of one population on to another. For example, a neuron becoming inhibitory even when starting from an excitatory value. Thus, in population models it is often common not only to interpret negative weights as inhibitory, but even to allow a domain crossing of such weight values. Such domain crossings certainly do not mean that excitatory receptors become inhibitory or vice versa. Learning with such models could describe developmental processes in which new synapses in the population might become active, or even new synapses being formed. In principle, one should no longer speak of synapses in population models, but the term has become common when describing contacts in neural networks.

In later chapters we will discuss common models with mixed population nodes. However, many population models do separate excitatory and inhibitory populations. We will later argue about the differences and appropriateness of these formulations using some specific examples, in particular in models of cortical maps in Chapter 8 and auto-associative memory models in Chapter 9. As with all models, the appropriateness has to do with the scientific questions that the model is designed to answer, as well as the ability to capture the effects under investigation sufficiently. The mixed population node is sufficient for most of the discussions in this book. Such models are typically more compact and easier to study analytically. In contrast, models with separate inhibitory and excitatory nodes are easier to relate to biological networks. Such models can also include properties not present in the simplified mixed population versions, but most mechanisms of brain process discussions in this book can be followed with exemplary models of mixed population nodes.

6.4   Synaptic scaling and weight distributions

Repeated application of additive association rules results in runaway synaptic values. Many modelling examples include a simple restriction of the range for synaptic values, either explicitly, or through a finite number of training steps used in the simulations. While such approximations are sometimes sufficient and appropriate in terms of the modelling objective, real neural systems need some balance and competition between synapses to allow stable learning in diverse sensory situations. We therefore have to consider competitive synaptic scaling. We start this section with example applications of some of the above rules and demonstrate some resulting weight distributions.

6.4.1 Examples of STDP with spiking neurons

Synaptic efficiencies are continuously changing as long as learning rules are applied. However, to study the consequences of these rules we can consider the distribution of weights, and how they change with time. In general, since we typically consider learning many random patterns, we can think of weight changes as stochastic processes. There have been many methods developed to analyse stochastic systems, such as Fokker–Planck equations which describe the time evolution of the probability density function of systems like the one considered here. Such methods can be used to describe the drift and possible equilibrium distributions of synaptic weights. Synaptic distributions can also be explored with direct applications of the plasticity rules in simulations, as shown next.

We will now consider the basic STDP rule of eqn 6.3 with kernel 6.4. It is clear that the strength of synapses that consistently drive the spiking of a postsynaptic neuron are increased with this rule. The learning of synapses can be supervised, as in experiments, if we force the postsynaptic spiking to be in close temporal relation to a presynaptic spike train. In contrast, spikes of presynaptic neurons that are uncorrelated with the postsynaptic spiking can occur before, or after, the postsynaptic spike. Such uncorrelated events can therefore elicit random events of potentiation or depression. If the overall effect of depression for such events is stronger than average potentiation, then synaptic weights decrease over time for patterns that should not be associated with the firing of the postsynaptic neuron. We thus expect a bimodal distribution for such basic association rules, with some synapses tending toward the maximal possible strength, while others decay to zero.

To demonstrate this in more detail, we will now follow work of Sen Song, Kenneth Miller, and Larry Abbott and study a single IF neuron with 1000 excitatory synapses that are individually driven by presynaptic Poisson spike trains with average firing rates of 20 Hz. When we start the simulations we set all the synaptic weights to large values. As a consequence, the postsynaptic neuron fires with large frequencies in a very regular manner because the average synaptic input exceeds the firing threshold of the neurons, as discussed in Chapter 5. We then apply an additive STDP rule with marginally stronger LTD than LTP. The average synaptic weight decreases under these conditions, resulting in neuronal responses with lower firing rates and an increased coefficient of variation, as illustrated in Fig. 6.12A. Interestingly, some synapses survive and become the major driving source of the neuron. The weight distribution resulting after 5 min of simulated time using the additive STDP rule is shown in Fig. 6.12B. There are many synaptic weights clustering around very small values, with a few synapses that have large synaptic weights approaching the upper limit imposed in the simulations. Analytical results also indicate that weight distributions with the additive Hebbian rule have bimodal distributions with peaks approaching the limiting values.

It is worth analysing the above experiments in more detail. In Chapter 5, we discussed the fact that IF neurons respond with regular firing to random spike trains if the synaptic efficiencies are strong enough so that the average current is larger than the firing threshold of the neuron (see Fig. 5.7). The firing time of the IF neuron in this mode is mainly determined by the average input current, so that each individual presynaptic spike is not solely responsible for a postsynaptic spike. We can quantify the average responsibility of presynaptic spike for a postsynaptic spike by measuring the

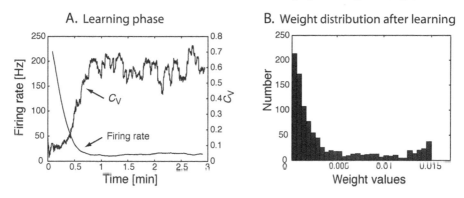

Fig. 6.12 (A) Firing rate and C_V, the coefficient of variation, of an IF neuron that is driven by 1000 excitatory Poisson spike trains while the synaptic efficiencies are changing according to an additive STDP rule with asymmetrical Gaussian plasticity windows. (B) Distribution of weight values after 5 min of simulated training time (which is similar to the distribution after 3 min). The weights were constrained to be in the range of 0–0.015. The distribution has two maxima, one at each boundary of the allowed interval. [These simulations follow closely the work of Song, Miller, and Abbott, *Nature Neuroscience* 3: 919–26 (2000).]

cross-correlation function between them. To do this, we define a quantity $s(\Delta t)$ that has the value $s = 1$ if a spike occurs in the time interval Δt, and is zero otherwise ($s = 0$). With this spike train representation it is straightforward to quantify the correlation between the presynaptic spikes and the postsynaptic spikes using the cross-correlation function,

$$C(n) = \langle s^{\mathrm{pre}}(t)s^{\mathrm{post}}(t + n\Delta t)\rangle - \langle s^{\mathrm{pre}}\rangle\langle s^{\mathrm{post}}\rangle, \qquad (6.22)$$

where the expressions enclosed in angular brackets denote the average over time of that quantity. The correlation is zero if the pre- and postsynaptic spike trains are independent (that is, $\langle s^{\mathrm{pre}}s^{\mathrm{post}}\rangle = \langle s^{\mathrm{pre}}\rangle\langle s^{\mathrm{post}}\rangle$). The correlation is larger than zero when there is, on average, more incidence of close relations between pre- and postsynaptic spikes. The quantity is negative if presynaptic spikes result in a consistent reduction of postsynaptic spikes (anti-correlation).

Measurements of such cross-correlations confirm that a single input spike train has little correlation with the output spike train when the IF neuron is in the regular firing regime. The measured average cross-correlations corresponding to the above simulation with initial weight values of $w = 0.015$ is shown in Fig. 6.13 with star symbols and interpolated with a dashed line. This resulted in regular firing of the postsynaptic neuron with a frequency of around 270 Hz. The average cross-correlation in these simulations is consistent with zero if we consider the results within their variance indicated by error bars. The similar values of the average cross-correlations for positive and negative time shifts, Δt, indicate that the occurrence of a presynaptic spike before a postsynaptic spike is equally as likely as the occurrence of a presynaptic spike after a postsynaptic spike. The equal average occurrence of presynaptic spikes before and after a postsynaptic spike means that, statistically, LTP occurs as much as LTD. The average behaviour of the neuron would thus never change if the effects of LTP and LTD were equal. However, if the effect of LTD is a little bit stronger than that of LTP, such that the area under the LTD branch of STDP (Fig. 6.7) is larger than the area under the LTP branch, then we get a reliable decrease of the weight values over time.

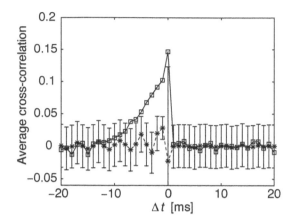

Fig. 6.13 Average cross-correlation function between presynaptic Poisson spike trains and the postsynaptic spike train (averaged over all presynaptic spike trains) in simulations of an IF neuron with 1000 input channels. The spike trains that lead to the results shown with stars were generated with each weight value fixed to 0.015. The cross-correlations are consistent with zero when considered within the variance indicated by the error bars. The squares represent results from simulations of the IF neuron driven by the same presynaptic spike trains as before, but with the weight matrix after Hebbian learning shown in Fig. 6.12. Some presynaptic spike trains cause postsynaptic spiking with a positive peak in the average cross-correlation functions when the presynaptic spikes precede the postsynaptic spike [see also Song and Abbott, *Neurocomputing* 32 & 33: 523–8 (2000)]. No error bars are shown in this curve for clarity.

The average cross-correlations between all presynaptic spikes and the postsynaptic spikes with the weights after learning, as shown in Fig. 6.12, are plotted in Fig. 6.13 with squares. These weights caused a much lower and more realistic frequency of the postsynaptic spike train around 18 Hz. The peak for small negative values of Δt in the cross-correlation curve indicates that some presynaptic spike trains were responsible for eliciting a postsynaptic spike. This increased correlation of some spike trains supports the LTP necessary to stabilize the corresponding synapses. Song and Abbott, who first elaborated the arguments outlined here, demonstrated that a steady state, with a reasonably large coefficient of variation, can be reached for different firing frequencies in the input spike trains. Of course, the time it takes to reach the steady state after changing the input frequency depends on the time it takes to modify the synaptic weights. Such biological details have not yet been determined experimentally. In the case of a very fast transition to a steady state, this would mean that the neuron could also adapt to a change in the firing frequencies of inputs, something that has been termed gain control. However, too rapid a permanent change of synaptic weights has other disadvantages for the stability of learning.

While the above results with spiking neurons are encouraging, there are still many questions concerning the biological details of the STDP rules, specifically with regard to scaling mechanisms and the form of weight dependence. Also, to consider the stability of the learning process further, we have to consider such learning rules in

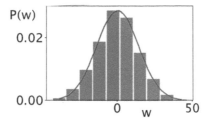

Fig. 6.14 Normalized histograms of weight values from simulations of 500 synapses on to a population node after training 1000 exponentially distributed random patterns with the Hebbian covariance learning rule 6.11. A fit of a Gaussian distribution to the data is shown as the solid line.

networks of neurons. Before turning to networks in the next chapter, we need briefly to discuss scaling in rate models.

6.4.2 Weight distributions in rate models

For some discussions later in this book, it is useful to know the weight distribution of the Hebbian covariance rule (eqn 6.11), which is the dominant rule in population or rate models. In many studies using this rule, random patterns are used to represent the input patterns of the presynaptic nodes. The random numbers for postsynaptic responses are assumed to be independent of these inputs, at least during the learning phase. This is a reasonable assumption since learning is aimed at establishing correlations between input and output pattern, and learning should cease when this correlation is established. We thus consider independent firing rates, r_i and r_j, for the pre- and postsynaptic nodes.

If we take the basic, additive, Hebbian covariance rule of eqn 6.11 and start with weight values of $w_{ij}^0 = 0$, then we can write the weight values after learning N_p patterns as

$$w_{ij} = \frac{1}{\sqrt{N_p}} \sum_\mu (r_i^\mu - \langle r_i \rangle)(r_j^\mu - \langle r_j \rangle). \tag{6.23}$$

Here, we have used a learning rate of $\epsilon = 1/\sqrt{N_p}$ so that the width of the weight distribution does not change with the number of training patterns, for reasons we will see shortly. After subtracting the mean from each random number for the pre- and postsynaptic firing rates, we end up multiplying random variables with zero mean and variance σ^2. Those new random variables are again random variables, which can have a different distribution than the distributions used to generate the firing pattern, as explained in Appendix 3.5. It is important here that the learning rule of eqn 6.23 is a sum over N_p independent random variables. Then, the central limit theorem tells us that the sum is a random variable whose distribution approaches a Gaussian distribution with mean zero and variance σ^2/N_p, at least for very large sums. This is the reason for the specific normalization in eqn 6.23, since the width of the Gaussian distribution is proportional to the square root of the variance.

A Gaussian distribution is indeed what we find in numerical simulations of this rule. An example program is in `weightDistribution.py` which also demonstrates how to fit a function in Python. This demonstrate uses exponentially distributed firing rates for the input and output patterns in a numerical experiment, somewhat mimicking physiological finding. However, different distributions, such as the frequently studied patterns made out of equally distributed binary numbers, produce similar results. The resulting frequency histogram of the weight values after 1000 learning steps with the covariance rule is shown in Fig. 6.14. We have included a fit of the simulated weight distribution to the Gaussian function that shows that the data are well approximated by a Gaussian distribution, as we predicted above.

Programs/weightDistribution.py

```
1  # Weight distribution of Hebbian synapses in rate model
2  import numpy as np
3  import matplotlib.pyplot as plt
4  from scipy.optimize import curve_fit
5
6  nn=100; npat=1000 # number of nodes and patterns
7
8  rPre = np.random.exponential(10,(nn,npat))
9  rPost = np.random.exponential(20,(nn,npat))
10 w=(rPost-np.mean(rPost))@(rPre--np.mean(rPre)).T/npat
11
12 # Histogram plotting
13 n, bins = np.histogram(w)
14 dx = bins[1]-bins[0]
15 n = n/(sum(n)*dx)
16 x = np.zeros(10)
17 for i in range(10):
18     x[i] = bins[i]+ dx/2
19 plt.bar(x,n,8)
20
21 # Fit normal ditribution to data
22 def func(x, mu, sig):
23     return 1/(np.sqrt(2*np.pi)*sig)*np.exp(-(x-mu)**2/(2*sig**2))
24
25 popt, pcov = curve_fit(func, x, n)
26 x = np.linspace(x[0],x[9],50)
27 plt.plot(x, func(x, *popt), 'r-')
28 plt.xlabel('w'), plt.ylabel('P(w)')
```

6.4.3   Competitive synaptic scaling and weight decay

The discussion above showed that we can constrain the width of weight distributions with small learning rates. Many demonstrations with computer simulations only use a small number of training patterns, so that runaway synapses are not a problem. However, maintaining a balance between synapses is extremely important to build reliable and responsive systems. We cannot discuss this topic in its entirety at this point, since network properties, such as inhibition, contribute. Here, we will discuss possible mechanisms for competitive synapses in single nodes. We discussed in Section 6.4.1 an example of synaptic scaling with additive STDP and restricted weights, where the number of strong channels is reduced for higher-frequency inputs. This is biologically realistic, as it has been found with fluorescent labelling that the number of active channels does vary in such situations. Some experiments have also demonstrated more directly that synaptic efficiencies depend on the average postsynaptic activity. For example, blocking some inhibitory channels of a neuron, which would increase its activity, scales down synaptic efficiencies, whereas forced reduction of postsynaptic activity leads to an increase of synaptic efficiencies. So far, the biological mechanisms of synaptic scaling are not completely understood. A simple implementation based on limited resources, which keep the summed synaptic strength constant, seems unlikely. However, there are new physiological findings that have the potential of solving the puzzle, such as regulation mechanisms of glial cells.

Although the precise biological mechanisms are not yet clear, we can model competitive synapses in various ways. Most of these mechanisms are mathematically equivalent to normalizing the weight vector. This normalization can be observed either strictly, or only dynamically on average (asymptotically). An example for a strict observation of the norm is to divide each weight value by the sum of all weights after each update,

$$w_{ij} \leftarrow \frac{w_{ij}}{\sum_j w_{ij}}, \tag{6.24}$$

which keeps the length of the weight vector to exactly one. This formula only holds when weight values are positive. In the case of positive and negative values, we need to divide by the square root of the sum of squares. In the formula, we used an arrow to indicate that the original weight values are replaced with the normalized values, instead of introducing a new symbol for the weights. The normalization in eqn 6.24 is an example of multiplicative (or divisive) scaling, since the rate of change depends on each weight value. While it is easy to implement in simulations, this normalization scheme is problematic since it is a non-local operation to sum all the weight values, which is computationally expensive and biologically unrealistic. Much more useable are dynamic implementations, which do not keep the weights strictly constant at each time step, but can enable useful scaling with local implementations.

The most direct way to model scaling is to include a separate weight dynamic on a time scale much longer than the synaptic plasticity discussed so far. For example, as recommended by Mark van Rossum, we can measure a running average, $a(t)$, of postsynaptic activity with a leaky integrator,

$$\tau_s \frac{da(t)}{dt} = -a(t) + \delta(t - t^{\text{spike}}), \tag{6.25}$$

where we used again the δ-function described in Appendix 3.3. The time constant, τ_s, of this process should be on the order of minutes, or more. This average amplitude can then be used to scale the weights in a multiplicative way, for example like

$$\frac{dw_{ij}(t)}{dt} = \beta w_{ij}(t)(a_{\text{goal}} - a(t)) + \gamma w_{ij}(t) \int_0^t dt(a_{\text{goal}} - a(t)), \tag{6.26}$$

where β and γ are constants. The first term on the right-hand side drives the weight toward a goal value, a_{goal}, and the second term minimizes the remaining error over time.

Another possibility, which is particularly elegant and useful for theoretical reasons, is to include such scaling dynamics together with the above-discussed plasticity in a form called weight decay. Such scaling mechanisms are particularly appropriate and useful in rate models since the independent variable is already a rate that we want to

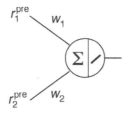

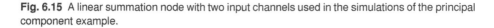

Fig. 6.15 A linear summation node with two input channels used in the simulations of the principal component example.

stabilize. Several decay terms have been discussed in the literature. For example, a simple weight decay can be added to the basic Hebbian rule,

$$\Delta w_{ij} = r_i r_j - c w_{ij}, \tag{6.27}$$

where the decay amplitude, c, has to be chosen appropriately. However, it is difficult to find a balance between appropriate reinforcement of this synapse and the constant decay term. It is therefore more appropriate to make this constant dependent on the rate of the output node. The Scottish neural network pioneer David Willshaw suggested the rule

$$\Delta w_{ij} = r_i (r_j - w_{ij}), \tag{6.28}$$

which often works quite well. This also looks similar to the basic Hebbian rule where w is the average postsynaptic rate that defines the postsynaptic plasticity threshold. Of course, it is possible to use other decay amplitudes, c, as functions of the postsynaptic rate, which can change how fluctuations around the mean are treated. For example, the Finnish scientist Erkki Oja suggested a quadratic form,

$$\Delta w_{ij} = r_i r_j - (r_i)^2 w_{ij}, \tag{6.29}$$

which is particularly useful, as discussed next. Weight decay terms can be derived from penalty terms in objective functions when deriving learning rules as minimizers of objective functions, as discussed in Chapter 7. Finally, as already mentioned, Bienenstock, Cooper, and Munro long ago suggested a scaling scheme that seems to have more biological realism. They pointed out that the threshold for LTP depends on the time-averaged recent activity of a neuron. Only postsynaptic activity that exceeds this threshold can induce LTP, otherwise LTD is induced.

6.4.4 Oja's rule and principal component analysis

The Hebbian rule with a weight decay term, as suggested by Oja (eqn 6.29), is particularly interesting as this not only normalizes the weight vector to unit length, but also has further theoretical advantages. Let us study the consequence of this rule on a linear node with two input channels (Fig. 6.15) that is driven by random input taken from a two-dimensional probability distribution with zero mean. The details of this computer experiment are outlined below. The training examples of the pairs $(r_1^{\text{pre}}, r_2^{\text{pre}})$ define points in the r_1^{pre}–r_2^{pre} plane. These training examples are shown as dots in Fig. 6.16. Before applying Oja's learning rule we initialized the weight vector with random values. The end point of the randomly chosen initial weight vector is shown as a cross in the figure. The trajectory of the end point of the weight vector during learning, when applying Oja's rule, is shown as the line extending from the cross that marks the initial weight values. At the end of the training session, after the network has been trained on a large number of sample points from the distribution, the weight vector converged to the point indicated in the figure as an arrow. The final weight vector has a length of $|w| = 1$.

While the weight normalization is important, as discussed above, Oja's rule also implements efficiently an algorithm called principal component analysis (PCA). The purpose of PCA is to describe high-dimensional data in a reduced yet meaningful way. Such data reduction can be illustrated with the example shown in Fig. 6.16. The direction of the largest variance of the data in this figure, which is the direction given by the weight vector after training, is called the first principal component. The variance in the perpendicular direction, which is called the second principal component, is less. In higher dimensions, the next principal components are in further perpendicular directions with decreasing variance along the directions. If one would be allowed to use only one quantity to describe the data, then one can choose values along the first principal component, since this would capture an important distinction between the individual data points. Of course, we lose some information about the data, and a better description of the data can be given by including values along the directions of higher-order principal components. Describing the data with all principal components is equivalent to a transformation of the coordinate system and thus equivalent to the original description of the data.

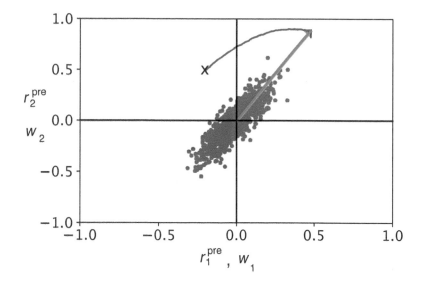

Fig. 6.16 Simulations of a linear node trained with Oja's rule on training examples (indicated by the dots) drawn from a two-dimensional probability distribution with mean zero. The weight vector with initial conditions indicated by the cross converges to the weight vector (thick arrow), which has length $|w| = 1$ and points in the direction of the first principal component.

Training a population node with Oja's rule results in a training vector along the first principal component. This is an example of the extraction of central tendencies, or prototypes, as mentioned in Section 6.1.4. The prototype is here the direction of the first principal component, and the values of individual data points along this direction distinguish each individual from the prototype. A single node can only express a single quantity describing the input data, but it is also possible to design networks in which other nodes represent further principal components. Principal component analysis is based on the assumption that the components of the data vectors are statistically independent. While this is true in the example shown in Fig. 6.16, since we chose the components independently in the program, components of natural patterns are often correlated. For example, let us think about the variables in the data sets as representing the age and height of children. The positive correlation between these values is apparent in the data, but we can also ask which combinations of these values provide independent quantities for describing the data. This form of analysis is called independent component analysis (ICA), and much progress has been made in implementing such an analysis with neural networks.

Programs/oja.py

```
1  # PCA a la Oja
2  import numpy as np
3  import matplotlib.pyplot as plt
4
5  w = np.array([[ -0.2,0.5]]).T; wTraj=w
6  a = -np.pi/6
7  rot = np.array([[np.cos(a),-np.sin(a)],
8                  [np.sin(a),np.cos(a)]])
9
10 # Training
11 for i in range(1000):
12     rPre = 0.05*np.random.normal([0,0],[1,4]);
13     rPre = rot@rPre
14     plt.plot(rPre[0],rPre[1],'b.')
15     rPost = rPre@w
16     w = w+0.1*rPost*(rPre-rPost*w.T).T
17     wTraj = np.append(wTraj,w,axis=1)
18
19 # Plotting results
20 plt.plot(wTraj[0,:],wTraj[1,:],'r')
21 plt.plot([0,w[0]],[0,w[1]],'k')
22 plt.plot([-1,1],[0,0],'k'); plt.plot([0,0],[-1,1],'k')
23 plt.axis([-1,1,-1,1])
```

The example of Fig. 6.16 is simulated with the program oja.py. The network for this particular two-dimensional problem has only one linear node with two input channels. This architecture is specified by the initial weight matrix with arbitrary values. A rotation matrix is then defined to, which is used in the generation of training examples. The training over 1000 training examples is done in the loop. In each of these training steps, a new training point is chosen in and plotted, the node output is calculated, and this postsynaptic value is in training with learning rule eqn 6.29

Note that the training data are first chosen from a two-dimensional Gaussian distribution with standard deviation of 4 in one direction, and standard deviation of 1 in the other direction. This produces this elongated shape of data points, which is rotated by using the rotation matrix. The trajectory of the weights is then plotted with a red line, while the end vector of the weight is plotted with a thick black line in Line 18. An arrowhead, a large X indicating the initial weight values, and some labels where added later.

6.5 Plasticity with pre- and postsynaptic dynamics

We have highlighted the effect of consistent causal relations between presynaptic and postsynaptic spike pairings. In this last section we want to give an example of a model that captures more detailed temporal factors of separate presynaptic and postsynaptic mechanisms as described by Costa, Froemke, Sjöström and van Rossum, (eLife, 2015). The model is another example of how to use coupled differential equations including leaky integrators in simulations. While the model does not describe the specific biophysical process underlying these changes, it does describe their consequences for the timing and spike-frequency dependence of plasticity that can explain several experimental findings.

The model considers a separate factor for the presynaptic component P and the postsynaptic component q of plasticity. These quantities change with discrete jumps at specific times as determined by the spike trains. More specifically, let us consider a presynaptic spike train

$$X(t) = \sum_t \delta(t - t_{\mathrm{pre}}) \tag{6.30}$$

and a postsynaptic spike train

$$y(t) = \sum_t \delta(t - t_{\mathrm{post}}) \tag{6.31}$$

$Y(t)$, where $\{t_{\mathrm{pre}}\}$ and $\{t_{\mathrm{post}}\}$ are the discrete times of the presynaptic and postsynaptic spikes, respectively. The base synaptic weight is then given by the Hebbian product

$$w = Pq. \tag{6.32}$$

The presynaptic and postsynaptic components change according three-factor models

$$\Delta P(t) = (-d_- y_-(t)y_+(t) + d_+ x_+(t - \epsilon)y_+(t))Y(t). \tag{6.33}$$

$$\Delta q(t) = c_+ x_+(t)y_-(t - \epsilon)Y(t) \tag{6.34}$$

Note that these quantities change at discrete times t determined by the spike occurrences, hence the use of the symbol Δ which does not include any time constants. The constants c_+, d_-, and d_+ specify the strength of how presynaptic and postsynaptic traces contribute to potentiation and depression. Specifically, there is a presynaptic potentiation trace, $x_+(t)$, a postsynaptic potentiation trace $y_+(t)$, and a postsynaptic depression trace $y_-(t)$, that are triggered by spikes according to

$$\tau_{x+} \frac{\mathrm{d}x_{+}}{\mathrm{d}t} = -x_+(t) + \tau_{x+} X(t) \tag{6.35}$$

$$\tau_{y+} \frac{\mathrm{d}y_+}{\mathrm{d}t} = -y_+(t) + \tau_{y+} X(t) \tag{6.36}$$

$$\tau_{y-}\frac{dy_-}{dt} = -y_-(t) + \tau_{y-}Y(t).\tag{6.37}$$

For the implementation of these equations it is good to note that the term $dtX(t)$ would be 1 if there is a spike occurrence and zero otherwise. Also note that we included a small term ϵ in equations (6.34) and (6.34) to indicate that this trace term refers to the value before the update by a possible spike occurrence.

While this three-factor model is already more detailed than the plasticity models before, the authors also included the Tsodyks-Markram model of short-term plasticity (PNAS, 1998), given by

$$\frac{dr}{dt} = \frac{1 - r(t)}{D} - p(t)r(t)X(t)\tag{6.38}$$

$$\frac{P}{dt} = \frac{P - p(t)}{F} + P(1 - p(t))X(t)\tag{6.39}$$

factor $r(t)$ describes the depletion of vesicles after transmitter release, and $p(t)$ is the effective presynaptic activity that determines the effective weight at time t,

$$w(t) = p(t)q(t)r(t).\tag{6.40}$$

The constants D and F determine the recovery time of the short-term plasticity process, whereas P determines the base strength of the synapses. This is the quantity that gets changed with the long-term plasticity factors above,

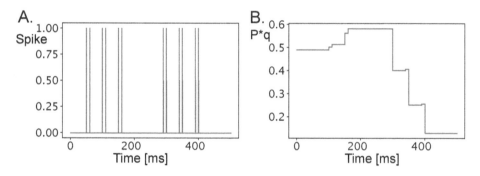
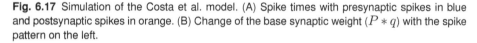

Fig. 6.17 Simulation of the Costa et al. model. (A) Spike times with presynaptic spikes in blue and postsynaptic spikes in orange. (B) Change of the base synaptic weight ($P * q$) with the spike pattern on the left.

The specific constant values that we used in the following simulation are noted in the program `CostaModel.py`. The values are thereby chosen to describe experimental findings of cortical pyramidal-to-pyramidal connections in layer 5. This program calculates the change in the synaptic weight value with each of the 6 spikes of a 60Hz presynaptic spike train where the first three spikes are followed by postsynaptic spikes with a 10 ms delay, and the next three pesynamptic spikes are preceded with postsynaptic spikes by 10 ms as shown in Fig. 6.5A. The resulting base synaptic strength without the presynaptic short-term depression factor is shown in Fig. 6.5B.

Programs/CostaModel.py

```
1  # Costa model of synaptic dynamics
2  import numpy as np
3  import matplotlib.pyplot as plt
4
5  tmax=500; dt=0.1
6  X = np.zeros(tmax*int(1/dt)); a=[500,1000,1500,3000,3500,4000]; X[a]=1
7  Y = np.zeros(tmax*int(1/dt)); b=[600,1100,1600,2900,3400,3900]; Y[b]=1
8
9  tauym = 32.7; tauyp = 230.2; tauxp = 66.6; D = 200; F = 50
10 cp = 0.0618; dp = 0.1548; dm = 0.1771
11 xp = np.array([0]); yp = np.array([0]); ym = np.array([0])
12 P = np.array([0.7]); q = np.array([0.7])
13 r = np.array([1]); p = np.array([P])
14
15 for t in range(0,tmax*int(1/dt)):
16
17     xp = np.append(xp,xp[t]+dt*(-1/tauxp*xp[t])+X[t])
18     yp = np.append(yp,yp[t]+dt*(-1/tauyp*yp[t])+Y[t])
19     ym = np.append(ym,ym[t]+dt*(-1/tauym*ym[t])+Y[t])
20
21     r = np.append(r,r[t]+dt*(1-r[t])/D - dt*X[t]*p[t]*r[t])
22     p = np.append(p,p[t]+dt*(P[t]-p[t])/F + X[t]*P[t]*(1-p[t]))
23
24     q = np.append(q,q[t]+Y[t]*cp*xp[t]*ym[t-1])
25     P = np.append(P,P[t]+X[t]*(-dm*ym[t]+dp*xp[t-1])*yp[t])
26     if P[-1]<0: P[-1]=0
27     if P[-1]>1: P[-1]=1
28     if q[-1]<0: q[-1]=0
29     if q[-1]>2: q[-1]=2
30
31 plt.plot(P*q)
```

III

Networks

7   Feed-forward mapping networks

In this chapter we explore the ability of basic neural networks that feed input form and input layer through possible layers of hidden notes to the output layer. We show that such neural networks can implement mapping functions. Mapping neural representations are important in many brain processes and have dominated models in cognitive science in the form of multilayer perceptrons. We start exploring the effects of choosing appropriate values for synaptic weights through learning algorithms. While feedforward networks are not enough to explain cognitive functions alone, they are an important ingredient of brain-style information processing and have contributed greatly to our understanding of adaptive systems. This chapter includes some review about concepts of machine learning and more recent developments such as deep learning. Such techniques are becoming increasingly important for industrial applications as well as analysing neuroscience data. However, we will largely focus on their relation to brain-style information processing.

7.1   Deep representational learning

To illustrate the abilities of networks introduced in this chapter, we follow an example of optical character recognition (OCR). OCR is the process of (optically) scanning an image of a hand-drawn or printed character, for example with a digital camera, and interpreting this digital image so that the computer 'understands' its meaning. For example, if we scan an image of a number 2, than we would like to store a binary number 00000010 in the computer. This binary number is a standard representation for encoding the number 2 in the American Standard Code for Information Interchange (ASCII). Once the letter is represented with this code, a computer program can use this code to infer meaning and use this to perform specific tasks, such as displaying a representation of the number on a computer screen, printing the number with different fonts on paper, or to search for this number in a text.

OCR is usually an easy tasks for humans and until recently humans typically outperform engineered systems. To discuss the example in more detail, it is useful to distinguish two processes in the perception of a letter, the physical sensing of an image of a letter, and attaching meaning to such an image. In the OCR example above this translates to a scanning phase, which converts the printed image into a binary representation of the sensory input, and an recognition phase, which relies on the transformation of a sensory representation into a semantic representation where some meaning is attached. This is essentially what we are doing right now while reading this text. When we read a character such as a number, each character has to be transformed from the representation on paper to a representation in the brain which can be interpreted by the brain.

Fundamentals of Computational Neuroscience. Third edition. Thomas P. Trappenberg,
Oxford University Press. © Oxford University Press 2023. DOI: 10.1093/oso/9780192869364.003.0007

Let's discuss the example of recognizing the hand-written number '2' as shown on the left side of Fig. 7.1. The first step towards perception of this letter is to get the signal into the brain. This is achieved by an optical sensor called eye with photoreceptors able to transduce light falling onto the retina into signals that are transmitted to the brain. We approximate this process with a simplified digitizing model retina of only $12 \cdot 12 = 144$ photoreceptors. Each of these photoreceptors transmits a signal with value 1 if the area covered by the receptor (its receptive field) is covered with a certain percentage by the image. In this way we end up with the digitized version of the image shown on the right side of Fig. 7.1.

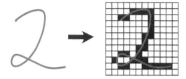

Fig. 7.1 (Left) A printed version of the number 2 and (right) a binary version of the same letter using a 12×12 grid.

This model is certainly a crude approximation of a human eye. The resolution in the human retina is much higher; a typical retina has around 125 million photoreceptors. Also, the receptors in a human retina are not homogeneously distributed, as in our example, but have highest density in the centre of the visual field called the fovea. In addition, it is well known that much more sophisticated signal processing goes on in a human eye through several neuronal layers with specialized neurons and elaborate connectivity pattern before a signal leaves the eye through the axons of ganglion cells. However, this crude model is simply intended to illustrate the idea of a basic representation.

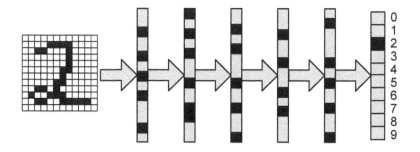

Fig. 7.2 A (relatively) deep neural network for the MNIST hand-written character recognition benchmark.

A sensory feature vector or array is the necessary input to any object recognition system. Given the sensory input, we can formulate the character recognition problem as the process of mapping this sensory feature vector into a new vector that represents the meaning of the object, $\mathbf{y}$ as

$$f : \mathbf{x} \in \mathbb{S}_1^n \rightarrow \mathbf{y} \in \mathbb{S}_2^m, \tag{7.1}$$

where n is the dimensionality of the sensory feature space ($n = 144$ in our example), and m is the dimensionality of the semantic object representation space ($m = 8$ if we consider the transformation to an ASCII code). $\mathbb{S}_1$ and $\mathbb{S}_2$ are the sets of possible values for each individual component of the vectors. For example, the components of the vector can consist of binary values ($\mathbb{S} = [0, 1]$), discrete values ($\mathbb{S} = \mathbb{N}$), or real values ($\mathbb{S} = \mathbb{R}$) such as the firing rates of neurons. Our OCR example is a mapping from a binary feature vector to binary vector of the ASCII code. Or, as illustrated in Fig. 7.2, could be a vector with components where the activation of a single component would indicate a specific number as shown on the right in Fig. 7.2. In the brain this would be the sensory firing pattern of retinal neurons to maybe the firing patterns of motor neurons that cause the physical response of articulating the meaning of the number visual.

In the implementation of such mapping functions it is now common to transform the sensory representation into a serious of intermediate representations, also called hidden representations as these activation are usually not observed. Of course, we can observe them in our computer simulations, or we could measure brain activity if we compare such models to brain processing. Of course, the critical question is how we find the transformations between the representations. We will outline in this chapter how this is done through learning connections parameters called weights between the elements of the network, which we conjecture represents the learning of synaptic connections between layers of neurons.

It is now common to use many hidden layers in applications of such mapping networks such as in computer vision. This is why such methods in AI are now called deep learning. Scaling up the networks with many layers and large number of neurons in each layer has been challenging for many years as the computational cost of such simulations does increase dramatically with increasing network size. Moreover, the number parameters in such model also increases dramatically, which demands an increase in training examples to prevent overfitting. The huge progress in the last several years has been due to, a combination of factors, among others the availability of large training sets, the efficient implementation of such networks on Graphical Processing Units (GPUs), and advancements in regularization techniques to prevent overfitting. The success of deep learning can be attributed to the fact that a lot of problems have an inherent hierarchical structure, like object recognition where objects are made up of combine basic features. A good way of thinking about deep learning is that it is mainly about learning representations. This then allows a difficult transformation to be broken up into simpler transformation as indicated in Fig. 7.2.

To discuss how representational learning and building a recognition system, we start with the smallest possible system called a perceptron which does not even have a hidden layer. We then move to a multilayer perceptron that has hidden nodes, and finally generalize this to more layers and also to slightly modified operations for each layer as common in deep learning applications. The general sequence of operations with such networks is thereby quite straight forward. Each of the receiving nodes in each layer takes a combination of the activation values of the previous layer, let's call them $r_{i,j}$ for the j-th note in layer i, to determine their activation value,

$$\textbf{Neuron activation function:} \quad r_{i+1,j} = f(\mathbf{r}_i; \mathbf{w},). \tag{7.2}$$

For example, the basic networks discussed next are simply adding up each of the

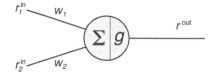

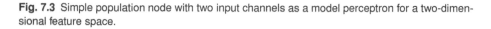

Fig. 7.3 Simple population node with two input channels as a model perceptron for a two-dimensional feature space.

activities of the previous nodes with corresponding weight values and maybe adding a non-linearity of this net input. This is the activation function of a neuron. The main task is then to find the parameters $\mathbf{w}$ so that the actual output of this network $\mathbf{r}^{\text{out}}$ is the same as the desired target output $\mathbf{r}^{\text{target}}$ such as provided by a teacher. The is provided by a learning rule that tell us how we should change the weight values in each learning step:

$$\textbf{Learning rule:} \quad \delta \Delta \mathbf{w} = l(\mathbf{w}, \mathbf{r}, \mathbf{r}^{\text{target}}). \tag{7.3}$$

The above mathematical functions only show two quite generic function that we have to specify in more detail below. The point here is just to highlight that there are these two steps of specifying the operations of the neural networks, one about how activation of the nodes are calculated, and one about how the parameters are learned. Eduardo Ceiianello called these the neuroninc equation and memonic equation in his influential 1961 paper. We will mainly use the population node as the neuron activation function, and we will in the following discussing a rule called error-backpropagation for the learning rule which has been very influential in training neural networks. In this rule, the difference between the actual output and the target output (error) is propagated backwards somewhat inverse to the neuron activation function in order to change the weight values with a Hebbian-like rule between a pre- and post-synaptic neuron. At the end of the chapters you should be able to write programs that can recognize handwritten digits.

7.2 The perceptron

7.2.1 The simple perceptron as boolean function

We demonstrate in this section that a population node, also called perceptron in this circumstance of a simple machine learning system, can represent certain types of vector functions. For this we set the firing rates of the input channels to

$$r_i^{\text{in}} = x_i. \tag{7.4}$$

The node in this simple perception system has to have at least n input channels, where n is the dimensionality of the feature space. We can illustrate the general idea with a single note that has only two binary input values, $r_1 = x_1$ and $r_2 = x_2$. Such a simple perceptron in a two-dimensional feature space would look like the one illustrated in Fig. 7.3. The firing rate of the output represents a function The output of this perceptron

Table 7.1 Boolean AND function

x_1	x_2	y
0	0	1
0	1	0
1	0	0
1	1	1

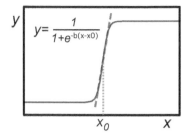

Fig. 7.4 The logistic function $f_l(x)$ as an example of a sigmoidal function. Historically, many perceptrons also used the related $\tanh(x) = 2 * f_l x - 1$ function.

can represent the function value

$$\tilde{y} = r^{\text{out}} = g(w_1 x_1 + w_2 x_2; \theta), \tag{7.5}$$

where g is an activation function that can have parameter θ such as the firing threshold, and w_1, w_2 are the weight values assigned to each input channel. Not that we can easily extend this to more input channels and even to systems with several output nodes,

$$\mathbf{r}^{\text{out}} = g(\mathbf{w}\mathbf{r}^{\text{in}}; \theta). \tag{7.6}$$

We used thereby a matrix notation (see eqn 6.20).

In order to specify the specific function we want the perceptron to learn, we have to give examples of the desired target output of the perceptron. In case of a Boolean function, we can specify all possible output values for every of the possible $n_c = 2^2 = 4$ different combinations of feature values, $\{(0,0), (0,1), (1,0), (1,1)\}$. A specific choice of a Boolean function, that of the Boolean AND function, is shown in Table 7.1. In order to approximate these possible output values, we chose as the perceptron gain function the sigmoidal function (logistic function)

$$g(x; \beta) = \frac{1}{1 + e^{-\beta x}} \tag{7.7}$$

as illustrated in Fig. 7.4.

Of course, this function gives us a strict value of 0 or 1 only asymptotically, but we can simply treat a value of r^{out} less than 0.5 as a zero and outputs larger than 0.5 as a 1. Also, this is a differentiable approximation of the threshold function in the sense that when the parameter β that describes the slope of the function around $x = 0$ goes to infinity, then the threshold function is recovered.

We are now ready to talk about the training of the perceptron. The idea is that we choose arbitrary numbers for the weight values and then calculate what the output of the

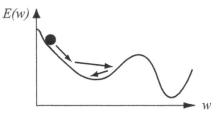

Fig. 7.5 Illustration of error minimization with a gradient descent method on a one-dimensional loss (error) surface $L(w)$.

perceptron is. We can then compare this to the target value, which represents the input of a teacher. Such learning is therefore called supervised learning. The comparison is quantified with an error function, also called a loss function in optimization. We choose here a common function in traditional neural networks, that of the mean square error function,

$$L(\mathbf{w}) = \frac{1}{2N} \sum_i \left(y^{(i)} - y(\mathbf{x}^{(i)}; \mathbf{w}) \right)^2. \tag{7.8}$$

N is thereby the number of example pairs $(\mathbf{x}^{(i)}, y^{(i)})$ used for training, and the bracketed index (i) indicates the index of the i-th training example in contrast to an exponent.

To find the parameters $\mathbf{w}$ that minimize the loos function (the difference between the actual and desired output of the perceptron), we use a computational technique called gradient descent. This method is an iterative procedure where we start with random choices of the parameters and iteratively improve them to give smaller loss values. This is illustrated in in Fig. 7.5 for a chase where we would only have one weight value. Since we have usually many weight values, this is more realistically a high dimensional function or error surface. To find the minimum of the loss function, we change the weight parameters along the negative slope of the function, which is the negative gradient if this is a function with more than one parameter,

$$w_j \leftarrow w_j - \alpha \frac{\partial L}{\partial w_j}. \tag{7.9}$$

The constant α is a learning rate.

More formally, to calculate the gradient in the gradient descent rule eqn (7.9) we have to recall two rules from calculus namely that the derivative of an exponent function is

$$\frac{\mathrm{d}}{\mathrm{d}x} x^n = n x^{n-1}, \tag{7.10}$$

and the derivative of the Euler function is

$$\frac{\mathrm{d}}{\mathrm{d}x} e^x = e^x, \tag{7.11}$$

which means that this function at every point is equal to its slope. Finally we need the chain rule

$$\frac{\mathrm{d}}{\mathrm{d}x} f(g(x)) = \frac{\mathrm{d}f}{\mathrm{d}g} \frac{\mathrm{d}g}{\mathrm{d}x}. \tag{7.12}$$

With these rule we get

$$\frac{\partial L}{\partial w_j} = \frac{1}{N} \sum_i \left((y^{(i)} - y(\mathbf{x}^{(i)}; \mathbf{w}))(-1) \frac{\partial y}{\partial w_j} \right). \tag{7.13}$$

The derivative of our model with respect to the parameters is

$$\frac{\partial y}{\partial w_j} = \frac{\partial}{\partial w_j} \frac{1}{1 + e^{-\sum_i w_i x_i}} = \frac{e^{-\sum_i w_i x_i}}{(1 + e^{-\sum_i w_i x_i})^2} \frac{\partial \sum_i w_i x_i}{\partial w_j}. \tag{7.14}$$

In the remaining derivative derivative over the sum only the term survives that contains the w_j. Hence this derivative is x_j. We can also write the some other portion of this equation in terms of the original function, namely

$$\frac{e^{-\sum_i w_i x_i}}{(1 + e^{-\sum_i w_i x_i})^2} = y(1 - y), \tag{7.15}$$

and hence

$$\frac{\partial y}{\partial w_j} = y(1 - y)x_j. \tag{7.16}$$

We can now collect all the pieces and write the whole update rule for the weight values as

$$w_j \leftarrow w_j - \alpha \frac{1}{N} \sum_i \left((y^{(i)} - y(\mathbf{x}^{(i)}; \mathbf{w}))y(\mathbf{x}^{(i)}; \mathbf{w})(1 - y(\mathbf{x}^{(i)}; \mathbf{w}))x^{(i)}_j \right) \tag{7.17}$$

The first part of in the sum is after called the delta term

$$\delta(\mathbf{x}^{(i)}; \mathbf{w}) = (y^{(i)} - y(\mathbf{x}^{(i)}; \mathbf{w}))y(\mathbf{x}^{(i)}; \mathbf{w})(1 - y(\mathbf{x}^{(i)}; \mathbf{w})), \tag{7.18}$$

or, if we write this without the arguments to better see the structure, it is

$$\delta^{(i)} = (y^{(i)} - y)y(1 - y) \tag{7.19}$$

We can thus write the learning rule as

$$w_j \leftarrow w_j + \alpha \frac{1}{N} \sum_i \left(\delta^{(i)}(\mathbf{x}^{(i)}; \mathbf{w})x^{(i)}_j \right) \tag{7.20}$$

This learning rule is called the delta rule as the change of the weight values is proportional to the difference between the desired and actual output often expressed as δ-term, $\delta = y_i - r_i^{\text{out}}$. For a linear perceptron, which is the perceptron with a linear activation function $f(x) = x$, this is simply given by $f' = 1$. The weight change for a linear perceptron is therefore

$$\Delta w_{ij} = \alpha(y_i - r_i^{\text{out}})r_j^{\text{in}}. \tag{7.21}$$

This rule, without the derivative of the activation function, was used previously for threshold perceptrons and is called the perceptron learning rule. Since the threshold function is not differentiable at the threshold, this function is formally not a gradient descent rule. However, it turns out that this rule still works for training the threshold perceptron on simple classification problems.

Also, note the similarity of the delta learning rule with Hebbian plasticity as discussed in Chapter 6 (eqn 6.10). This learning rule has now two Hebbian terms. The weights are increased by an amount proportional to the product of the presynaptic node (input value) r_j^{in} and the desired postsynaptic value y_i. This is a supervised Hebbian learning term. However, the weights are also decreased by the product of the input value r_j^{in} and the actual postsynaptic value r_i^{out}. This term is like unlearning the actual response of the perceptron when the perceptron does not give the right answer. Learning ceases when the actual output is equal to the desired output, since the δ-term is then zero. The algorithm of the delta rule is summarized with general activation functions in Table 7.2.

Table 7.2 Summary of delta-rule algorithm

Initialize weights arbitrarily
Repeat until error is sufficiently small
Apply a sample pattern to the input nodes: $r_i^0 = r_i^{\text{in}} = \xi_i^{\text{in}}$
Calculate rate of the output nodes: $r_i^{\text{out}} = g(\sum_j w_{ij} r_j^{\text{in}})$
Compute the delta term for the output layer: $\delta_i = g'(h_i^{\text{out}})(\xi_i^{\text{out}} - r_i^{\text{out}})$
Update the weight matrix by adding the term: $\Delta w_{ij} = \epsilon \delta_i r_j^{\text{in}}$

The program implementation of the simple perceptron in Python is given in program `PerceptronOr.py`. The program starts with defining the training problem (the training dataset) in feature arrays X and desired label vector Y. The columns of the matrix X correspond to the feature vector of each sample, and the columns therefore represent all the training samples. We then introduce and initialize some variables, specifically the number of input nodes Ni and output nodes No, the weight matrix to the output nodes wo is initialized randomly, dwo are the changes (gradients) of the weights, and do is the delta term of the output node.

Programs/PerceptronOr.py

```
1  import numpy as np
2  import matplotlib.pyplot as plt
3
4  X=np.array([[0,0,1,1],
5              [0,1,0,1],
6              [1,1,1,1]])
7  Y=np.array([[0,1,1,1]])
8
9  # model specifications
10 Ni=3; No=1;
11
12 #parameter and array initialization
13 Ntrials=100
14 wo=np.random.randn(No,Ni); dwo=np.zeros(wo.shape)
15 error1=np.array([])
16 error2=np.array([])
17
18 for trial in range(Ntrials):
```

```
19    y = 1/(1+np.exp(−wo@X)) #output for all pattern
20    do = y*(1−y)*(Y−y)  # delta output
21    # update weights with momentum
22    dwo = 0.9*dwo+do@X.T
23    wo = wo+0.5*dwo
24    error1 = np.append(error1,np.sum((Y−y)**2))
25    error2 = np.append(error2,np.sum(1−(abs(Y−y)<0.1)))
26
27  plt.plot(error1); plt.plot(error2/4)
```

An example learning curve where we show the absolute difference between the desired output and the actual output of the network is shown on the left in Fig. 7.6 by the blue line. Overall, the error is getting smaller, indicating that some learning takes place. The error does not, however, reach 0. This comes from the fact that we use a sigmoid function which approaches a value of 1 only asymptotically. However, we can introduce another post-processing step in which we apply a threshold function. This corresponds to the error that we calculate in the above program. The corresponding learning curve is shown on in orange on the left graph in Fig. 7.6. This demonstrates that this perceptron can solve the Boolean OR function with this post-processing step. The error function such as the loss used for training is somewhat useful as it shows that there is continuous progress during learning even when the thresholded value stays constant, although the values themselves do not tell the whole story. The thresholded values give us some indication of how many patterns are recognized, but it would be better to check every pattern separately, something which we omitted to keep the program short. It is very useful to always calculate error numbers that can be interpreted in terms of the performance that a user is looking for, which is not necessarily the loss function used for the gradient descent.

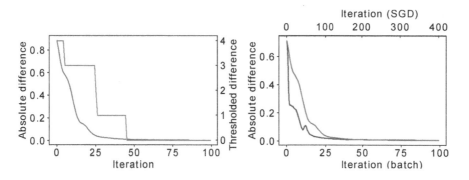

Fig. 7.6 Learning curve of sigmoid perceptron trained on the Boolean OR function. The graph of on the left-hand side shows the learning curve for batch learning. The blue curve shows the absolute difference between the desired output and the sigmoidal activation of the output node. The orange line shows the thresholded difference. The right-hand graph compares the batch learning curve (blue) from the left graph to the SGD learning curve (red).

We have already discussed batch versus online learning in the linear case and it might be good to review this again for backpropagation. We have derived here the learning rule based on the mean square error over all the training points. This corresponds to applying all the training examples and calculating the average gradient

Table 7.3 BooleanXOR function

x_1	x_2	y
0	0	1
0	1	0
1	0	0
1	1	1

before updating the weight values based on this average. This is batch training, since we use the whole batch of training examples for each weight update step. In contrast, we use one training example at a time, $(\mathbf{x}^{(i)}, y^{(i)}$, and calculate the gradient for this point, and use this gradient to update the weight value after the application of each data point. This is an online learning method since the point is to use each incoming data point for one update and there is no need to store anything. Of course, in reality we want to perform several iterations so that we must keep each training point. In the implementation below, we chose a random sample from the training pattern. If the training patterns are random, then this method is the stochastic gradient descent (SGD). An example of such a learning curve is shown as red line in the right-hand graph of Fig.7.6.

What is the advantage or disadvantage of the different methods? The batch algorithm guarantees that the average training error decreases. So if we plot this curve and see that the training error is increasing we know that there must be something wrong. By contrast, when we change the weights based on the last training example it is expected that the performance of the other training points get worse and we need to reduce the pace of the learning rate. Note that here we showed performance curves in the training set. We must, of course, study the generalization, which is difficult to show in this sized example.

As usual in machine learning, different methods will perform differently in different situations. However, it is now common to have large data sets where an online approach is more appropriate. Also, there are benefits of SGD in that this approach produces stochastic paths through the weight space which might help avoid local minima or shallow areas. This is even more important in the non-linear case as the linear case corresponds to a convex optimization problem with no local minima. Again, it is now common with large datasets to use mini-batches. This will help in the processing for keeping a smaller dataset in memory before loading new mini-batches. Within each mini-batch we can still learn in a batch or SGD way.

7.2.2 Multilayer perceptron (MLP)

Let us now consider the XOR function which is $y = 1$ if both arguments are the same and 0 otherwise as shown in Table 7.3.

It is interesting to try and learn this case using the perceptron program as this does not seem to work. Indeed, this function cannot be learned by the perceptron as the XOR function is not linearly separable. This lead to the demise of perceptrons in the 1970s although it was clear that more elaborate perceptrons with multiple layers could solve this problem. Frank Rosenblatt started to build such networks out of the simple neuron models and wrote a book about them. He even started to build neural computers based on such perceptrons and trained them similar to the algorithm shown below. It seems that due to Rosenblatt's early death and Marvin Minsky's strong opposition to perceptrons that the many researchers in this area were made believe that learning was problematic with these more elaborate structures. Thus, multilayer perceptrons only became popular again when effective training was rediscovered and made popular in 1986s by Rumelhart, Hinton, and Williams.

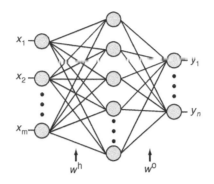

Fig. 7.7 The standard architecture of a feedforward multilayer network with one hidden layer, in which input values are distributed to all hidden nodes with weighting factors summarized in the weight matrix $\mathbf{w}^h$. The output values of the nodes of the hidden layer are passed to the output layer, again scaled by the values of the connection strength as specified by the elements in the weight matrix $\mathbf{w}^o$.

We will now consider networks of simple sigmoidal neurons to build up what are commonly called artificial neural networks since the perceptron is basically just one neuron. We will first consider a network structure as shown in Fig. 7.7. The network has a layer of m input nodes, a layer of h hidden nodes, and a layer of n output nodes. The input layer merely represent the input values, while the hidden and output layer perform active calculations specified earlier with perceptron neuron (egn 7.7). The term hidden nodes comes from the fact that these nodes do not have connections to the external world such as input and output nodes. The network is a graphical representation of a non-linear function of the form

$$\mathbf{y} = g(\mathbf{w}^o g(\mathbf{w}^h \mathbf{x})). \tag{7.22}$$

It is easy to include more hidden layers in this formula. For example, the activation rule for the output of a four-layer network with three hidden layers and one output layer can be written as

$$\mathbf{y} = g(\mathbf{w}^o g(\mathbf{w}^{h3} g(\mathbf{w}^{h2} g(\mathbf{w}^{h1} \mathbf{x})))), \tag{7.23}$$

where each layer uses the same activation function. Let us discuss a special case of a multilayer mapping network where all the nodes in all hidden layers have linear activation functions ($g(x) = x$). Eqn 7.23 then simplifies to

$$\mathbf{y} = \mathbf{w}^o \mathbf{w}^{h3} \mathbf{w}^{h2} \mathbf{w}^{h1} \mathbf{x}$$
$$= \tilde{\mathbf{w}} \mathbf{x}. \tag{7.24}$$

In the last step we have used the fact that the multiplication of a series of matrices simply yields another matrix, which we labelled $\tilde{w}$. Eqn 7.24 represents a single-layer network as discussed earlier. It is therefore essential to include non-linear activation functions, at least in the hidden layers, to take advantage of the computational advantages of hidden layers that we are about to discuss. Note that it is also possible to build more diverse networks, such as by including connections between different hidden layers, not just between consecutive layers as shown in Fig. 7.7. However, the basic layered structure is sufficient for the following discussions and we will come back to this point later in the book.

Since the perceptron was not able to represent some Boolean functions, we should now ask which functions can be approximated by multilayer perceptrons. The answer is, in principle, any. A multilayer feedforward network is a universal function approximator. This means that, given enough hidden nodes, any mapping functions can be approximated with arbitrary precision by these networks. While this can be proven formally, it is also easy to comprehend why this is the case. Each hidden nodes adds another factor with its own free parameters to the function that is represented by the network. For example, with the combination of two sigmoidal nodes that have the opposite weights and different offsets, one can build a local function like the one shown on the left in Fig. 7.8. With such local functions, that can be tunes in size and location of the bump, one can build up arbitrary non-linear functions in as much precision as one wants.

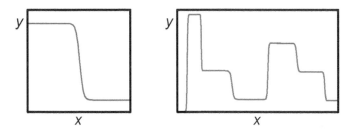

Fig. 7.8 Left: A basis function in form of a sigmoid function. The right-hand function is made up of the basis function by simply adding scaled, shifted, and reflected copies of the basis function.

The remaining problems involve knowing how many hidden nodes we need, and finding the right values for the weights. Also, the general approximator characteristics does not tell us if it is better to use more hidden layers or just to increase the number of nodes in one hidden layer. These are important concerns for practical engineering applications of those networks. These questions are related to the bias-variance trade-off since more nodes will increase the complexity of the model and can hence increase the potential for high variance (overfitting), while too few terms have the potential to introduce a bias (underfitting).

To train these networks, we consider again minimizing MSE. The learning rule is then given by a gradient descent on this error function,

$$w_j^l \leftarrow w_j^l - \alpha \frac{\partial E}{\partial w_j^l}, \tag{7.25}$$

with $l \in \{h, o\}$.

Specifically, the gradient of the MSE error function with respect to the output weights is given by

$$\frac{\partial E}{\partial w_{ij}^o} = \frac{1}{2} \frac{\partial}{\partial w_{ij}^o} \sum_k (\mathbf{y}^{(k)} - \mathbf{y})^2$$

$$= \frac{1}{2} \frac{\partial}{\partial w_{ij}^o} \sum_k \left(\mathbf{y}^{(k)} - g(\mathbf{w}^o g(\mathbf{w}^h \mathbf{x}^{(k)})) \right)^2$$

(7.26)

Let's call the activation of the hidden nodes $\mathbf{y}^h$,

$$\mathbf{y}^h = g(\mathbf{w}^h \mathbf{x}). \tag{7.27}$$

Then we can continue with our derivative as,

$$\frac{\partial E}{\partial w_{ij}^o} = \frac{1}{2} \frac{\partial}{\partial w_{ij}^o} \sum_k \left(\mathbf{y}^{(k)} - g(\mathbf{w}^o \mathbf{y}^h) \right)^2$$

$$= - \sum_k g'(\mathbf{w}^h \mathbf{x}^{(k)})(y_i^{(k)} - y_i) y_j^h$$

$$= \delta_i^o y_j^h, \tag{7.28}$$

Eqn 7.28 is just the delta rule as presented earlier because we have only considered the output layer. The calculation of the gradients with respect to the weights of the hidden layer again requires the chain rule as they are more embedded in the error function. Thus we have to calculate the derivative

$$\frac{\partial E}{\partial w_{ij}^h} = \frac{1}{2} \frac{\partial}{\partial w_{ij}^h} \sum_k (\mathbf{y}^{(k)} - \mathbf{y})^2$$

$$= \frac{1}{2} \frac{\partial}{\partial w_{ij}^h} \sum_k \left(\mathbf{y}^{(k)} - g(\mathbf{w}^o g(\mathbf{w}^h \mathbf{x}^{(k)})) \right)^2. \tag{7.29}$$

After some battle with indices (which can easily be avoided with analytical calculation programs such as MAPLE or MATHEMATICA), we can write the derivative in a form similar to that of the derivative of the output layer, namely

$$\frac{\partial E}{\partial w_{ij}^h} = \delta_i^h x_j, \tag{7.30}$$

when we define the delta term of the hidden term as

$$\delta_i^h = g^{h\prime}(h_i^{in}) \sum_k w_{ik}^o \delta_k^o. \tag{7.31}$$

The error term δ_i^h is calculated from the error term of the output layer with a formula that looks similar to the general update formula of the network, except that a signal is propagating from the output layer to the previous layer. This is the reason that the algorithm is called the error-backpropagation algorithm.

Table 7.4 Summary of error-back-propagation algorithm

Initialize weights arbitrarily
Repeat until error is sufficiently small
Apply a sample pattern to all input nodes: x_i
Propagate input through the network by calculating the rates of
nodes in successive layers l: $y_i^l = g(\sum_j w_{ij}^l y_j^{l-1})$
Compute the delta term for the output layer:
$\delta_i^o = g'(y_i^{o-1})(y_i^{desired} - y_i^o)$
Back-propagate delta terms through the network:
$\delta_i^{l-1} = g'(y_i^{l-1}) \sum_j w_{ji}^l \delta_j^l$
Update weight matrix by adding the term: $\Delta w_{ij}^l = \alpha \delta_i^l y_j^{l-1}$

In this derivation we used the MSE over all the training patterns. Since all the training patterns are used at once, this algorithm is again a batch algorithm. Using a batch algorithm is generally a good idea, but it also takes up a lot of memory with large training sets and we have mentioned that an online version when new data points arise in a random order can help with avoiding local minima. This is called stochastic gradient descent. The online version of this algorithm is summarized in Table 7.4. This algorithm is commonly applied to random mini-batches at a time.

The basic multilayer perceptron implementation in Python for the XOR problem is illustrated in program MLPxor.py. As already discussed in the simple perceptron implementation before, the program starts by defining the training problem (the training dataset) in feature arrays X and desired label vector Y. We then introduce and initialize some variables which now include the activation of the hidden nodes h and the weights to the hidden nodes wh, as well as the corresponding gradient dwh and delta term dh. We then iterate over trials. We implemented here the batch version where we propagate forward all samples from the training set and update the weights. This code is very compact, using matrix notations. In general, is it useful to think about the layers of the neural network for performing operations such as building the dot product between the input vector and the weight matrix. This compact formulation helps a great deal with building complex models.

Programs/MLPxor.py

```
1  #MLP for the xor function
2  import numpy as np
3  import matplotlib.pyplot as plt
4
5  X=np.array([[0,0,1,1],
6              [0,1,0,1],
7              [1,1,1,1]])
8  Y=np.array([[1,0,0,1]])
9
10 # model specifications
11 Ni=3; Nh=4; No=1;
12
13 #parameter and array initialization
14 Ntrials=1000
15 wh=np.random.randn(Nh,Ni); dwh=np.zeros(wh.shape)
16 wo=np.random.randn(No,Nh); dwo=np.zeros(wo.shape)
```

```
17  error=np.array([])
18
19  for trial in range(Ntrials):
20      h=1/(1+np.exp(-wh@X)) #hidden activation for all pattern
21      y=1/(1+np.exp(-wo@h)) #output for all pattern
22
23      do=y*(1-y)*(Y-y)  # delta output
24      dh=h*(1-h)*(wo.transpose()@do)  # delta backpropagated
25
26      # update weights with momentum
27      dwo=0.9*dwo+do@h.T
28      wo=wo+0.1*dwo
29      dwh=0.9*dwh+dh@X.T
30      wh=wh+0.1*dwh
31
32      error=np.append(error,np.sum(abs(Y-y)))
33  plt.plot(error)
```

An example learning curve where we show the absolute difference between the desired output and the actual output of the network appears on the left of Fig. 7.9, while on the right is shown the error when using a threshold post-processing as we did with the perceptron. This demonstrates that the MLP can solve the Boolean XOR function.

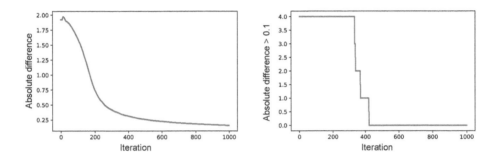

Fig. 7.9 Learning curve of an MLP trained on the Boolean XOR function. The graph on the left-hand side shows the learning curve of the absolute difference between the desired output and the sigmoidal activation of the output node. The graph on the right shows an example of the performance when we use the rounded value of the output node as prediction.

7.2.3 MNIST with MLP

Most of the Multi-layer perceptron techniques have been known at least since the late 1960s, although they became only more widely recognized in the mid 1980s. While there was at this time much excitement, scaling these networks up to larger problem sizes turned out to be in practice more challenging than expected. For example, when simply replacing the above XOR pattern with the MNIST data set turns out to be difficult train. Another problem when training even deeper network, MLPs with more hidden layers, is the vanishing gradient problem that was realized by Sepp Hochreiter and Jürgen Schmidhuber. The essense of this problem is that the gradients can be getting very small, such as in the tails of the sigmoid function, and backpropagating such small gradients is further diluting them. Their solution led Schmidthuber and Hochreiter to the proposal of Long Short Term Memory (LSTM) that will be discussed further in Chapter 9. We will simply show that the problem is somewhat relieved by using a leaky-rectified-linear grain function,

$$g(x) = \begin{cases} x & \text{if } x > 0 \\ 0.1 & \text{otherwise} \end{cases} \tag{7.32}$$

instead of the sigmoid function. While this function is differential at $x = 0$, we can simply take a one-sided derivative at this point. Furthermore, we will also change the output function to a function that is more appropriate for probabilistic multi-class classification. First we demand that the output vector is normalized so that the sum of the vector elements is equal to one.

$$\mathbf{y} \leftarrow \frac{\exp(\mathbf{y})}{\sum \exp(\mathbf{y})}. \tag{7.33}$$

We will see that this is appropriate when viewing classification in a probabilistic framework. We will discuss this further in Section 7.4. We will there also show that the negative cross-entropy

$$L = \sum_j Y^{(j)} \log y^{(j)} \tag{7.34}$$

is appropriate for classification. The derivative of this loss function is also simple,

$$\frac{\mathrm{d}L}{\mathrm{d}y} = Y - y. \tag{7.35}$$

Finally, a very important aspect of the application of a gradient method is to use some form of randomness in the process to avoid local minima or shallow areas in the loss surface. An elegant simple way is to use random mini-batches during learning. That is, we are taking only a certain number of random training examples for each gradient step. This so-called stochastic gradient descent (SGD) method has become the standard for practical application of such artificial neural networks and deep learning. An example program that includes these changes for the MNIST example is given below.

Programs/MNISTmlp.py

```
 1  import numpy as np
 2  import matplotlib.pyplot as plt
 3  import pandas as pd
 4
 5  df = pd.read_csv('mnist_784.csv')
 6  X = df.iloc[:,0:784].values/255
 7  Y1 = df.iloc[:,784].values
 8
 9  Y=np.zeros((10,70000))
10  for i in range(70000): Y[Y1[i],i]=1
11  X=np.append(X.T,np.array([np.ones(70000)]),axis=0)
12
```

```
13
14 # model specifications
15 Ni=785; Nh=128; No=10
16
17 #parameter and array initialization
18 Ntrials=100
19 wh=np.random.randn(Nh,Ni); dwh=np.zeros(wh.shape)
20 wo=np.random.randn(No,Nh); dwo=np.zeros(wo.shape)
21 error=np.array([])
22
23 for trial in range(Ntrials):
24     i=np.random.permutation(range(1000))
25     for batch in range(10):
26         Xtrain=X[:,batch*100:(batch+1)*100]
27         Ytrain=Y[:,batch*100:(batch+1)*100]
28
29         h=wh@Xtrain; h=np.where(h<0,0.1*h,h)
30         y=np.exp(wo@h); y=y/np.sum(y,0)
31         do=(Ytrain-y)
32         dh=wo.T@do
33
34         # update weights with momentum
35         dwo=0.9*dwo+do@h.T
36         wo=wo+0.001*dwo
37         dwh=0.9*dwh+dh@Xtrain.T
38         wh=wh+0.001*dwh
39
40         error=np.append(error,np.sum(abs(Ytrain-y)))
41 plt.plot(error)
```

7.2.4 MLP with Keras

While we have implemented the MLP from scratch in order to explain all the details of the model, there are now many software packaged which make their implementation much simpler. For example, the Python package called sklearn is a comprehensive machine learning library that is easy to use and contains many useful routines, including multilayer perceptrons. This is a useful library to explore as it contains many modern data analytics routines. While we will not do this further here, we will directly jump to a library called Keras that was invented to provide deep learning routines in a sklearn style. This library is useful as this can run programs with the help of graphic processor units (GPUs) that can speed up the processing of such models considerably. Indeed, GPUs are commonly is essential for deep learning as the size of the models for advanced applications are commonly applied to large data sets. GPUs are processors that are optimized for array operations such as operations to generating graphics. Most of our operations around neural networks can take advantage of these specialized processors as neural networks are based on matrix or tensor operations, including additions, multiplications and convolution operations that we will discuss further below. Indeed, the discussion and implementation of convolutional neural networks below are another motivation to introduce this library here.

Let us discuss the basic example of a deep network in Keras. A deep neural network here is simply a network that has several layers. We can use this to finally return to the example of recognizing hand-written digits. In particular, we will use the famous MNIST (Modified National Institute of Standards and Technology) database that has driven a lot of developments in deep learning. The data set consists of digitized examples of hand-written numbers from 0 to 9. Each image consist of 28*28 pixels. The first 14 examples from this data set are shown in Fig. 7.10.

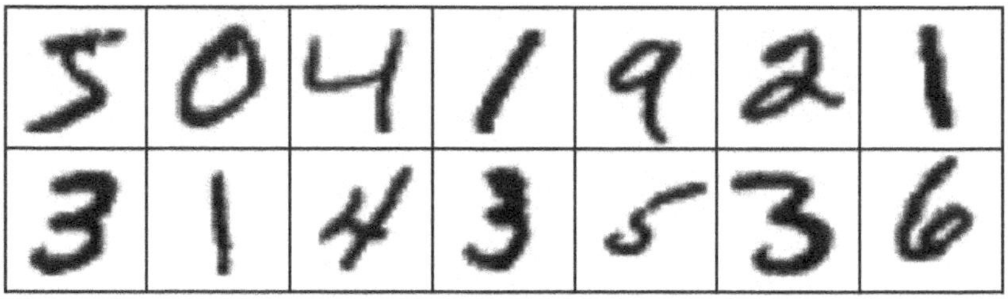

Fig. 7.10 The first 14 examples from the MNIST dataset of hand-written digits.

A network with 6 layers as outlined at the beginning of this Chapter in Fig. 7.2 is implemented in program MLPmnist.py. The first part of the program is concerned with the preparation of the data in the appropriate format such as gathering all the pixels in the image into a large vector of size 784 (= 28*28) and rescaling it to a range of $[0, 1]$. We will later discuss why such a normalization is useful. Also, we change the labels into a 1-hot representation which is vector of length equal to the number of classes with zeros in all components except the position that indicates the label of this class. For example, with three classes we could have $1 \rightarrow [1, 0, 0], 2 \rightarrow [0, 1, 0], 3 \rightarrow [0, 0, 1]$. We can use the Keras function to_categorical() for this purpose.

Programs/MNISTmlpKeras.py

```
1  import numpy as np
2  import matplotlib.pyplot as plt
3  from keras import models, layers, optimizers, datasets, utils
4
5
6  (x_train, y_train), (x_test, y_test) = datasets.mnist.load_data()
7
8  x_train = x_train.reshape(60000, 784)/255
9  x_test = x_test.reshape(10000, 784)/255
10 y_train = utils.to_categorical(y_train, 10)
11 y_test = utils.to_categorical(y_test, 10)
12
13 inputs = layers.Input(shape=(784,))
14 x = layers.Dense(128, activation='relu')(inputs)
15 x = layers.Dense(128, activation='relu')(x)
16 x = layers.Dense(128, activation='relu')(x)
17 x = layers.Dense(128, activation='relu')(x)
18 x = layers.Dense(128, activation='relu')(x)
19 outputs= layers.Dense(10, activation='softmax')(x)
20
21 model = models.Model(inputs=inputs, outputs=outputs)
22
23 model.compile(loss='categorical_crossentropy',
24               optimizer='Nadam', metrics=['accuracy'])
25
```

```
26| history=model.fit(x_train, y_train,
27|              batch_size=128,
28|              epochs=10,
29|              validation_data=(x_test, y_test))
30| score = model.evaluate(x_test, y_test)
31| print('Test loss:', score[0],'Test accuracy:', score[1])
```

The interesting part here is how the neural network can be specified in Keras. Keras provides two principle ways to specify models, one called sequential model which is limited to purely sequential models with single inputs and outputs, and the more general functional model which can be used to assemble more complex models. The functional model notation is not much more difficult and even slightly more sensible so that we will use this mode right away. A functional model in Keras is specified by specifying a general input, then specifying functions for layers and connecting them by specifying their individual inputs, and finally to collect a single model by calling a function Model() in which we specify the input and output of the entire model. Note that a function with two bracket pairs, like Dense()(), means that the first function returns a function which is then called with the second argument list.

The MLP is characterized by a fully connected layer where each neuron of the previous layer is connected to every neuron in the receiving layer. Such layers are now commonly called dense layers. We have to specify the activation function for each layer if it is not linear, which is here the rectified linear function (relu)

$$g(x_i) = \begin{cases} x_i & \text{if } x_i > 0 \\ 0 & \text{otherwise} \end{cases} \qquad (7.36)$$

except the last layer for which the activation function is a softmax function

$$g(x_i) = \frac{e^{-x_i}}{\sum_j e^{-x_j}}. \qquad (7.37)$$

The model has to be compiled which is necessary to that the program is prepared for execution on GPUs if available. Most of the examples in this book are prepared to be small enough so that a GPU is not required. In the compilation step we specify which loss function to use, which optimizer we will use, and also which metric we use to evaluate the results. Of course, we have to discuss these choices in more detail, but for now we want to show that such networks with these popular choices can do remarkable well. It is common that this simple model results in a test accuracy of around 98% on the MNIST dataset. In contrast, a comparable Support vector machine (SVM), which was a popular method before deep learning, achieves around 91% on the MNIST dataset.

The performance of the model after learning is important for us. However, it is also very instructive and important for the development of the models to monitor the performance of the model during learning. We call such graphs learning curves. We can draw different type of curves, either evaluated on the training set or evaluated on the validation set. It is easy to plot such curves in Keras as the fit function already includes a history of evaluations as a callback function, and Keras provides the framework to code your own callback function. Other deep learning frameworks also commonly include a way to visualize the progress during learning. In the code above we assigned the returned pointer of the fit function to dictionary list variable `history`. The `key()` function lists the key names for the included values, which results in the graph shown in Fig. 7.11. We can see that the validation accuracy, is fairly consistent around 0.975, while the training accuracy is increasing, which might be a sign of overfitting. The behaviour of such curves is quite useful observe when developing the model. It can provide some diagnostic values when the model is not learning properly.

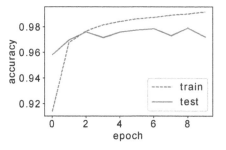

Fig. 7.11 Example of the learning curves. The blue dotted line corresponds to the accuracy over the training data, while the red solid line corresponds to the accuracy over the validation data.

7.2.5 Some remarks on gradient learning and biological plausibility of MLPs

MLPs have taught us many lessons for network processing such as representational learning their ability to implement complex mapping functions. These lessons seems invaluable when considering the functionality of the brain. However, arguing on the biological plausibility depends very much on the context and the level that these models are aimed at. For example, some people have criticized MLPs as biologically unrealistic since neurons spike and have therefore a binary response function. However, as we argued already in Chapter 5, the model neurons here might be better characterized as modelling population of neurons. However, then there is some uncertainty over the interpretation of the weights that we often equate with synaptic efficacies.

There has been ongoing debates on the biological plausibility of error-backpropagation learningn if this training is intended to model the dynamics of biological learning based on synaptic plasticity. The back-propagation of error signals seems difficult to realize in cortical networks. While some form of information exchange between postsynaptic and presynaptic neurons is possible, the wide use of such mechanisms for a back-propagation of errors through the whole network seems challenging. For example, a neuron would have to gather the back-propagated errors from all the other nodes to which it projects. This not only raises synchronization issues, but also has disadvantages for true parallel processing in the system. The inclusion of derivative terms in the delta signals is also problematic. The back-propagation of inaccurate derivative terms can quickly lead to inaccurate updates of the weights in the network. Finally, it has never been resolved how a forward propagating phase of signals can be separated effectively from the back-propagation phase of the error signals. However, there are also several proposals how such an algorithm could be implemented biologically in different ways. This ranges from back-propagating action potentials to network configurations of feedback connections that will achieve error-backpropagation in principle. Regardless of the direct biological implementation, the value of being able to find solutions to a mapping problem is in itself an important contribution to enable building functional network models, regardless of the possibility of finding solutions with different methods.

However, caution of applying MLP models for fitting neuroscientific data is also important. We mentioned above that feedforward mapping networks are universal function approximators, which necessitates caution when interpreting them in computational neuroscience. For example, in experiments we often measure some response function as a function of some parameters controlled experimentally. A multilayer mapping network, as universal approximator, will be able to approximate every such function arbitrarily well with the right choice of parameters in the network. When such networks are used to fit experimental data one might be tempted to claim that these systems represent models of the brain, on the basis that the processing nodes in the network resemble neurons. Just being able to fit some experimental relations can thus have limited scientific use. A good model sheds light on possible explanations, and the explanatory value of a model is therefore something to always keep in mind.

In practice, there are also many challenges to apply large neural network models to data fitting. It is well recognized that simple gradient descent optimization can get stuck in local minima and that there are advanced methods. This includes using momentum terms for the gradients that keeps some memory of previous updates. This also includes higher-order derivative terms that can approximate better non-linear optimization manifolds. Regularization techniques are becoming increasingly important with the growing size of network models, and many other techniques have been instrumental in making deep networks applicable to industrial applications. This area of machine learning is very active, and some inspiration from and for neuroscience have been derived. However, we will continue to focus on illustrating the fundamentals of computational neuroscience.

7.3 Convolutional neural networks (CNNs)

7.3.1 Invariant object recognition

Humans are able to recognize objects even though they vary in form, size, location, and viewing angle, etc. For example, take a cup and move it in front of your eyes, rotate it, or view it from different distances. Recognizing the cup does not crucially depend on the viewing conditions. While we have seen that neural systems can learn to recognize objects through supervised learning in mapping networks, such recognition processes are quite sensitive against changes in the input vector, and the changes in the viewing condition of the cup result in very different activation patterns of the retina. Invariant object recognition has hence puzzled neuroscientists and engineers alike for a long time. Solving invariant object recognition can be achieved in hierarchical networks.

Much of the human brain is involved in visual processing to some degree, and vision research is a strong domain within neuroscience. Here we outline briefly a hypothesis of how invariant visual object recognition is achieved within the ventral visual pathway of the brain (see discussion of the what-and-where pathways in Section 10.1.2). Kunihiko Fukushima already advanced such invariant object recognition models in 1979, a hierarchical, multilayered artificial neural network which was motivated by studying the visual system of monkeys. We outline here briefly the more physiological model called VisNet as suggestions by Edmund Rolls, Simon Stringer, and collaborators before discussing popular incarnations of invariant networks with convolutions neural networks that have been advanced by Yann LeCun and colleagues.

A. Ventral visual pathway   B. Layered cortical maps

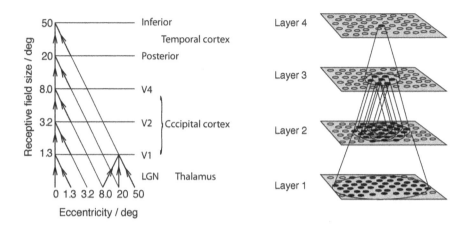

Fig. 7.12 (A) Illustration of the increase of receptive field sizes in the ventral visual pathway. (B) Layered model called VisNet of the ventral visual pathway, which consists of competitive layers where each node in a layer is connected to a restricted area of nodes in the previous layer [adapted from Stringer and Rolls, *Neural Networks* 21: 888–903 (2008), and references therein].

The hierarchical levels in the ventral visual pathway are outlined in Fig. 7.12A. After some preprocessing of visual patterns in the retina, where important functions are implemented, such as adaptation to brightness, the patterns are mapped into the lateral geniculate nucleus (LGN) of the thalamus, which is the major target of the optic nerves from the eyes. Then, the signal reaches the primary visual cortex V1, and is then passed to higher cortical areas. In VisNet, these areas are typically associated with V2, and then areas in the posterior and inferior-temporal cortex. VisNet is therefore represented with four cortical layers, as shown in Fig. 7.12B. A crucial component of the model is that each node in a layer is connected to a spatially restricted area of nodes in the layer below. As a consequence, the receptive fields of the nodes, which is the area of the visual fields to which they can respond, increases with each level. The receptive fields in the inferior-temporal cortex are large and effectively cover the entire visual field.

Each layer in the model is a competitive map, where competition is implemented through adjustment of the firing threshold of nodes until a predefined sparseness is reached in each layer, as discussed in Section 8.5.1. The model is trained on sequences of patterns from movements of objects in the visual field, such as translation or rotations of objects. Weights between the layers are adjusted with Hebbian learning proportional to the activation of pre- and postsynaptic activity. Early versions of the model used a form of Hebbian learning with a trace rule, where some memory in the neural activity (trace) was used for Hebbian weight changes. Such rules use temporal associations between moving objects. However, recent simulations also showed that similar results can be achieved without a trace when objects in consecutive time steps have some overlap with previous neural representations. These rules thus use spatial associations. Simulations have shown that VisNet is able to learn invariant object recognition, including invariance to translation, rotation, and size. Recent studies also showed that multiple objects can be trained simultaneously. VisNet clearly demonstrates how a hierarchical, competitive network with increasing sizes of receptive field and corresponding increasing abstraction representations, from an early image-based representation to an later object-based representation, can achieve invariant object recognition. Since this is a common architecture of cortical processing, the results should also hold for other sensory modalities.

7.3.2 Image processing and convolutions filters

In deep learning, the use of additional layers with learned parameters allows for the learning of hierarchical features. Increasing the number of layers has allowed successful applications of neural networks to more complex problems. Models with tens or even hundreds of layers are now not uncommon. The question is then how we can make the neural networks scalable as it not only takes more computer time to process the models, but also increases the demand on training examples to learn the increased number of parameters of more complex models. One set of advancements we can make is building-in some assumptions into our network architecture. Here we discuss a particular important case, that of building-in a position invariance of features. By this we mean that the recognition of a digit in our OCR system should not depend on the position where the character was presented in our visual field. In contrast, if we have a feature vector such as values indicating specific medical tests such as the blood pressure or the blood sugar level, then it matters very much where this related number is noted in the feature vector.

For the following discussion it is useful to realize that neurons can represent detectors or filters for specific features, meaning that neurons become maximally activated for specific input patterns. This is easily understood in vision applications. Most of the success in deep neural networks have been demonstrated with image processing and involve convolutional neural networks. In this section we will first review an important mathematical operation called a convolution before incorporating this into our feedforward network structures. We will discuss this again with the example of the MNIST hand-written digits.

Let us start by define the mathematical operation called convolution for a 1-dimensional discrete signal,

$$(f * s)(t) = \sum_{t'=0}^{T} f(t')s(t + t').$$
(7.38)

We used here the notation of t for the running variable as this is often applied to time series. Of course, this is only a notation and we could chose any symbol we like. This formula describes how to apply a filter f to a signal $s(t)$. Lets say we have a signal given by

$t =$	0	1	2	3	4	5	6	7	8	9
$s =$	0	0	0	0	0	1	1	1	1	1

Let us convolve this signal with a small filter $f = [-1, 1]$. This is done by placing the filter over the first part of the vector, then multiplying the elements together, and then summing the resulting elements to calculate the first element of the filtered image. In our case this is $(f * s)(0) = f(0) * s(0) + f(1) * s(1) = 0$. We then do a similar calculation starting at the second place of the signal, $(f * s)(0) = f(1) * s(1) + f(2) * s(2) = 0$. If we apply the filter to all possible start positions of the original signal, we get the nine-component vector for the filtered image $(f * s) = [0, 0, 0, 0, 1, 0, 0, 0, 0]$. If we apply the filter only to every second entry as starting place, then we would get the resulting filtered signal $(f * s) = [0, 0, 1, 0, 0]$. Shifting the filter by a certain value is called a stride. Using a filter with a stride other than 1 results in compressed signals. In any case, it might be interesting to note that the resulting filtered signal for this particular example filter is actually extracting the change in the original signal.

Note that the filtered signal even with a stride of 1 has one less position than the original vector. This is because the filter we used had two components so that I can only apply the filter to the second last place to not run over the bound of our original signal vector. There are several tricks to force the filtered signal to be the same size as the original signal. For example, we could just add an arbitrary value of s=0 at the time following our last entry. The filtered values are then of course a little bit biased, but sometimes it is convenient to keep the size the same. This is called zero padding. Alternatively, we could repeat values from the beginning of the signal, which is called periodic padding. In any case, these are just some technical tricks.

Before proceeding, it is appropriate to make a few technical remarks about our specific choice of a convolution definition. We used here a definition of a convolution that is common in machine learning. In engineering, a common alternative definition of a one-dimensional discrete convolution is

$$\text{Alternative definition:} \quad (f * s)(t) = \frac{1}{T} \sum_{t'=0}^{T} f(t')s(t - t'). \quad (7.39)$$

In this notation, the filter is reversed (flipped) compared to our original definition above. In machine learning circles the plus sign seems now to be the dominant way of formulating the convolution, and because we are later learning the values of the filter anyhow, this part of the definition does not influence the results. We also included more properly some normalization in this definition which is usually a good idea. However, this only adds an overall normalization constant to the convolution operations that can be absorbed in a learning process when we use such operations in a trainable network. Hence, our simplified definition seem more appropriate within our applications domain. Finally, we can also express a convolution for a continuous signals mathematically as

$$(f * x)(t) = \int_{-\infty}^{\infty} f(t')x(t + t')dt'. \tag{7.40}$$

A function like the filter appearing in an integral as above are mathematically called a kernel function.

It is straight forward to generalize a convolution to n-dimensional data. Mathematically, a complete n-dimensional convolution can be written as

$$(f * g)(x_1, ..., x_n) = \int_{-\infty}^{\infty} \cdots \int_{-\infty}^{\infty} f(x_1', ..., x_n')g(x_1 - x_1', ..., x_n - x_n')dx_1'...dx_n', \tag{7.41}$$

where we used the letter g for the signal. g is here an n-dimensional array. Such an n-dimensional structure with the corresponding rules of operations is mathematically called a tensor. For example, a three-dimensional tensor would be a cube, and convolving them with another three-dimensional tensor (cube) would result in another three-dimensional tensor (cube). The discrete two-dimensional case can be written as

$$(f * g)(u, v) = \sum_{u'=0}^{U} \sum_{v'=0}^{V} f(u', v')g(u + u', v + v'). \tag{7.42}$$

We used here the nomenclature u and v for the coordinates of the signal. These letters are often used for the pixel space of digital cameras. In this convolution operation, we place the upper-left corner of the filter f at a position (u, v) of the image g, multiplying the overlapping components with each other, and then summing the resulting values to arrive at the value for the position (u, v) of the filtered image.

It is now common that software packages have already function implementations for convolution operations. It might be useful to note that most implementations are based on the convolution theorem which states the convolution of two tensors becomes a point-wise multiplication in Fourier space. Hence, one first applies a FFT (Fast Fourier Transform) to the tensors, multiplies the results pointwise, and then use an inverse FFT to get the corresponding convolution.

Let us apply a convolution to filter our MNIST images. Specifically, let us apply a 2×2 filter with −1s on the left column and 1s on the right column,

$$\begin{pmatrix} -1 & 1 \\ -1 & 1 \end{pmatrix}$$

The resulting convolution is shown in Fig. 7.13. As can be seen, this filters highlights vertical edges. More specifically, a grey value there indicates that there are no edges. The darker pixels show where there are transitions from a smaller value to a higher gray-scale value in the original image, where as a lighter pixel indicates where there are horizontal transitions between a higher and smaller value in the original image. Horizontal edges are suppressed, although we could design a similar filter for vertical edges or even more complicated transitions.

Of course, our filter is very small and only shows edges with significant changes between two consecutive edges. There are therefore better designs of edge detectors, such as the Canny edge detector. These techniques combine such gradient filters with Gaussian smoothing and removal of some spurious cases. Also, a continuous version

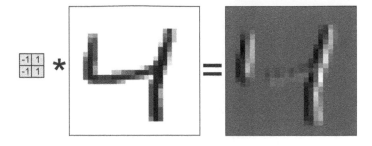

Fig. 7.13 An example of small edge detector applied to a digit of 4 from the MNIST dataset.

of edge filters is for example described by Gabor functions such as the ones shown in Fig. 7.14A and B. A Gabor function is described by a sinusoidally modulated Gaussian,

$$f(u,v) = e^{-\frac{u^2 + \gamma v^2}{2 * \sigma^2}} \cos(\frac{2\pi}{\lambda} u + \varphi). \tag{7.43}$$

The example of a 64^2 pixel filter with parameters $\gamma = 0.5$, $\sigma = 10$, $\lambda = 32$, and $\varphi = \pi/2$ is shown in Fig. 7.14A. This filter can be rotated with a rotation matrix

$$\begin{pmatrix} x \\ y \end{pmatrix} \leftarrow \begin{pmatrix} \cos(\varphi) & \sin(\varphi) \\ -\sin(\varphi) & \cos(\varphi) \end{pmatrix} \begin{pmatrix} x \\ y \end{pmatrix} \tag{7.44}$$

as shown in Fig. 7.14B for $\varphi = \pi$. Interestingly, such functions describe some of the neurons in the primary visual cortex of primates. Detecting edges seems therefore a good first step to process images, a fact that we will encounter again in later discussion.

A. Gabor function with $\varphi = \pi/2$ B. Rotated version of A

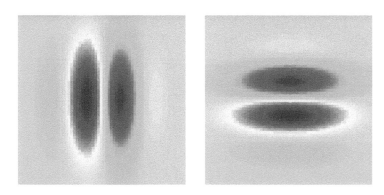

Fig. 7.14 Example of Gabor functions for (A) vertical and (B) horizontal edge detection.

7.3.3 CNN and MNIST

The idea of designing position invariant feature detectors in neural networks was first described by Fukushima in 1980. Fukushima worked at this time for NHK, the

Japanese public broadcaster, together with physiologists as NHK was interested to understand the mechanisms of human vision. It was well known since the early 1960s from experiments by Hubel and Wiesel that some neurons in the primary visual cortex, the first stage of visual processing in the cortex, are edge detectors, and that such features detectors must be combined in a way so that object recognition becomes invariant to the location in space.

Edge detectors are the workhorse of traditional computer vision, and we discussed in Chapter 2 how such filters are implemented with convolutions. The neural networks that we discussed before had to learn individual weights for each pixel location. Even if this network would learn to represent an edge detector, separate detectors have to be learned for each location in an image since edges can appear in all locations. Another way of thinking about convolution is that a neuron (specific filter) is applied to every possible location in the image. This leads us to the idea of weight sharing and convolutional neural networks (CNNs).

To discuss the implementation of this network type with Keras we go back to the MNIST benchmark example. The basic idea of a convolutional network is to replace the dense connections of regular networks, that are implemented with a matrix multiplication $h = wx$ with that of a convolution $h = w * x$. So the network can look a lot like the one shown in Fig. 7.2. While such a convolutional network has much less parameters than a dense network, implementing the convolution and running it efficiently on a computer is challenging. It is therefore that we need to use graphics processing units (GPUs). GPUs are special purpose processors that are designed for efficient matrix operations, and these processors have been very helpful in deep learning. In particular, NVIDIA has added specific support for deep learning operations, and it is such lower-level support on which we rely in the following. While there are specific frameworks that even support directly the programming with GPUs, such as Tensorflow or Theano, we chose here to apply Keras that is itself utilizing backends like Tensorflow and Theano, as well as other support on GPUs, to implement the operations we need in deep learning. Hence, as long as your programming environment is implemented to take advantage of GPUs, we can ignore the details and work on a higher level with system architectures. If you do not have a GPU than I recommend running the following MNIST examples on a smaller training set.

Programs/MNISTcnn.py

```
 1  import numpy as np
 2  import matplotlib.pyplot as plt
 3  from keras import models, layers, optimizers, datasets, utils, losses
 4
 5  (x_train, y_train), (x_test, y_test) = datasets.mnist.load_data()
 6  print(np.shape(x_train))
 7  plt.matshow(255-x_train[5,:,:], cmap='gray')
 8
 9  x_train = x_train.reshape(60000, 28, 28, 1)/255
10  x_train = x_train[:1024,:,:,:]
11  x_test = x_test.reshape(10000, 28, 28, 1)/255
12  y_train = utils.to_categorical(y_train[:1024], 10)
13  y_test = utils.to_categorical(y_test, 10)
14
15  inputs = layers.Input(shape=(28, 28, 1,))
16  x=layers.Conv2D(32, kernel_size=(3, 3), activation='relu')(inputs)
```

```
17  x=layers.Conv2D(64, (3, 3), activation='relu')(x)
18  x=layers.MaxPooling2D(pool_size=(2, 2))(x)
19  x=layers.Dropout(0.25)(x)
20  x=layers.Flatten()(x)
21  x=layers.Dense(128, activation='relu')(x)
22  x=layers.Dropout(0.5)(x)
23  outputs=layers.Dense(10, activation='softmax')(x)
24
25  model = models.Model(inputs=inputs, outputs=outputs)
26
27  model.compile(loss=losses.categorical_crossentropy,
28                optimizer=optimizers.Adadelta(),
29                metrics=['accuracy'])
30
31  model.fit(x_train, y_train,
32            batch_size=128,
33            epochs=2,
34            verbose=1,
35            validation_data=(x_test, y_test))
36  score = model.evaluate(x_test, y_test, verbose=0)
37  print('Test loss:', score[0])
38  print('Test accuracy:', score[1])
```

The Keras program to apply a CNN to the MNIST data is given in MNISTcnn.py. The program starts by linking the required libraries and reading the data as we did before for the dense network (MLP). The only difference is that we now reshape the input data into a two-dimensional array instead of the one-dimensional feature vector for each example. Actually, the data are already in the form of 28×28 for each sample, but since Keras expects the number of channels we have still to reshape it into the form $28 \times 28 \times 1$. The model is then defined with Keras functions for convolutional layers. The model starts with a convolutional layer that produces filtered images with 32 channels where each channel is the result of filtering with a separate filter. The size of the filter is specified with the kernel_size parameter. We used a rectified linear (relu) activation functions that is common for deep networks. We then add another convolution layer. Since the output size is defined by the previous we don't have to include the input size. In this layer we expand the representation to 64 channels.

The next layer is a new type of layer that is produced by a fixed kernel type defining an operation that is called max pooling. Max pooling takes a consecutive patch of pixels, in this case a pooling size of (2,2), and replaces this with one pixel of the maximum of this patch. This will shrink the image size, in this example case by 1/2 in each direction. Shrinking the image is important as we eventually want to get away from details of a picture to a more high-level (semantic) description of the input. Replacing some image patch with only the max value of its pixels seems to be a rather drastic way of doing this, and some other proposals have been proposed. For example, we could take the average of the pixels. Such an average pooling is in practice not so much different than the max pooling operation. To reduce the signal size we could also shift the filter by more than one pixel every time it is applied. The number of pixels for which the filter is moved every time during a convolution operation is called a stride. Much more advanced techniques have been proposed, such as capsule networks, but this is beyond our discussion at this point.

The next layer we add is a dropout layer. This is actually not really a new layer but a post-processing of the current layer so turn off randomly some of the nodes. The probability of a neuron to be turned off is set to 25% in our example. Dropout is a common technique to prevent overfitting. Overfitting in neural networks can happen when individual neurons become very sensitive to specific training examples, and turning neurons off randomly during training forces a more distributed representation. This can be seen as a type of data augmentation as the next layer has to learn noisy versions of the patterns and hence cannot specialize on single sharp features. Dropout is only turned on during training as we want all the neuron active during predictive recalls. Since dropout affects the training accuracy it is possible that the training accuracy is lower than the accuracy of the test set.

At the end we feed this new representation of the image into a classification network which is an MLP in itself. The function `layers.Flatten()` does flatten the features into a one-dimensional vector that is the input to the MLP. The rest of the code specifies to train this network and to evaluate it similar to our previous examples.

CNNs do improve the MNIST recognition even further and are now at the point where they can recognize most examples in the test set. Running this network in a reasonable time requires a GPU, but it is easy to get accuracies above 99%. Indeed, we are getting to a point where the few mistakes of the network can even be questioned to be real mistakes. For example, an interesting variant of such networks has been studied by Jürgen Schmidhuber's lab using a design with several parallel CNN streams that resemble an ensemble method similar to classification forests discussed in Chapter 3. They showed that such a network is able to recognizes all but 32 examples. These examples are shown in Fig. 7.15 together with their 'correct' label shown in the upper right corner and the first and second choice produced by the network at the bottom of each image. I leave it to the reader to judge for themselves if these labels are sensible.

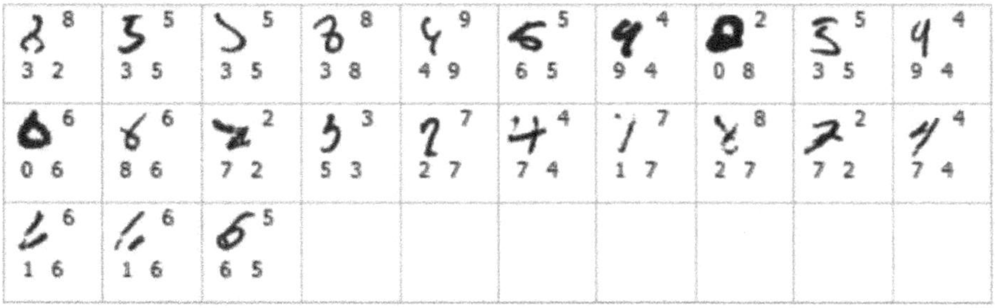

Fig. 7.15 The examples of the MNIST test set that were misclassified in the networks [from Dan Ciresan, Ueli Meier, and Jürgen Schmidhuber, Multi-column Deep Neural Networks for Image Classification: Technical Report Number IDSIA{04-12, p. 4, Figure 2b, © The Authors, 2012].

7.4 Probabilistic interpretation of MLPs

The focus of the above sections of this chapter were concerned with the important realization of feedforward neural networks as function approximators and classifiers. We will elaborate in this section on their embedding in a probabilistic interpretation, which is important in the context of a brain theory that emphasizes a model for an uncertain world.

7.4.1 Probabilistic regression

We have previously stressed that a MLP can be seen as a universal function approximator. We have also used them, together with there convolutional cousins, as a classifier. We will now discuss their useful interpretation in probabilistic regression and classification. This is not only relevant for a deeper understanding of such models, but also for our understanding of the role of brain processing. The challenge in modelling the world is taking uncertainty into account, and describing such models in terms of uncertainty or probability is therefore valuable if not essential.

Let us illustrate the problem with a linear regression problem where data are normally distributed around a linear function $y = wx$ as illustrated in Fig. 7.16. More precisely, the probability of a data point having a value of y given the feature value x is

$$p(y|x; \mathbf{w}) = N(wx, 1) \tag{7.45}$$

$$= \frac{1}{\sqrt{2\pi}} \exp\left(-\frac{1}{2}(y - wx)^2\right). \tag{7.46}$$

This functions specifies the likelihood (probability) of values for y, given an input x and the model with parameter w. While we demonstrate this here with this simple one-dimensional function, the general principle can immediately be generalized to high-dimensional non-linear functions like the ones implemented by MLPs. Specifying a model with a density function is an important step in modern modelling and machine learning. In this type of thinking, we treat data from the outset as fundamentally stochastic. That is, data can be different even in situations that we have identical inputs.

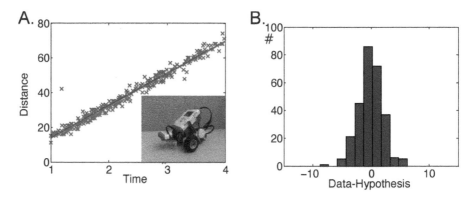

Fig. 7.16 (A) distances traveled of a small robot that is going back and forth in front of a wall and measures the distances with an ultrasonic sensor. (B) The distribution of data points around the red regression line in (A).

The question of learning is now how to determining the parameters of the model from example data. In a probabilistic framework we seek the parameters which would make the example data most likely under the model. This maximum likelihood principle is implemented by considering how likely each given training point is. If the training samples are independent of each other, then the probability encountering all m values is the product of the probability of each data point,

$$p(y^{(1)}, y^{(2)}, ..., y^{(m)} | \mathbf{x}^{(1)}, \mathbf{x}^{(2)}, ..., \mathbf{x}^{(m)}; w) = \Pi_i^m p(y^{(i)} | \mathbf{x}(i); w). \tag{7.47}$$

Inserting the values of the given data point results in a function of the parameters. This function is called the likelihood function

$$L(w) - \Pi_i^m p(w; y^{(i)}, x^{(i)}). \tag{7.48}$$

Since this function it is not a probability density function, we replaced the notation of the vertical bar '|' with the semi-colon ';'. Instead of evaluating this large product, it is common to use the logarithm of the likelihood function, so that we can use the sum over the training examples,

$$l(w) = \log L(w) = \sum_i^m \log(p(w; y^{(i)}, x^{(i)})). \tag{7.49}$$

The logarithmic function increases monotonically. Hence, the maximum of L is also the maximum of l. The maximum (log-)likelihood can thus be calculated from the training data as

$$\boldsymbol{w}^{\mathrm{MLE}} = \mathrm{argmax}_w l(w; x^{(1)}, y^{(1)} ..., x^{(m)}, y^{(m)}). \tag{7.50}$$

In case of the Gaussian example above, this is given by

$$l(w) = \log \Pi_{i=1}^m \frac{1}{\sqrt{2\pi}} \exp\left(-\frac{(y^{(i)} - wx^{(i)})^2}{2}\right) \tag{7.51}$$

$$= \sum_{i=1}^m \left(\log \frac{1}{\sqrt{2\pi}} - \frac{(y^{(i)} - wx^{(i)})^2}{2}\right) \tag{7.52}$$

$$= -\frac{m}{2} \log 2\pi - \sum_{i=1}^m \frac{(y^{(i)} - w\mathbf{x}^{(i)})^2}{2}. \tag{7.53}$$

Here you can see why the log is a good choice as we can look at a sum instead having a long product of potentially very small numbers. Since the first term in the expression in eqn 7.53, $-\frac{m}{2} \log 2\pi$, is independent of w, maximizing the log-likelihood function is equivalent to minimizing (because of the minus sign) a quadratic error term. So, in general, with Gaussian distributed data around a non-linear and potentially high-dimensional hypothesis function $h(\mathbf{x}; \mathbf{w})$, maximizing the likelihood of data is equivalent to minimizing the least mean square (LMS) error function.

$$E = \frac{1}{2}(y - h(\mathbf{x}; \mathbf{w}))^2. \tag{7.54}$$

So using the LMS in neural networks has some important probabilistic justification. However, we also see that there is room for optimizing models when the statistical assumptions differ.

7.4.2 Probabilistic classification

In a similar way, we can consider classification as probabilistic logistic regression. In classification, features are mapped to a finite number of possible categories, and the simplest example for this is binary classification. A probabilistic version of this is the Bernoulli model in which a random number takes the value of $y = 1$ with probability ϕ, and the value $y = 0$ with probability $1 - \phi$. Let us consider the case of classification when the parameter ϕ, depends on an attribute in a non-linear way such as

$$p(y) = \phi(\mathbf{x}; \mathbf{w})^y 1 - \phi(\mathbf{x}; \mathbf{w})^{1-y}. \tag{7.55}$$

The corresponding log-likelihood function is the cross-entropy

$$l(\mathbf{w}) = \sum_{i=1}^{m} y^{(i)} \, log(\phi(\mathbf{x}; \mathbf{w})) + (1 - y^{(i)}) \, log(1 - \phi(\mathbf{x}; \mathbf{w})). \tag{7.56}$$

To find the corresponding maximum we can use the gradient ascent algorithm,

$$\mathbf{w} \leftarrow \mathbf{w} + \alpha \nabla_{\mathbf{w}} l(\mathbf{w}). \tag{7.57}$$

To calculate the gradient we can calculate the partial derivative of the log-likelihood function with respect to each parameters,

$$\frac{\partial l(\mathbf{w})}{\partial w_j} = \left(y \frac{1}{\phi} - (1 - y) \frac{1}{1 - \phi} \right) \frac{\partial \phi(\mathbf{w})}{\partial w_j} \tag{7.58}$$

where we dropped indices for better readability.

Let us apply this to logistic regression. An example of 100 sample points of two classes (crosses and stars) are shown in Fig. 7.17. The data suggest that it is far more likely that the class is $y = 0$ for small values of x and that the class is $y = 1$ for large values of x, and the probabilities are more similar in between. Thus, we put forward the hypothesis that the transition between the low and high probability region is smooth and qualify this hypothesis as parameterized density function known as a logistic function or sigmoid function

$$\phi(\mathbf{x}; \mathbf{w}) = \frac{1}{1 + \exp(-\mathbf{w}^T \mathbf{x})}. \tag{7.59}$$

As before, we can treat this density function as function of the parameters $\mathbf{w}$ for the given data values (likelihood function), and use maximum likelihood estimation to estimate values for the parameters so that the data are most likely. The density function with sigmoidal offset $w_0 = 2$ and slope $w_1 = 4$ is plotted as solid line in Fig. 7.17.

We can now calculate the derivative of the hypothesis function ϕ with respect to the parameters for the specific choice of the logistic functions. This is given by

$$\frac{\partial \phi}{\partial w} = \frac{\partial}{\partial w} \frac{1}{1 + e^{-wx}} \tag{7.60}$$

$$= \frac{1}{(1 + e^{-wx})^2} e^{-wx}(-x) \tag{7.61}$$

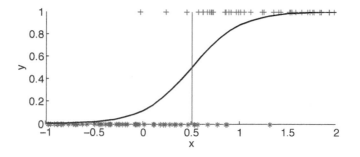

Fig. 7.17 Binary random numbers (stars) drawn from the density $p(y = 1) = \frac{1}{1+\exp(-w_1 x - w_0)}$ (solid line).

$$= \frac{1}{(1 + e^{-wx})}(1 - \frac{1}{(1 + e^{-wx})})(-x) \tag{7.62}$$

$$= -\phi(1 - \phi)x \tag{7.63}$$

Using this in eqn 7.58 and inserting it into eqn 7.57 with the identity

$$\left(y\frac{1}{\phi} - (1 - y)\frac{1}{1 - \phi}\right)\phi(1 - \phi) = y(1 - \phi) - (1 - y)\phi \tag{7.64}$$

$$= y - y\phi - \phi + y\phi \tag{7.65}$$

$$= y - \phi \tag{7.66}$$

gives the learning rule

$$w_j \leftarrow w_j + \alpha \left(y^{(i)} - f(\mathbf{x}^{(i)}; \mathbf{w})\right) x_j^{(i)} \tag{7.67}$$

This is equivalent to the perceptron learning rule we discussed before. Our derivation shows that this learning rule relates to assumptions of a probabilistic model.

7.4.3 Maximum a posteriori (MAP) and regularization with priors

Before moving to more complex multivariate models, this is a good opportunity to discuss regularization in from of weight decay in a probabilistic (Bayesian) framework. Maximum likelihood estimation is the workhorse of probabilistic supervised learning, though it is useful to put this even into a wider context of probabilistic modelling. In the probabilistic sense, choosing parameters values, given data, should be based on a model of the parameters themselves,

$$p(\mathbf{w}|\mathbf{x}, y). \tag{7.68}$$

Let us assume we can know this conditional distribution. For example, let us assume it looks like the one-dimensional example shown in Fig. 7.18. If we know this distribution we can pick a parameter value that we like. For example, we could pick the value w_1, which is the most probable value given the specific data. This is called the maximum a posteriori (MAP)

$$\mathbf{w}^{\mathrm{MAP}} = \mathrm{argmax}_{\mathbf{w}} p(\mathbf{w}|\mathbf{x}, y). \tag{7.69}$$

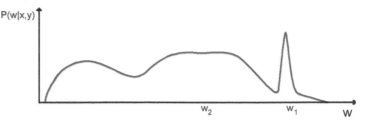

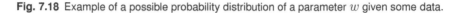

Fig. 7.18 Example of a possible probability distribution of a parameter w given some data.

The main difficulty with MAP or using another procedure based on the distribution $p(\boldsymbol{w}|\mathbf{x}, y)$ is that we usually do not know this distribution a priori. Instead, our approach has been to formulate a probabilistic model in the form of a parameterized density function like

$$p(y|\mathbf{x}; \mathbf{w}). \tag{7.70}$$

We will now discuss the relation of these density functions. To start with, in the probabilistic model of eqn 7.70, we assumed that the feature data are magically given, but we could also consider how we select data values in a randomized fashion so that we can again consider the more general case

$$p(y, \mathbf{x}|\mathbf{w}) = p(y|\mathbf{x}; \mathbf{w})p(\mathbf{x}|\mathbf{w}). \tag{7.71}$$

Again, if we pick the training data uniformly, so that the marginal distribution over the features is just a constant, then

$$p(y, \mathbf{x}|\mathbf{w}) \propto p(y|\mathbf{x}; \mathbf{w}). \tag{7.72}$$

Next, we can use Bayes's theorem to relate the posterior $p(\mathbf{w}|\mathbf{x}, y)$ to the data model, namely

$$p(\mathbf{w}|\mathbf{x}, y) = \frac{p(y, \mathbf{x}|\mathbf{w})p(\mathbf{w})}{\int_{\mathbf{w}' \in W} p(\mathbf{x}, y|\mathbf{w}')p(\mathbf{w}')d\mathbf{w}'}, \tag{7.73}$$

where W is the domain of the possible parameter values.

This expression can be used to estimate the most likely values for the parameters. For this we should notice that the denominator, which is called the partition function, does not depend on the parameters $\mathbf{w}$ as we are integrating (summing) over all possible values. The most likely values for the parameters can thus be calculated without this term and are given by the maximum a posteriori (MAP) estimate,

$$\boldsymbol{w}^{\mathrm{MAP}} = \mathrm{argmax}_\mathbf{w} p(\mathbf{x}, y|\boldsymbol{w})p(\boldsymbol{w}). \tag{7.74}$$

The name of the method comes from the fact that we modify our prior knowledge of parameters, which is summarized as prior distribution $p(\boldsymbol{w})$ by combining this to measurements $(\mathbf{x}, y)$ from specific realizations of the parameters, which is given by the likelihood function $p(\mathbf{x}, y|\boldsymbol{w})$. The resulting posterior distribution should then be a better estimate of the probability of values for the parameters. The function $\mathrm{argmax}_x(f(x))$ picks the argument x for which the function $f(x)$ is maximal. The argument of the function is the set of parameters that is, in a Bayesian sense, the most likely value for the parameters, where, of course, we now treat the probability function as a function of the parameters (e.g., a likelihood function). For a uniform prior, $p(\mathbf{w}) = const$, we get

$$\mathbf{w}^{\text{MAP}} = \mathbf{w}^{\text{MLE}}. \tag{7.75}$$

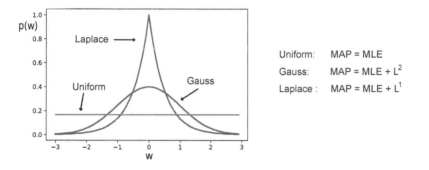

Fig. 7.19 Three distribution commonly used as priors for the parameters when learning together with a maximum likelihood estimate.

While a uniform prior of the parameters has been an easy first choice, we can think of other priors. For example, let us assume that the values of the parameters should more likely be small rather than large. More specifically, let's assume that we think they should be normal distributed around 0. Then we can write the MAP estimate (eqn 7.74) as

$$\boldsymbol{w}^{\text{MAP}} = \text{argmax}_{\mathbf{w}} p(\mathbf{x}, y | \boldsymbol{w}) \mathcal{N}(0, \sigma^2). \tag{7.76}$$

As usual, we maximize the logarithm of the corresponding likelihood functions instead, which leads to

$$\boldsymbol{w}^{\text{MAP}} = \text{argmax}_{\mathbf{w}} \log(p(\mathbf{x}, y | \boldsymbol{w})) + \alpha ||w||^2, \tag{7.77}$$

with

$$\alpha = \log \frac{1}{2\sigma^2}. \tag{7.78}$$

This is also called a L^2 regularization that hence corresponds to a Gaussian prior on the weights. Similarly, L^1 regularization correspond to a prior of a isotropic Laplace distribution

$$p(\mathbf{w}) = \frac{1}{2b} \exp\left(-\frac{|\mathbf{w}|}{b}\right), \tag{7.79}$$

which is more peaked towards 0 as can be seen by a comparison of these distributions in Fig. 7.19. Hence the L^1 regularization forces more weights towards 0 compared to the L^2 regularization. This is another example showing how a probabilistic interpretation sheds some light on techniques that have been originally introduced more heuristically. A simple summary of the three priors and their resulting equivalence between MLE and MAP is shown in the table on the right of the figure.

Finally, while we have discussed the common quantities of MAP and MLE in machine learning, it is good to realize that both learning methods only give us a point estimate, a single answer for the most likely values of the parameters given a specific data set from which this likelihood has to be estimated. A point estimate is commonly used to make decisions about which actions to take. However, it is possible that other sets of parameter values might only have a little smaller likelihood value, and the situation could quickly change with a few more data points. It is therefore much more prudent to consider also other values. For example, looking again at the example in Fig. 7.18, another strategy might be to pick a weight value in a range where variations in this value would not change the probability considerably in some range, such as values around w_2.

Moreover, in a Bayesian sense, all other choices should be taken into account with their corresponding likelihood. This is particularly true when estimating our confidence for an estimation. In a Bayesian sense, we need to combine all possible estimates with their likelihood. Thus, a limit of the maximum estimation methods discussed earlier, which are dominating much of the current practices in machine learning applications, is that they do not take distribution of answers into account. Some people thus distinguish machine learning from more advanced probabilistic programming. While such advanced probabilistic modelling techniques can give us answer to much deeper questions, the machine learning methods discussed in this book with point estimates are commonly easier to apply to high-dimensional problems.

7.4.4 Mapping networks with context units

The study of cognitive abilities of humans reveals that our behaviour, for example the execution of particular motor actions, often depends on the context in which we encounter a certain situation. For example, we might encounter an equivalent situation on two consecutive days, such as seeing a person in front of a house who is apparently studying the building in some detail. On the first day we might just think that this person is interested in architecture and we will likely proceed without acting further on this encounter. In the morning of the second day we might read in the newspaper about an increase in burglaries in the area, and seeing the person of the previous day again studying a house might very well prompt us to enquire about his or her intentions.

A simple architecture that demonstrates some form of contextual processing was proposed by Jeffrey Elman and is sometimes called an Elman-net. An example is outlined in Fig. 7.20, which illustrates a mapping network with four input nodes, three hidden nodes, and four output nodes. In addition to the standard feedforward mapping components, the network has context nodes. The three context nodes shown in the figure contain the activation of the hidden nodes of the previous time step. Furthermore, the activations of the context units are fed back into the system as internal inputs (rather than external inputs) for the next time step. The architecture therefore includes a new class of projections that feed into cells which, in turn, can influence the sending node at a later time. The network is therefore said to be recurrent. This type of physical back-projection should not be confused with the information flow that is used during training the networks, such as in the error-back-propagation algorithm discussed above.

The network in Fig. 7.20 is only one example of this class of networks, where we have included context nodes that receive inputs from the hidden nodes. We can also include context units that receive inputs directly from output or input nodes. The latter remember the input of the previous time step, and such a mechanism is often termed

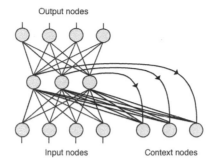

Fig. 7.20 Recurrent mapping networks as proposed by Jeffrey Elman consisting of a standard feedforward mapping network with four input nodes, three hidden nodes, and four output nodes. However, the network also receives internal input from context nodes that are efferent copies of the hidden node activities. The efferent copy is achieved through fixed one-to-one projections from the hidden nodes to the context nodes that can be implemented by fixed weights with some time delay.

short-term memory. We will discuss related but distinct forms of short-term memory as used in the physiology and psychology literature in Chapter 9.

The context units in the example of Fig. 7.20 are designed to contain the activity of the hidden nodes at the previous time step. This can formally be achieved with linear units and setting the weight values to one while assuming some delay in the projections. The network functions as follows. For each input to the network, consisting of the external input from the input nodes and from the context nodes (which memorized the previous firing rates of the hidden nodes), we calculate the activation of the hidden nodes and then the activation of the output nodes. The activation of the hidden nodes is also copied to the context nodes. All this can be thought of as a basic time step of the network. Thus, we can treat the network at each time step as a standard feedforward mapping network and can thus use the back-propagation algorithm discussed before. However, the function of the network now has inherent time dynamics in that there is a new input to the hidden nodes at the next time step (even with the same external input from the input nodes as in the previous time step). To take into account the context during training we have to train the network on whole sequences of inputs. The advantage is that the network can generate sequences of outputs, and we can thus use those models in a wider context. In particular, these networks can learn to predict the next output in a sequence of symbols, and they have been used primarily in this context.

7.5 The anticipating brain

Most of this chapter was dedicated to the discussion of the capabilities of multilayer perceptrons as function approximators and their ability for hierarchical representational learning. In general, such networks are capable to perform complex transformations, something that is clearly needed for advanced information processing. However, while the information-processing principles of neural networks are fundamentally important, it does not seem the only necessary mechanisms to realize minds. To end this chapter, we take the idea of neural mapping and representational networks a bit further with an architecture that seems to describe better brain organizations and processing.

Central to this emerging brain theory is the view of the brain as an anticipating memory system or a generative model of the world. We will also incorporate several processing principles that seem essential in realizing cognitive functions.

1. The brain can develop a model of the world, which can be used to anticipate or predict the environment.
2. The inverse of the model can be used to recognize causes by evoking internal concepts.
3. Hierarchical representations are essential to capture the richness of the world.
4. Internal concepts are learned through matching the brain's hypotheses with input from the world.
5. An agent can learn actively by testing hypothesis through actions.
6. The temporal domain is an important degree of freedom.

The remainder of this chapter is a discussion of the anticipating brain hypothesis and related model implementations. We start with a general overview of the anticipating brain which should show more clearly how the points above are related. We then outline some specific models and discuss their relation to statistical methods of generative density estimation.

7.5.1 The brain as anticipatory system in a probabilistic framework

To formalize the thesis we need to introduce some notations which help to discuss the systems in a compact way. We start by denoting a sensory state with a vector $mathbf s$, where the components can be any relevant quantity, such as spikes or firing rates of primary sensory neurons. Also, these sensory states can describe any kinds of sensations, including olfaction, touch, vestibular senses, proprioreceptive feedback, and vision. Sensory states are caused by physical processes in the environment, and we can formalize this by writing the sensory state as a function of a causal state, $\mathbf{c}$,

$$\mathbf{s} = g(\mathbf{c}). \tag{7.80}$$

The function g describes the physical process of generating the sensory response. We can refine this notation further by recognizing that the brain can respond with changing patterns to stimulations from the world. The reasons for different responses include noise somewhere in the system and/or the dependency of the system on hidden variables. In any case, it is thus appropriate to consider the probability that a certain sensory state is evoked by a given causal state,

$$p(\mathbf{s}|\mathbf{c}). \tag{7.81}$$

This describes the conditional probability (or conditional probability density) of having a sensory state given a specific set of causes. Thus, a sensory state, as considered here, can be different for identical presentations of a sensory scene. Only the probability of finding a specific sensory state depends on the environmental condition.

While we alluded here to the physical causes of a specific sensory state, the key idea is that the brain represents a model of the world that can represent the causes internally and is hence able to generate corresponding generative states. This is hence a generative model

$$\text{Generative brain model:} \quad p(\mathbf{s}|\mathbf{c}; \theta). \tag{7.82}$$

We have used here the same symbol c of the causes although these are really the causes as represented in the brain and as re hence a function of the firing of neurons, $\mathbf{c}(\mathbf{r})$. The distinction of the model causes and real world causes can easily be made from the notion that the model density function has parameters θ. Before we move to outlining how to learn such models, we want to stay a bit longer at this high level to discuss the big picture.

While it is likely that everyone understands, to some extent, what is meant by the word 'cause', it is interesting to realize that there can be different opinions on the causes inferred by different agents. For example, imagine sitting in a concert hall and listening to a symphony. What are the causes of our experience in this situation? Or, more precisely, on which level should we define causes? Should the orchestra as a whole be considered a cause, or an individual player, or her instrument, or even parts of the instrument? While it might seem a bit niggling to contemplate this issue, resolving it is central to our thesis and highlights two important functions of brain processing. First, we propose that one of the major goals of the brain is to learn what causes are by forming internal concepts. Second, the brain must learn concepts at different levels of abstraction, from some concrete representations of sensory states, such as edges of objects or sound fragments, to more abstract representations such as going to a concert. Learning concepts and predicting causes in our environment is thus central to the thesis developed here.

When considering learning of concepts which can explain causes, it will be important to consider systems that can explore the environment actively. The notation of 7.81 would only be appropriate for a passive observer. Instead, we should explicitly consider that the carrier of the brain, called an agent in the following, can interact with the environment. For example, the agent could direct its gaze to specific locations in space, or the agent could touch an object or pick it up to test some hypothesis about the object or the environment. We denote an action of the agent with a vector $\mathbf{a}$ to allow for distributed representations of motor output. We thus consider the probability of sensory states, given causes in the environment, and specific actions of the agent by writing:

$$p(\mathbf{s}|\mathbf{c}, \mathbf{a}). \tag{7.83}$$

The central conjecture followed now is that the brain is trying to match sensory input with internally generated states. The internal representations of sensory states in primary sensory cortex are denoted by $\mathbf{s}'$. While these states depend on input from the environment, they also depend on expectations from higher cortical areas. More specifically, the distribution of the cortical sensory states, s', depends on the primary input from the environment, s, and some states, c', of higher cortical areas:

$$p(\mathbf{s}'|s, c'). \tag{7.84}$$

We call these higher-order cortical representations concepts. Concepts on a certain level of cortical representations depend in turn on concepts of higher-order cortical representations, c'', c''', etc., which in turn are influenced by input from lower cortical areas.

On an abstract level, we see the brain as a generative model of the world, G, which can generate probability distributions of concepts on different levels, ultimately generating expectations of sensory states:

$$p(\mathbf{s}'; G). \tag{7.85}$$

The inverse of the model can be seen as a recognition model, Q, which evokes internal concepts from causes in the environment. The world model, which is embedded in the central nervous system, is dissected according to the above discussion in Fig. 7.21 with a layered structure that includes the necessary bidirectional connections. Such related models have been termed deep belief networks; 'belief networks' for their ability to generate expectations, and 'deep' for their layered architecture. At this stage it is not easy to clearly separate the generative model from the recognition model, since the whole system is highly interactive, but the distinction of a generative and recognition model can sometimes be made explicit, as discussed below.

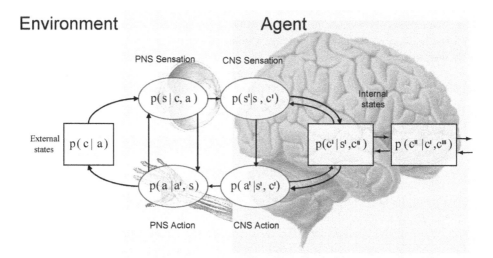

Fig. 7.21 Illustration of an agent–environment system with probabilistic notations describing various components of the system. The illustration includes the environment which causes sensory experiences of the agent. The interface between the environment is illustrated as the peripheral nervous system (PNS) with exemplary sensory and action components. The central nervous system (CNS) is a predictive memory system with layered representations [extended from Friston, *Philosophical Transactions of the Royal Society* B 360, 815–36 (2005)].

The concepts at different levels of cortical representation have to be learned in n self-supervised way through the interaction with the environment and ingrained into a memory system. For example, the early visual system can learn to recognize different sequences of retinal patterns. Sequences of these concepts can then be learned by higher-order cortical areas. In turn, higher-order concepts that are evoked by specific sensory input can influence the expectations of concepts in lower cortical representations, ultimately anticipating specific patterns of sensory input. We discuss below a more concrete system that shows some of these abilities.

Testing how good the world model is can only be achieved though interactions with the environment. This can be seen as hypothesis testing, or inference, of the world model with environmental data. We presented the state of the environment, $p(\mathbf{c}|\mathbf{a})$ as a probabilistic quantity, which does not only mean that causes are noisy, but incorporates that causes are changing beyond our control. The conditional probability on the actions generated by the agent describes that the world states can be influenced by actions generated by the agent. Thus, hypothesis testing by the agent is somewhat different from common inference techniques in statistics in that the agent seems to be able to actively interact with the environment. Activation of specific concepts can guide specific actions, which, in turn, can manipulate the environment in a specific way, which in turn can guide further learning. For example, when whistling to a child, he might first recognize the funny face and unusual shape of the mouth. The child might then form a hypothesis that the mouth has something to do with the whistling sound and might touch the mouth to verify this hypothesis. Such active learning might be necessary to reduce the demands on learning in large systems.

7.5.2 Variational free energy principle

A key way of formulating and realizing these ideas is the concept of variational free energy introduced by Karl Friston. Making sense of the world would mean that we know what the causes are of a given sensory information, of course in a probabilistic sense,

$$\text{True recognition (posterior):} \quad p(\mathbf{c}|\mathbf{s}) = \frac{p(\mathbf{c}, \mathbf{s})}{p(\mathbf{s})}. \tag{7.86}$$

Now, measuring and modelling $p(\mathbf{c}, \mathbf{s})$ might not be too bad as we have just to record a lot of combinations between causes and sensory states, but evaluating all possible sensory states to calculate the marginal $p(\mathbf{s})$ is usually not tractable. To solve this problem, let us introduce a recognition model

$$\text{Recognition model:} \quad q = p(\mathbf{c}|\mathbf{s}; \mathbf{w}) \tag{7.87}$$

with parameters $\mathbf{w}$. This model is useful if we minimize the difference between this model and the true posterior

$$q^* = \text{argmin}_w KL(p(\mathbf{C}|\mathbf{s}; \mathbf{w}).p(\mathbf{s}|\mathbf{c})). \tag{7.88}$$

We used here the Kulbach-Leibler divergence for the difference measure as mentioned in Chapter 3.5.6, though other measures could be used as well. Now, this does not help us too much so far as we do not know the true posterior $p(\mathbf{s}|\mathbf{c})$. However, we can also modify the KL divergence with Bayes's rule,

$$KL(q, p) = KL(q, \frac{p(\mathbf{s}), \mathbf{c}}{p(\mathbf{s})}) \tag{7.89}$$

$$= KL(q, p(\mathbf{s}, \mathbf{c})) + \ln(p(\mathbf{s})) \tag{7.90}$$

$$\leq KL(q, p(\mathbf{s}, \mathbf{c})) = F \tag{7.91}$$

The last line defines the variational free energy, which is hence an upper bound on the difference between true and model posterior. Minimizing this upper bound will

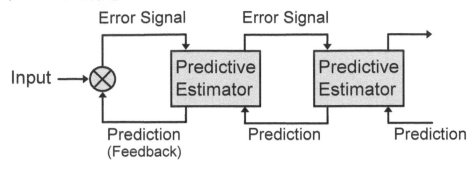

Fig. 7.22 Illustration of a predictive coding neural network where the hierarchical neural network can predict visual input by minimizing the prediction error in the input and on each level of representations. This minimization takes place on a short time scale for recognition and on a longer time scale for learning.

minimize this difference. This still leaves us with the joined probability of causes and sensory data, and this is where the generative brain model comes in handy. We can use this model together with a prior probability of causes in the model, $p(\mathbf{c}; \theta)$.

$$\text{generative + prior:} \quad p(\mathbf{c}, \mathbf{s}|\theta) = p(\mathbf{s}|\mathbf{c}; \theta)p(\mathbf{c}; \theta). \tag{7.92}$$

So we have now to estimate (learn) two sets of parameters, the recognition model weights $\mathbf{w}$ and the generative model weights θ. To do this we use a scheme called EM which stands for expectation maximization where we fix one parameter set to learn the other by minimizing the free energy and visa versa.

$$\mathbf{w}_{t+1} = \text{argmin}_{\mathbf{w}} F(\mathbf{w}, \theta_t) \tag{7.93}$$
$$\theta_{t+1} = \text{argmin}_{\theta} F(\mathbf{w}_t, \theta). \tag{7.94}$$

Thus, we can build complex models that explains the environment by learning through minimizing the variational free energy. This will minimize the surprise, maximizing the likelihood of observed data.

7.5.3 Deep sparse predictive coding

The above discussion seems abstract, and it is useful to discuss the influential example of the realization of such a model as given by Rajesh Rao and Dana Ballard in 1999 in which they showed that these kind of models can explain some interesting details of receptive fields. As outlined above, the brain activity should be able to generate sensory input that can match the real world. In this way of thinking, we would turn the direction of the perceptron around, making higher-order neural activity predict lower-order activity until it can match sensory input. The reverse information flow can then carry the prediction error to be minimized by learning. Minimizing the prediction error is thereby equivalent to minimizing the variational free energy for Gaussian models.

The architecture is illustrated in Fig. 7.22 from the seminal work of Rao and Ballard from 1999. Thus, we consider now image I that should be closely matched by combining basis vectors $\mathbf{w}_i^1$,

$$I = g(\sum_i \mathbf{w}_i^1 r_i^1) + \nu^1 \tag{7.95}$$

$$= g(\mathbf{w}^1 \mathbf{r}^1) + \nu^1. \tag{7.96}$$

We used here again the symbol w for the parameters instead of the generative model parameters θ above as we do now consider again the model implementation with neural networks. Also, in the equation above, we allowed for some small deviation of the image I and the reconstruction $g(\mathbf{w}^1 \mathbf{r}^1)$ that we counted for with a noise term ν^1. For a good generative model, we want to minimize two things. The first one is that we want a small reconstruction error. We can measure this objective with the square error between the image and the reconstruction,

$$E = \frac{1}{(\sigma^1)^2} ||I - g(\mathbf{w}^1 \mathbf{r}^1)||^2. \tag{7.97}$$

Before discussing our second desired constraint, we want to make this generative model hierarchical so that we can extend this to deep learning. This is easily done by repeating the idea that a higher-order neural activation predicts the lower-level activity like

$$r^1 = g(\sum_i \mathbf{W}_i^2 r_i^2) + \mu^2 \tag{7.98}$$

$$= g(\mathbf{w}\mathbf{r}) + \mu^2. \tag{7.99}$$

The objective function to be minimized should then be the error term from both levels,

$$E = \frac{1}{(\sigma^1)^2} ||I - g(\mathbf{w}^1 \mathbf{r}^1)||^2 + \frac{1}{(\sigma^1)^2} ||I - g(\mathbf{w}^1 \mathbf{r}^1)||^2. \tag{7.100}$$

As we outlined above, this objective function has an important probabilistic interpretation as it represents the minimization of the log-likelihood in a model that represents events within a Gaussian uncertainty. This probabilistic interpretation allows to an elegant formulation of the additional constraint that we want to pose onto our biological predictive network.

More specifically, beside the minimization of prediction error, there seems to be a second important factor to optimize in order to explain physiological findings in the brain. This factor is sparse coding. The idea of sparse coding in the brain has been advanced for many years by Horace Barlow (1961), and it was finally widely recognized in the modelling field with the beautiful demonstration by Olshausen and Field (1997). An efficient code is hereby considered to be a sparse vector $\mathbf{r}$ where only a small number of the coefficients r_i are non-zero. More specifically, even though we have a large number of neurons that can be active, only a small number of neurons should be active at a specific moment in time to represent one specific image. We can incorporate this constraint elegantly through a prior on the neural activity, such as $p(\mathbf{r}^1)$. For example, we could assume that the activations are distributed with a Gaussian around zero. This would be equivalent to a log-likelihood of $||\mathbf{r}^1||^2$. Other common choices are a Cauchy distribution with a log-likelihood of $\log(1 + ||\mathbf{r}^1||^2)$, or an exponential distribution with a log-likelihood of $||\mathbf{r}^1||$. Finally, we will also consider the priors of the filters corresponding to the weight matrices. If we also assume Gaussian priors for those, we reach the final objective function of

$$E = \frac{1}{(\sigma^1)^2}||I - g(\mathbf{w}^1\mathbf{r}^1)||^2 + \frac{1}{(\sigma^1)^2}||I - g(\mathbf{w}^1\mathbf{r}^1)||^2 - \frac{\alpha}{2}||\mathbf{r}^1||^2 - \frac{\beta}{2}||\mathbf{W}^1||^2 \quad (7.101)$$

with regularization parameters α and β.

As we outlined above, the weights can then be learned by following the gradient of this objective function, dE/dw_{ij}^1. While we are familiar with this gradient approach to learning synaptic weights, Rao and Ballard also used this objective function to derive the dynamic of the neuron activities by minimizing the objective function along the corresponding gradient dE/dr_i^1. In this equation we see that the activity of the neurons appear on the left-hand side and the right-hand side of the equation. This makes it formally a recurrent network as discussed and analysed more formally in Chapter 9. We will there see again that the activation dynamic of a neural network can be seen as a result of traversing along an energy surface.

The interpretation of brain processes as sparse predicitve coding has opened many explanations of neurophysiological findings. For example, receptive fields of early layer representations are matching physiological findings of Huble and Wiesel in the primary visual cortex. This includes the Gabor-shaped filters represented by the receptive fields as already discussed before, but also less-known effects such as surround suppression or end-stop cells.

7.5.4 Predictive coding of MNIST

We demonstrate here only a very simple implementation with one neural layer with program MNISTpredCode.py. Note that we only read in the images and do not use the labels in this program. This program is therefore an example of self-supervised training. We are only using 100 images in this example.

Programs/MNISTpredCode.py

```
1  import numpy as np
2  import matplotlib.pyplot as plt
3  import pandas as pd
4
5  df = pd.read_csv('mnist_784.csv')
6  X = df.iloc[:,0:784].values/255
7  X=np.append(X.T,np.array([np.ones(70000)]),axis=0)
8
9  # model specifications
10 N0=785; N1=128
11
12 #parameter and array initialization
13 Ntrials=100
14 w=np.random.randn(N1,N0)
15 error=np.array([])
16
17 for trial in range(Ntrials):
18     e=0
19     for i in range(100):
20         r=np.random.randn(N1)
21         for t in range(10):
```

```
22          dI=X[:,i]—w.T@r/N1
23          r=r+0.1*w@dI.T
24       w=w+0.1*np.outer(r,dI)
25       e=e+dI@dI
26    error=np.append(error,e)
27 plt.plot(np.sqrt(error))
```

Each of the 100 images is read in and compared with the prediction of the model. Since the weights are randomly chosen at the beginning, this is not a very good reproduction of the images. The error between the image and the prediction is then used to update the activations of the representational neurons according to the dynamics derived from the energy function. In this simple example we just took the prediction error with no further regularization term, and the normalization is choosen ad hoc instead of the estimated variance. The update is done with a step size of 0.1 for these 10 update steps. After this, we use the predicition error after the 10 activity iterations to update the weight values with a learning rate of 0.1. Since the weight updates are only done after the activation updates, the effective rate of change of the weights is therefore 10 times smaller than the update of the activations.

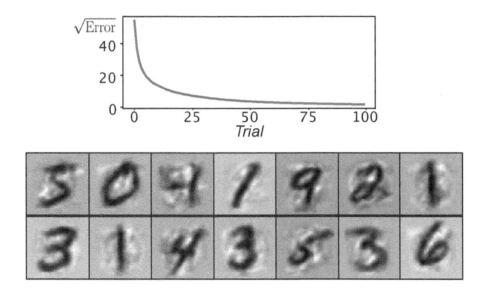

Fig. 7.23 The reconstruction of the first 14 examples from the MNIST dataset of hand-written digits (see Fig. 7.10).

The program prints out the evolution of the prediciton error at the end of the 10 activation iterations after each trial. This is shown in Fig. 7.23 on top. As can be seen, this prediction error diminishes which indicates learning. The reconstruction of the first 14 images of the MNIST data set are shown below which can be compared to the original images as shown in Fig. 7.10.

8 Feature maps and competitive population coding

This chapter is about representing information with maps, and about competitive dynamics in neuronal tissue. The chapter starts with an outline of a basic model of a hypercolumn in which neurons respond to specific sensory input with characteristic tuning curves. Such features are often represented in topographically organized maps in the brain. We discuss how such topographic feature maps can be self-organized. We then study the dynamics of activating such maps and model this with dynamic neural field theory. We discuss several examples of how signatures of such competitive dynamics can be seen in a variety of examples from different parts of the brain. This chapter includes some more formal discussions of population coding, as well as some extensions of the basic models including dynamic updates of internal representations through path-integration.

8.1 Competitive feature representations in cortical tissue

Neurons can represent features with tuning curves that represents their activation level with different feature values. Moreover, feature representations in the brain are are commonly organized topographically in the sense that neighbouring feature values are represented in adjacent neural tissue. A well-known example is that of orientation tuning curves in the primary visual cortex, as discovered by Hubel and Wiesel. We now put these observations together in a basic model of a hypercolumn. This model, shown in Fig. 8.1A, consists of a line of population nodes, each responding to a specific orientation. This orientation selectivity can be achieved by combining input from spatially selective cells, as indicated for some of the nodes. This model implements a specific hypothesis of cortical organization, namely, that the input to the orientation-selective cells is focal in the sense that it is very selective to a specific orientation and that the broadness of the tuning curves is primarily the result of lateral interactions indicated by arrows in the model.

Fig. 8.1C is a graph that shows the activity of nodes during a specific experiment. We used 100 population neurons for this demonstration that we call nodes in the following, but we will see later that this number of nodes is not essential. Each node corresponds to a certain orientation shown with the scale of degrees on the right. In this experiment, the response of the nodes was probed by externally activating a very small region, a narrow Gaussian essentially covering only one node, for a short time. After this time, the next node was activated, probing the response to consecutive orientations during this experiment. The nodes that receive external input for a specific orientation became very active. However, neighbouring nodes are also activated through lateral interactions

Fundamentals of Computational Neuroscience. Third edition. Thomas P. Trappenberg, Oxford University Press. © Oxford University Press 2023. DOI: 10.1093/oso/9780192869364.003.0008

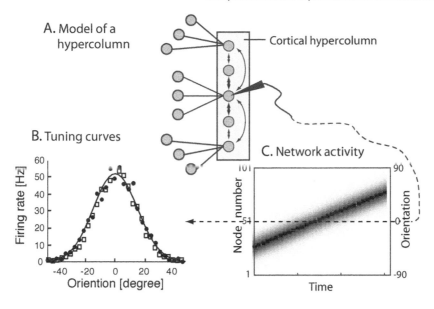

Fig. 8.1 (A) Basic model of a hypercolumn in which a lateral line of nodes is topographically organized to respond to specific orientations of line segments in the visual field. (B) The experimental data by Henry et al. (1974), as discussed in Section 5.4, are shown as solid circles, whereas recordings from the model are shown as open squares. (C) The evolution of the activity in the neural field during the experiment.

in the network. We call this consecutively active area an activity packet, although it is often simply called a bubble. The activation of the middle node, which responds maximally to an orientation of zero degrees, is plotted against the input orientation with open squares in Fig. 8.1B. The dots represent corresponding experimental data. The simulations also included noise proportional to the activation, not shown in Fig. 8.1C. As can be seen, the model data match the experimental data reasonably well.

Several assumptions and specific hypotheses are incorporated in this basic hypercolumn model. Specifically, we assumed in this model that orientation preference of hypercolumn nodes is systematically organized. The next section explores basic mechanisms leading to such organizations. The lateral interactions within the hypercolumn model are organized such that there is more excitation to neighbouring nodes, compared to more distant nodes, and there is inhibition between nodes that are even more remote. This lateral interaction in the model leads to dynamic properties of the model, which we study more formally in Section 8.3. Competition between features is often observed in physiological studies and has a multitude of behavioural consequences. The remainder of this chapter explores different applications and extensions of such models to demonstrate that this model captures basic brain processing mechanisms.

8.2 Self-organizing maps

Topographic maps in the brain have two major characteristics, namely that there is some order in feature space such that neighbouring areas represent neighbouring features, and that features with enhanced sensory resolution are over-represented with larger cortical space while preserving relations between feature values. The formation of such organizations is experience-dependent, since the formation of such maps can be disrupted in very young animals by sensory deprivation. While the formation of these maps is often viewed as a developmental process, there is increasing evidence that cortical maps can change dramatically even in mature age when given the opportunity. As discussed in Chapter 6, the models of Hebbian plasticity in this book describe changes of synaptic weight values in general and do not distinguish between developmental and functional plasticity. The models in this subsection can be seen as general models for activity-driven structural changes in neural maps, either during development or later in the life of an organism. Such maps are called self-organizing maps, or SOMs for short.

Note that the models discussed here are based on changes of neuronal responses based on Hebbian plasticity and long-range competition within the cortical sheet. There is some debated whether long-range topographical maps, such as the somatosensory homunculus shown in Fig. 1.7D, can be explained through synaptic organization mechanisms alone as it is also known that cortical development is guided by extracellular chemical substances. It is hence possible that ongoing topographic plasticity is guided by similar chemical processes. However, regardless of this physical implementation, the models here can be seen as an abstract level of activity-dependent organization.

8.2.1 The basic cortical map model

The model described here is based on a seminal paper by David Willshaw and Christoph von der Malsburg in 1976. We consider a two-dimensional cortical sheet, as illustrated in Fig. 8.2A. The nodes in this cortical sheet are population nodes with leaky integrator dynamics, as discussed in Chapter 5. However, we now consider these nodes in a network resembling a neural sheet. To simplify the notations, we write the following equations for a one-dimensional model with N nodes, as shown in Fig. 8.2B. It is straightforward to generalize the model to two or higher dimensions by using more indices (e.g. $i \rightarrow i_1 i_2 i_3$) or treating the index i as a vector (e.g. $i \rightarrow \mathbf{i}$). The change of the internal activation, u_i, of node i is given by:

$$\tau \frac{du_i(t)}{dt} = -u_i(t) + \frac{1}{N} \sum_j w_{ij} r_j(t) + \frac{1}{M} \sum_k w_{ik}^{in} r_k^{in}(t), \tag{8.1}$$

where τ is a time constant, w_{ij} is the lateral weight from node j to node i, w_{ik}^{in} is the connection weight from input node k to cortical node i, $r_k^{in}(t)$ is the rate of the input node k, and M is the number of input nodes. The activity of input nodes represents specific feature values, whereas the rate $r_i(t)$ of the cortical node i is related to the internal activation via an activation function. In this chapter we will primarily use the sigmoid function, with gain parameter β and offset parameter α,

$$r_j(t) = \frac{1}{1 + e^{\beta(u_j(t) - \alpha)}}. \tag{8.2}$$

Eqns 8.1 and 8.2 are the most fundamental equations used in many parts of this book. They were introduced in a slightly more general form by Stephen Grossberg in the late 1950s, and have since dominated many neural network models.

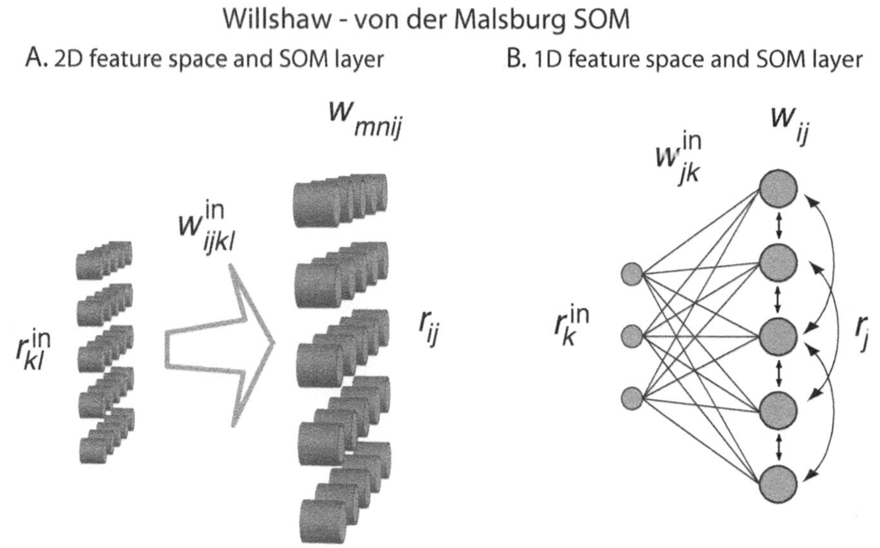

Willshaw - von der Malsburg SOM

A. 2D feature space and SOM layer   **B.** 1D feature space and SOM layer

Fig. 8.2 Architecture of self-organizing maps according to Willshaw and von der Marlburg in (A) two dimensions and (B) one dimension. The left layer of nodes represents sensory units and the right layer represents a cortical sheet. The purpose of the model is to illustrate learning experience based organization of input weights, while the weights in the cortical sheet have a fixed organization of short-distance excitation and long-distance inhibition.

The basic model defined by equations 8.1 and 8.2 distinguishes between two sets of weight values, the weight values of the input connections, w_{ik}^{in}, and the lateral weights in the cortical sheet w_{ij}. In this section we are concerned with learning the topographic mapping between input and output nodes while keeping the lateral weights fixed. Learning of the lateral weights will be considered later in this chapter. Here we set them to depend only on the distance between two nodes, with positive values (excitatory) for short distances and negative values (inhibitory) for large distances. Specifically, we chose a shifted Gaussian for most of the demonstrations,

$$w_{ij} = A_{\text{w}} \left(e^{-((i-j)*\Delta x)^2 / 2\sigma^2} - C \right), \tag{8.3}$$

with parameters A_{w}, σ, and C. To minimize boundary effects, we consider the model with periodic boundaries, so that the nodes form a ring (or a torus in higher dimensions).

The part considered next is the learning of input weights, w^{in}. We start with a random weight matrix so that no specific order is present before training. The learning follows general Hebbian philosophy. A specific feature is randomly selected, and the corresponding area around this feature value is activated in the input map. This activity triggers some response in the cortical map, likely at different places. However, an important feature of the dynamic in the cortical sheet with the lateral weights considered here is that this sheet functions as a kind of winner-takes-all (WTA) network in that it develops a dominating activity packet (as in Fig. 8.1C) through short-distant cooperation and long-distant competition. This will be discussed in more detail in Section 8.3 . Thus Hebbian learning of the input rates results in an increase of weights between the activated input nodes and the winning activity packet in the cortical sheet.

8.2.2 The Kohonen model

While Willshaw and von der Malsburg have demonstrated that the model leads to topographic organizations, we will demonstrate this with a much more efficient model introduced by Teuvo Kohonen. This model makes a number of simplifications that are appropriate for the following discussions and consistent with our philosophy of minimalistic modelling. The first simplification is that the representation of the input feature is changed. While a specific feature value is represented by the activation of a specific node in the previous model (e.g. by a coordinate of the activated node), the new model represents this feature value as activation value of one node in the one-dimensional model, or d input nodes in the d-dimensional case. A two-dimensional version of this model is shown in Fig. 8.3A and a one-dimensional version in Fig. 8.3B. With this feature representation, the values of the input connections should be interpreted as representing the preferred feature value (the preferred orientation in the case of V1 tuning curves) of the receiving nodes. To indicate this different interpretation of the connection values, we use the letter c for these connections (centres of the tuning curves). The activation of the cortical sheet, when activated with input r^{in}, is then given by

$$r_{ij} = \mathrm{e}^{-\sum_k (c_{ijk} - r_k^{\mathrm{in}})^2 / 2\sigma_{\mathrm{r}}^2},\tag{8.4}$$

where σ_{r} sets the width of the activated area. This activation function resembles the tuning curves discussed above, and networks with such activation functions are called radial-basis function (RBF) networks.

The next simplification is with respect to the dynamics of the recurrent cortical sheet. We mentioned already that the dynamics of the model led to responses of the neural sheet in the form of a tuning curve as shown in Fig. 8.1, at least in the situation of single feature inputs. It was also shown that the site of this tuning curve is determined by competitive mechanisms. The strongest active area will inhibit other activities in the network. The dynamics in the cortical sheet are therefore approximated with a WTA procedure. The activation of the cortical sheet after competition is set to the Gaussian (eqn 8.4), around the winning node. Thus, only the active area around the winning node participates in Hebbian learning, as outlined above. The learning of the input projections is therefore intended to make the current preferred feature of the winning node closer to the training example. Since neighbouring nodes in the cortical sheet are also activated, although less, these projections update in a similar way, but with less influence of the training example. Specifically, we use the learning rule:

$$\Delta c_{ijk} = \epsilon r_{ij}^*(r_i^{\mathrm{in}} - c_{ijk}),\tag{8.5}$$

which makes the connections to nodes around the winning node (labelled with a '*') more similar to the input example. The parameter ϵ specifies the learning rate.

The development of the centres of the tuning curves, c_{ijk}, in such a network with a cortical layer of 10×10 nodes is demonstrated in Fig. 8.4. In these figures, the

Kohonen SOM

A. 2-d feature space and SOM layer

B. 1-d feature space and SOM layer

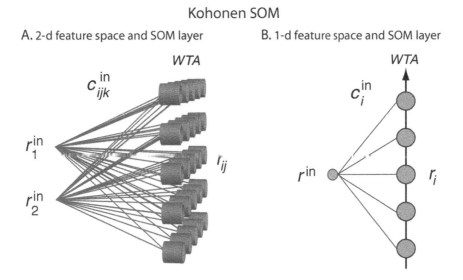

Fig. 8.3 Architecture of self-organizing maps according to Kohonen in (A) two dimensions and (B) one dimension. The WTA represents the procedure of finding the node with the maximal response for a given input feature.

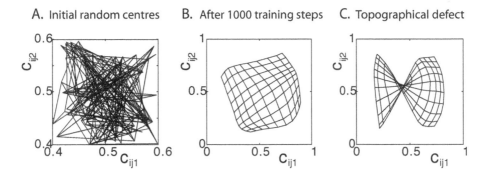

A. Initial random centres   B. After 1000 training steps   C. Topographical defect

Fig. 8.4 Experiment with two-dimensional self-organizing feature maps. (A) Initial map with random weight values. (B) and (C) Two examples of the resulting feature map after 500 random training examples with different random initial conditions.

locations of centres in feature space are plotted for each node as an intersection of lines, where the lines connect neighbouring nodes in the cortical sheet. The simulations were started with random values, as shown in Fig. 8.4A, so that no orderly relationship was present. The network was then exposed to equally distributed random examples within a unit square. After several training examples, we get a relatively homogeneous representation of the feature space as shown in Fig. 8.4B. The network has learned to represent the feature values of the training set in a topographic map in which neighbouring nodes represent neighbouring feature values. The form of the maps can differ dramatically depending on the initial conditions and the precise sequence of examples. In Fig. 8.4C, we show another example of the same simulations with a different initial state. A twist, or fold, in the representation occurred as different parts of the grid started organizing independently. Such results are not uncommon in simulations. They are sometimes called topographic defects and are stable in the sense that it is nearly impossible to unfold these twists. However, these can be avoided by, for example, using initially large σ values.

A program like som.py was used to produce the simulation plots in Fig. 8.4. As usual, we define some constants at the beginning. The constant sig2 is a shorthand notation of the denominator in the exponential of eqn 8.4. It is wise to define such reoccurring calculations with constants at the beginning of the program to save valuable computer time later. We also define constant matrices X and Y with the help of the numpy function meshgrid(). X is a matrix that contains the 'i' index of a node, and Y is a matrix that contains the 'j' index of a node. We need this later in the program to plot the mesh.

Programs/som.py

```
1  # Two dimensional self-organizing feature map al la Kohonen
2  import numpy as np
3  import matplotlib.pyplot as plt
4
5  nn = 10; lr = 0.02; sig = 2; sig2 = 1/(2*sig**2); ntrial = 0
6
7  x, y = np.meshgrid(np.arange(0, nn), np.arange(0, nn))
8
9  # Initial centres of prefered features:
10 c1=np.random.rand(nn,nn)
11 c2=np.random.rand(nn,nn)
12 #c1=0.05+x/nn
13 #c2=0.05+y/nn
14 # training session
15 for trial in range(10000):
16     if (np.mod(trial,100)==0): # Plot grid of feature centres
17         plt.axis([0,1,0,1]);
18         plt.plot(c1,c2,'k'); plt.plot(c1.T,c2.T,'k');
19         plt.show()
20
21     r_in=[np.random.rand(),np.random.rand()]
22     r=np.exp(-(c1-r_in[0])**2-(c2-r_in[1])**2)
23     winner = np.unravel_index(np.argmax(r, axis=None), r.shape)
24     r=np.exp(-((x-winner[0])**2+(y-winner[1])**2)*sig2);
25     c1=c1+lr*r*(r_in[1]-c1)
26     c2=c2+lr*r*(r_in[0]-c2)
```

After choosing random centres as starting values for the preferred stimuli of the neurons, we set up a long loop for learning. Before training, and after every 100 training examples, programmed as a condition with the numpy mod() function, we plot the mesh by connecting neighbouring nodes. We then choose a random stimuli and calculate the corresponding activation of the cortical map. We did not include the variance term in this line as the activation calculated there is only used to find the winner in the next line. The activation of the winning node is then calculated correctly in line, which is then used to update the centres according to eqn 8.5.

8.2.3   Ongoing refinements of cortical maps

Every new training example changes the map, and one is often faced with what Grossberg coined the plasticity–stability dilemma, in that we want to stabilize a map while still being able develop the map. In many technical applications, one starts the training with a large learning rate and gradually reduces this to small values. This is sometimes compared to developmental processes in mammals with critical periods in early postnatal periods. However, the brain also has the ability to adapt at high ages when given the opportunity. To demonstrate this we show another simulation in Fig. 8.5.

We started this network with perfectly organized centres (see graph for $t = 0$) to avoid topographic defects, since we are not interested here in the initial organization, but rather in the development of the maps in response to new exposures. The organized initial centres, as shown in the figure, were produced with:

```
for i in range(n_out)
    for j in range(n_out)
        c1[i,j]=i/n_out
        c2[i,j]=j/n_out
```

During the following adaptation steps, the network is first exposed to random training vectors in the unit square, as before. The representation did not change much after 1000 updates; only some small distortions were introduced caused by the updates of the weight matrix with the training examples. After 1000 training examples we changed the training vectors presented to the network. The new training examples consisted of random values similar to the previous ones, and, in addition, training examples with components $1 \le r_i^{in} < 2$, with random examples from each of the two quadrants. The simulation results after 100 and 1000 training episodes with these new training examples are shown in the last two graphs in Fig. 8.5. The topographic map branched out to reach representations of the additional feature values, although the representation is not as good as the representation of the initial training set even after some considerable time.

The simulations above demonstrate that SOM networks can learn to represent new domains of feature values, although the representation seems less fine-grained compared to the initial feature domain. The simulation results lead to some interesting conclusions if we speculate that the formation of cortical representation is driven by similar mechanisms. For example, it seems best to be exposed early in life to training examples from a broad feature space, including examples from all the features for which a fine-grained representation is desirable. This suggests that it is important to be exposed to different languages early in life to be able to achieve some high-level of sound discrimination ability in different languages.

Based on the above model we can suggest some training strategies that might be useful when exploring new domains. It seems possible to create a 'smart' training set that can help to adapt to new representations much better than a random training set. It might thereby be advantageous to include at first only training examples that are close to the feature domain originally learned and then slowly to increase the difference of the feature values. The model suggests that we can move and expand the whole feature representation in this way much more smoothly compared to the case in which we adapt to some extreme cases first and have then only a limited number of nodes available

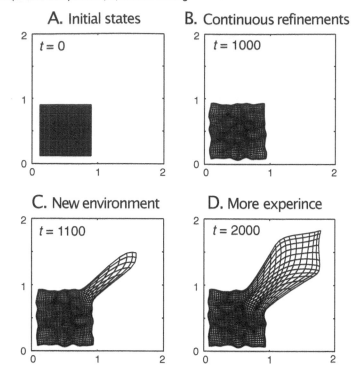

Fig. 8.5 Another example of a two-dimensional self-organizing feature map. In this example we trained the network on 1000 random training examples from the lower left quadrant. The next training examples were chosen randomly from the lower-left and upper-right quadrants. The parameter t specifies how many training examples have been presented to the network.

to represent the new feature domain. Also, constraining examples from highly trained areas is beneficial, and maybe even essential, in efficient learning. It is possible that we can develop better therapeutical treatments in rehabilitation based on such ideas.

A nice demonstration of representational plasticity in adult mammals is shown in Fig. 8.6 from experiments by Xiaoming Zhou and Michael Merzenich. They raised rat pups in a noisy environment that severely impaired the development of tonotopicity (orderly representations of tones) in the primary auditory cortex (A1), which lasted into adulthood. An example of such a map in an adult rat is shown in Fig. 8.6A. The diagonally dashed areas represent areas with neurons that showed pure frequency tuning. These rats were not able to recover normal tonotopic representation in A1 even though they were stimulated in adulthood with sounds of different frequencies. However, when the same sound patterns were used to train the rats in a discrimination task, which they had to solve to get a food reward, the developmentally degraded rats were able to recover a normal tonotopic maps, as shown in Fig. 8.6B. This example demonstrates that some goal-directed learning must take place in the animal. Also, traditional SOM models, as discussed in this section, are entirely driven by input data in a bottom-up way, and it is unlikely that such models are sufficient to explain these experimental results. Thus, top-down processing, such as guidance of the development of early sensory maps by goals and attention, seems important, and we will return to

A. Passively stimulated rat   B. Trained rat

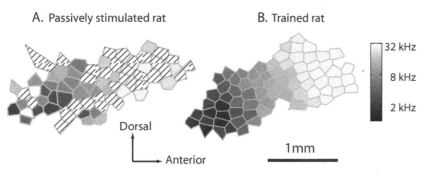

Fig. 8.6 (A) Frequency map in A1 of a rat that was developmentally degraded by being raised in noisy environments. The diagonally dashed areas contain neurons with poor frequency tuning. (B) Tonotopic map of an adult rat that recovered with training on a frequency discrimination task. [Data courtesy of Zhou and Merzenich, *Proceedings of the National Academy of Science USA* 104: 15935–40 (2007)].

the discussion of top-down processing in later chapters.

8.3   Dynamic neural field theory

We now turn to the other issue of cortical and, as we will see, some subcortical maps, that of the dynamics of the cortical sheet for a given topographic organization. The continuous time dynamic equation has already been introduced for a discrete set of nodes in eqn 8.1. We stated in the example of orientation tuning curves that the number of nodes does not really matter as long as there is a sufficient number of nodes to represent the feature space with sufficient granularity. Also, the feature of 'orientation' is really a continuous variable, and many concepts that the brain has to learn are of continuous nature. Indeed, cognitive processes are mostly of a continuous nature in space and time, and the following model is very successful in explaining many behavioural findings. It is therefore natural, and mathematically very convenient, to write eqn 8.1 in a spatially continuous form,

$$\tau \frac{\partial \mathbf{u}(\mathbf{x}, t)}{\partial t} = -\mathbf{u}(\mathbf{x}, t) + \int_{\mathbf{y}} \mathbf{w}(\mathbf{x}, \mathbf{y}) \mathbf{r}(\mathbf{y}, t) \mathrm{d}\mathbf{y} + I^{\mathrm{ext}}(\mathbf{x}, t) \qquad (8.6)$$

$$\mathbf{r}(\mathbf{x}, t) = g(\mathbf{u}(\mathbf{x}, t)), \qquad (8.7)$$

with a general activation function $g(\mathbf{u})$. We replaced the external input to this map with a general form $I^{\mathrm{ext}}(\mathbf{x}, t)$, as we will mainly study the dynamics of the neural field as topographically organized input. We used the term 'neural field' since the quantities $u(\mathbf{x}, t)$ and $r(\mathbf{x}, t)$ depend on continuous spatial coordinates and are called fields in physics. We wrote the equations for arbitrary spatial dimensions, although we will use mostly a one-dimensional version of this model to simplify the discussions. In a one-dimensional model we can replace the vector quantities, $\mathbf{x}, \mathbf{y}, \mathbf{u}, \mathbf{r}$, with real valued variables, x, y, u, r. We also use periodic boundary conditions to minimize boundary effects. Thus the feature space is formally a ring in one dimension, and we frequently use feature values in $(0, 2\pi]$ for demonstration purposes. When implementing the model for computer simulations we need to discretize the model with:

$$x \rightarrow i\Delta x \tag{8.8}$$

$$\int dx \rightarrow \Delta x \sum . \tag{8.9}$$

We recover the discrete model used above, eqn 8.1, when we identify the correspondences $u(i\Delta x, t) = u_i(t)$ and $\Delta x = 1/N$. Notice the scale factor in the last equation, which can easily be forgotten when replacing the integral with a sum.

8.3.1 The centre-surround interaction kernel

We studied the training of input weights for a fixed interaction kernel, $\mathbf{w}$, in the previous section. We now discuss the formation of $\mathbf{w}$ with fixed topographic input. We will use a one-dimensional example in which we call the feature that is represented by the cortical sheet the 'direction'. Each location of the cortical sheet represents a specific direction, but it also responds, to some extent, to neighbouring directions in the form of a Gaussian,

$$r(x - x^{\mathrm{P}}) = e^{-(x-x^{\mathrm{P}})^2/2\sigma_r^2}, \tag{8.10}$$

where x^{P} is the preferred direction of a location in the cortical sheet. With periodic boundaries we should replace the distance between x and x^{P} with,

$$|x - x^{\mathrm{P}}| \rightarrow \min(|x - x^{\mathrm{P}}|, 2\pi - |x - x^{\mathrm{P}}|). \tag{8.11}$$

We now use the continuous version of the basic Hebbian learning (eqn 6.10) to train an initial zero weight kernel on one example of every possible direction,

$$\mathbf{w}^{\mathrm{E}}(x, y) = \int_0^{2\pi} r(x - x^{\mathrm{P}})r(y - x^{\mathrm{P}})dx^{\mathrm{P}}. \tag{8.12}$$

This convolution integral is itself a Gaussian,

$$\mathbf{w}^{\mathrm{E}}(|x - y|) = A_w e^{-(x-y)^2/4\sigma_r^2}, \tag{8.13}$$

with a width that is a factor $\sqrt{2}$ larger than the width of the training patterns, and a scaling factor, A_w, that depends on the strength of the training pattern and a learning rate. This weight kernel is only a function of the distance between nodes and is always positive (excitatory), hence the label E. However, we also need inhibition in the network. We therefore consider a pool of inhibitory nodes which are activated by excitatory activations in the network and inhibit in turn the neural field globally. This can be incorporated in the network by shifting the excitatory kernel by an amount $A_w C$, where the constant C describes the relative amount of inhibition. The final weight kernel can be written as continuous version of eqn 8.3,

$$\mathbf{w}(|x - y|) = A_w \left(e^{-(x-y)^2/4\sigma_r^2} - C \right). \tag{8.14}$$

In this example we have derived the Gaussian weight kernel from training a recurrent

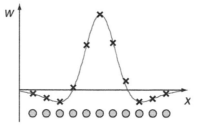

Fig. 8.7 Illustration of a Mexican-hat function. The crosses indicates the values that are used in a discrete version of a dynamic neural field model with nodes as indicated at the bottom.

network systematically on training examples with Gaussian shape. However, most of the behaviour discussed in the following holds also for models that are trained on different pattern shapes, as long as the resulting weight functions depend only on the distance (shift invariance), and have short-distance excitation and long-distance inhibition. For example, the commonly used Mexican-hat function, which can be calculated from the difference of two Gaussians, is illustrated in Fig. 8.7. This function is very similar to the shifted Gaussian above when the extent of the Mexican hat is on the order of the periodic cortical maps discussed here.

Various physiological examples suggest an effective interaction structure, with short-distance excitation and long-distance inhibition, in the brain. Such evidence influenced, for example, Cowan and Wilson to study neocortical models with such interaction structures in 1973. Another example was found in the intermediate layer of the superior colliculus, a midbrain area that is an important integration stage for many cortical and subcortical pathways that guide the direction of gaze. An example of the interaction structures within the superior colliculus from cell recordings in monkeys is shown in Fig. 8.8. In this figure we plotted the results for two sample neurons. The figure shows the influence of activity in other parts of the colliculus on the activity of each neuron. This influence has the characteristics of short-distance excitation and long-distance inhibition, and a model of the superior colliculus based on these characteristics was able to reproduce many behavioural findings for the variations in the time required to initiate a fast eye movement as a function of various experimental conditions.

8.3.2 Asymptotic states and the dynamics of neural fields

The cortical sheet is formally a dynamic system (recurrent network), and we can study the trajectories and asymptotic states in the state space of the network, as will be done more formally below. Here, we summarize some principal regimes of such models with local cooperation and global competition, which are important in the following discussions. These different regimes depend on the level of inhibition C, and can be categorized as follows.

1. **Growing activity:** When the inhibition is weak compared to the excitation between nearby nodes, so that the model is dominated by excitation, the dynamics of the model are governed by positive feedback. The whole map will eventually become active in this regime, which is therefore undesirable for brain processes.

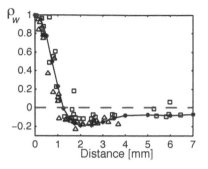

Fig. 8.8 Data from cell recordings in the superior colliculus in a monkey, which indicate the interaction strength ρ_w between cells in this midbrain structure. The solid line displays the corresponding measurement from simulations of a CANN model of this brain structure [from Trappenberg et al., *Journal of Cognitive Neuroscience* 13: 256–71 (2001)].

2. **Decaying activity:** When the inhibition is strong compared to the excitation, then the dynamics of the model are dominated by negative feedback. The neurons will respond to sufficiently strong input, but the activity of the map decays after removal of external input. Nevertheless, this regime is interesting from an information precessing point of view since it can facilitate competition between external inputs.

3. **Memory activity:** In an intermediate range of inhibition, which we will specify further below, an active area can be stable in the map, even when an external input is removed. This regime can therefore represent memories of feature values through ongoing activity in the network.

The regimes can easily be explored numerically with the program detailed below. An example of such a simulation is shown in Fig. 8.9A where we plotted the firing rates of the nodes in a network of 100 nodes on a grey-scale during the evolution of the system in time. All nodes are initialized to have medium firing rates, and a strong external stimulus to nodes number 40–50 was applied at time $t = 0$. The stimulated nodes, as well as some neighbouring nodes to the stimulated site, respond with an increase in their firing rate due to the excitatory weights to nearby nodes. Nodes far from the stimulated site decrease their firing rates due to inhibition. As mentioned above, we call the collection of nodes that are active compared to their background rate an activity packet, but in some of the literature it is also called a bubble, or bump.

The external stimulus was removed at $t = 10\tau$. The overall firing rates in the network decreased slightly following this removal of the external stimulus, and the activity packet became lower and a bit broader. However, the most interesting effect is that a group of neighbouring nodes with the same centre as the external stimulus, stayed active asymptotically. The dynamic of the cortical sheet is therefore able to memorize a feature with ongoing activity in the cortical map. We will argue below that this corresponds to a form of working memory as seen in physiological data. The activity packet can be stabilized at any location in the network depending on an initial external stimulus. The attractor is therefore a continuous manifold in the neural field limit, and the dynamic neural field (DNF) model is sometimes called a continuous

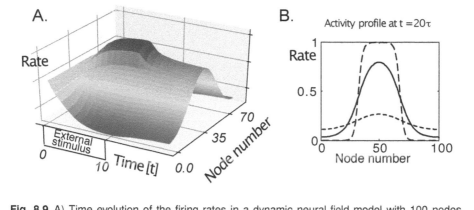

Fig. 8.9 A) Time evolution of the firing rates in a dynamic neural field model with 100 nodes. Equal external inputs to nodes 40–60 were applied at $t = 0\tau$. This external input was removed at $t = 10\tau$ (parameters of the models as in program `dnf.py`). B) The solid line represents the firing rate profile of the simulation shown in Fig. 8.9 at $t = 20\tau$. The dashed line shows similar results with increased weights $A_w = 10$. The dotted line shown results form a decaying activity packet with increased inhibition ($C = 0.7$).

attractor neural network (CANN). This is a special case of more general attractor neural networks (ANNs) discussed in Chapter 9. A new activity packet can be established at a new location by applying another external stimulus centred around a different node. The externally activated nodes, however, still receive inhibitory activity from the other activity packet in the network, and the external input has to be of sufficient strength and duration to ensure that the new activity packet becomes dominant in the network.

The rate profile at time $t = 20\tau$ is shown as a solid line in Fig. 8.9B. In these simulations we used an inhibition constant of $C = 0.5$ and an weight strength of $A_w = 4$. Using a larger weight strength, $A_w = 10$, results in a more rigid activity packet with sharper boundaries and rates of the nodes deep inside the activity packet nearly reaching the rate limit. Similar effects can be seen when using larger gains in the sigmoidal activation function or when using less inhibition. Using threshold functions as activation functions results in a box-shaped rate profile. We will utilize this finding in the following analysis. The active area decays with large inhibition constants, such as with $C = 0.7$ in the example. However, the decay process can take some time, so that a trace of the evoked area can still be seen at $t = 20\tau$, as shown with the dotted line in Fig. 8.9B.

An implementation of the DNF model in Python for Fig. 8.9 is given in program `dnf.py`. We are here using the numberical integrator provided in SciPy as outline in Chapter 3.4 for which we define the dynamic equations in function `udot()`. We then define parameters includes the number of nodes. While we set this number to `nn=100` in this example, it is important that our results do not depend on this number, and it is good to check whether simulation results are unchanged when using a different number (please try). The number of nodes will only change the resolution in feature space, `dx`. The variable `sig` influences the standard deviation of the weight matrix, and the constant C sets the inhibition.

Programs/dnf.py

```
1  import numpy as np
2  import matplotlib.pyplot as plt
3  from matplotlib import cm
4  from matplotlib.ticker import LinearLocator
5  from scipy.integrate import odeint
6
7  def udot(u, t, w, I_ext, dx, tau):
8      r=1/(1+np.exp(-u))
9      I_int=w@r*dx;
10     return tau*(-u+I_int+I_ext)
11
12 # Parameters
13 nn = 100; dx = 2*np.pi/nn; sig = 2*np.pi/10; C=0.5; tau=1
14
15 # Training weight matrix with Hebbian learning and scaling
16 i = np.arange(nn)
17 pat = np.zeros((nn,nn))
18 for loc in range(nn):
19     dis = np.fmin(abs(i-loc),nn-abs(i-loc))
20     pat[:,loc] = np.exp(-(dis*dx)**2/(2*sig**2))
21 w = pat@pat.T; w = w/w[0,0]; w = 4*(w-C)
22
23 # Update with input (central activation)
24 I_ext = np.zeros(nn); I_ext[int(nn/2-nn/10):int(nn/2+nn/10)] = 1
25 t = np.arange(10)
26 u0 = np.zeros(nn)  # Initial state
27 u = odeint(udot, u0, t, args=(w, I_ext, dx, tau))
28
29 # remove input
30 I_ext = np.zeros(nn)
31 t2 = np.arange(10,20)
32 u0 = u[-1,:]  # Initial state
33 u2 = odeint(udot, u0, t2, args=(w, I_ext, dx, tau))
34
35
36 # plot results
37 fig, ax = plt.subplots(subplot_kw={"projection": "3d"})
38 X = np.append(t,t2); Z = np.append(u,u2,axis=0).T
39 Y = np.arange(nn)/nn*2*np.pi
40 X, Y = np.meshgrid(X, Y)
41 ax.plot_surface(X,Y,Z,cmap=cm.coolwarm,linewidth=0,antialiased=False)
```

It is common in the application of the DNF model to set the components explicitly with a function such as the difference of two Gaussians. However, in this example we chose to train the excitatory part of the weight matrix with Hebbian training on Gaussian patterns. The pattern matrix `pat` contains `nn` patterns, each is a Gaussian centred around one of the nodes in the network. We then use the Hebbian learning rule in matrix form (see eqn 6.21 and its following comments) and is normalized to the maximal element (each diagonal element is equal and maximal). The resulting value is then shifted by the inhibition constant and again scales up with a factor of 4. Such a scaling factor can be related to the learning rate or other forms of normalization.

We then start the experiment with external input with non-zero elements for the 21 nodes around the central node and update the activity by integrating until $t = 10$. We then remove the input and integrate for another 10 time steps. The rest of the codes shows how to plot the neural fields in a 3d plot.

8.3.3 Examples of competitive representations in the brain

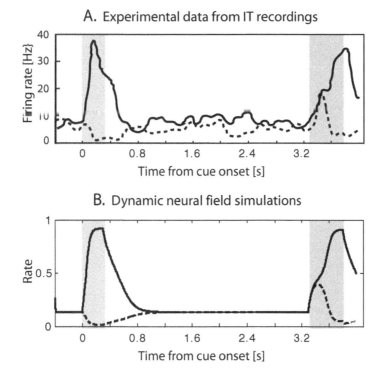

A. Experimental data from IT recordings

B. Dynamic neural field simulations

Fig. 8.10 (A) Example of responses of IT neurons from experiments by Chelazzi, Miller, Duncan, and Desimone, *Nature* 363: 345–7 (1993). Response to a 'good' object is shown as solid line, the response to a 'bad' object as a dotted line. (B) Simulations of the DNF model with moderately strong inhibition. The solid line is a recording from the central 'good' location, the dotted line from the 'bad' location [for details see Trappenberg, in *Computational modelling in behavioural neuroscience*, Heinke and Mavritsaki (eds), Psychology Press (2009)].

The tuning curves discussed in Section 8.1 only show maximal responses of a neuron during each stimulus presentation. We turn now to some other examples from different brain areas to demonstrate that such mechanisms capture fundamental aspects of brain processing.

Higher cortical areas represent increasingly complex features beyond orientation selectivity of V1 neurons, but we can still think of these representations in terms of neural fields. The only difference is that the represented feature value (orientation in V1) should be replaced by another feature value to which the other cortical area responds. However, the arguments discussed in this section do not crucially depend on the feature choice as long as the neurons show significant modulations with these feature values. Note that we do not want to leave the impression that specific cortical areas process only the specified features. Indeed, these features are somewhat biased by experimental conditions. Even neurons in V1 respond to other features. The 'true features' processed in a cortical area might be a complicated mix of features defined

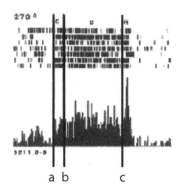

Fig. 8.11 Demonstration of physiological working memory through the maintenance of delay activity in physiological experiments. A target was presented between times a and b, and the location of the target had to be remembered until an action was required at time c [detail from Funahashi, Bruce, and Goldman-Rakic, *Journal of Neurophysiology* 61: 331–49 (1989)].

by the experimenter.

For example, the inferior-temporal (IT) cortex in monkeys is quite selective in responding to specific complex objects. Some data from recordings in this area by Chelazzi and colleagues are shown Fig. 8.10A. In their experiment they showed different objects to monkeys and selected objects to which the recorded IT cell responded strongly (good objects) and weekly (bad objects). In the illustration of Fig. 8.10A, the average firing rate of an IT cell to a good stimulus is shown as solid line. The period when the cue stimulus was presented is indicated by the grey bar in this figure. The response to a 'bad' object is illustrated in the figure with a dashed line. Instead of increasing the rate during the cue presentation, this neuron seems to respond with a firing rate below the usual background rate. At a later time, the monkey was shown both objects, and asked to select the object that was used for cueing. The IT neuron responds initially in both conditions, but the response is quite different at later stages.

Several aspects of the experimental data are captured by simulations of the DNF model as shown in Fig. 8.10B. The solid line represents the activity of a node within the response bubble of the neural field. In these simulations, a fairly large inhibition constant was used so that the activity declines after the external stimulus is removed. The activity of the dashed line corresponds to the activity of a node outside the activity bubble. The activity of this node is weakened as a result of lateral inhibition during the stimulus presentations. Also, when both objects are used as input, activity at both locations will initially rise. Only later will the slightly larger activity package, such as when modelled by additional support from working memory, dominate the dynamics and actively inhibit the other activity packet.

Another important issue is that of demonstrating physiological working memory by ongoing firing in the brain. The maintenance of neural activity over a delay period has been observed experimentally. An example of such an experiment by Funahashi, Bruce, and Goldman-Rakic is shown in Fig. 8.11. These researchers trained a monkey to maintain its eyes on a central fixation spot until a 'go' signal, such as a tone, indicated that it should move the eyes and focus on one of several possible targets peripheral to

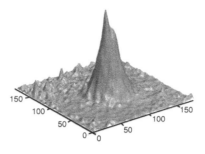

Fig. 8.12 Neuronal response from many hippocampal neurons in a rodent that responded to the subject's location (places) in a maze. The figure shows the firing rates of the neurons in response to a particular place, whereby the neurons were placed in the figure so that neurons with similar response properties were placed adjacent to each other [Samsonowich and McNaughton, *Journal of Neuroscience* 17: 5900–20 (1997)].

the fixation spot. The choice of the target to which the eyes should be moved in each trial was indicated by a short flash, between the first two vertical bars in the figure, but the subject was not allowed to move its eyes until the 'go' signal indicated by the third vertical bar in the figure. Thus, the target location for each trial had to be remembered during the delay period. The experimenters recorded from neurons in the dorsolateral prefrontal cortex (area 46) and found neurons that were active during the delay period. These neurons were sensitive to the particular target direction (the shown neuron only responded when the target was at 270 degrees), and this neuron could therefore indicate by its delayed activity to which target the eye should be directed after the delay period. It is possible that such ongoing activity of neurons is supported by intracellular mechanisms such as activation of ion channels with high reversal potentials. However, a more common explanation is that such working memory activity is sustained through lateral reverberating neural activity as captured by the DNF model. This model is attractive for several reasons, such as the ability to simulate interactions with other memories, as discussed later.

The final example illustrates the representations of space in the archicortex. Some neurons in the hippocampus of rats fire in relation to specific locations within a maze in which the rat is freely moving. In some experiments, the activity of many neurons has been recorded while a rat could freely run in a maze. When the firing rates of the different neurons are plotted on a map reflecting their physical location in the hippocampus, the resulting firing pattern looks like a randomly distributed code. A specific topography of neurons within the hippocampal tissue with respect to their maximal response to a particular place has not been found. However, if the plot is rearranged so that neurons that fire maximally in response to adjacent locations are plotted adjacent to each other, then a firing profile like the one shown in Fig. 8.12 can be seen. This is an example of a two-dimensional activity packet.

Since hippocampal place cells do not display a regularity in the physical space of the brain tissue, a hardwired (for example, genetically coded) connectivity pattern is likely not employed in this structure. However, we saw the regularities in the above models when organizing the nodes according to the feature values they represented. Discovering this organization in the functional map would have been difficult otherwise. This is demonstrated in Fig. 8.13 with a one-dimensional example, where we have labelled the nodes and indicated the relative strengths of weights between the different nodes with lines of different widths, corresponding to the relative strengths of the connections. Before learning, illustrated in Fig. 8.13A, we can assume that all nodes have equal weights relative to each other. The dimensionality of this model can be regarded as high when we take the number of neighbours, the number of nodes to which each node is relatively strongly connected, as a measure. Unlike the previous model, we have assigned each node randomly to a preferred direction where it fires maximally. After training we therefore get weights in the 'physical' space of the nodes, as indicated in Fig. 8.13B, that look rather random. The order in the connectivity only becomes apparent when we finally reorder the nodes so that strongly connected nodes are adjacent to each other. After doing so (Fig. 8.13C), we see that it has a one-dimensional structure which reflects the one-dimensional structure of the feature space that was used for training this network.

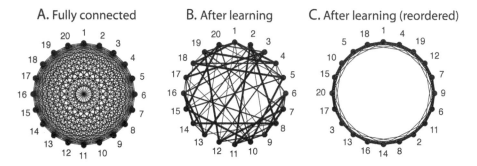

Fig. 8.13 A recurrent associative attractor network model, where the nodes have been arbitrarily placed in the physical space on a circle. The relative connection strength between the nodes is indicated by the thickness of the lines between the nodes. Each node responds during learning with a Gaussian firing profile around the stimulus that excites the node maximally. Each node is assigned a centre of the receptive field randomly from a pool of centres covering the periodic training domain. (A) Before training, all nodes have the same relative weights between them. (B) After training, the relative weight structure has changed, with a few strong connections and some weaker connections. (C) The regularities of the interactions can be revealed by reordering the nodes so that nodes with the strongest connections are adjacent to each other.

We reduced the dimensionality of the initial network to a one-dimensional connectivity pattern. If we had trained the initial network with examples from a two-dimensional feature space we would have produced a two-dimensional structure in the weight matrix, although this might only be visible after rearranging the nodes accordingly. The rearrangement of nodes we used is equivalent to the rearrangement of hippocampal neurons discussed above and explains why this had to be done to see the 'regularity' in the firing pattern. From this we can see that the network self-organizes to reflect the dimensionality of the feature space. The network 'discovers' the dimensionality of the underlying problem from activity dependent co-activation of neurons, which is the basic feature of Hebbian learning, as discussed in Chapter 6.

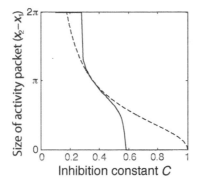

Fig. 8.14 Size of the activity package as function of the inhibition constant C. The dotted line corresponds to the solutions of eqn 8.17, whereas the solid line shows results from simulations.

8.3.4 Formal analysis of attractor states ◇

The dynamic neural field model in the form presented here was introduced by Sun-ichi Amari in 1977, when he also studied the solutions of such models in detail. We follow here some of the basic ideas in his analysis. For simplicity, we assume a threshold activation function, $g(x) = \theta(x)$, which makes the firing rates within the activity packet equal to one while setting the firing rates outside the activity packet to zero. As we will see, this choice is convenient. The results with a threshold activation function are a good approximation for networks with smoother activation functions, because the activity packets can be sharp even with a smooth sigmoidal activation function. The threshold activation function is useful because the stationary state ($\partial u/\partial t = 0$) of the dynamic eqn 8.6, without external input ($I_{\text{ext}} = 0$), can then be written as:

$$u(x) = \int_{x_1}^{x_2} w(x, y)\mathrm{d}y, \tag{8.15}$$

where x_1 and x_2 are the positions of the boundaries of the activity packet. This must be true for all x, including the boundaries for which $u(x_1) = u(x_2) = 0$, so that the following equation must also hold,

$$\int_{x_1}^{x_2} w(x_1, y)\mathrm{d}y = 0. \tag{8.16}$$

For the Gaussian weight kernel, eqn 8.14, the above equation can be solved with the error function (see eqn 3.54),

$$\sqrt{\pi}\sigma_r\mathrm{erf}(\frac{x_2 - x_1}{2\sigma_r}) = C(x_2 - x_1). \tag{8.17}$$

This equation can be solved numerically and is illustrated in Fig. 8.14 as a dotted line. Corresponding simulations of the DNF model are shown in Fig. 8.14 as a solid line. The analytical solution describes the stable regime quite well, but deviates somewhat from numerical solutions in the transition range between the different regimes.

What about the stability of the activity packet with respect to movements? To answer this question we calculate the velocity of the boundaries. A movement of the

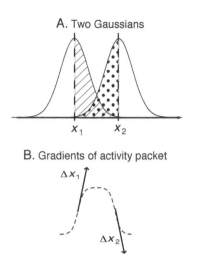

A. Two Gaussians

x_1 x_2

B. Gradients of activity packet

Δx_1

Δx_2

Fig. 8.15 (A) Two Gaussian bell curves centred around two different values x_1 and x_2. The size of the striped and dotted areas are the same due to the symmetry of the bell curve. The integrals from x_1 to x_2 over the two different curves are therefore the same. This is not true if the two curves are not symmetrical and have different shapes. (B) The dashed line outlines the shape of an activity packet from a simulation. The symmetry of this activity packet makes the gradients of boundaries equal except for a sign.

activity packet without external input can only result from forces generated by the shape of the activity packet itself. The force is then proportional to the gradient of the activity packet, and the velocity is

$$\frac{\mathrm{d}x}{\mathrm{d}t} = -\Delta x \frac{\mathrm{d}u}{\mathrm{d}t}, \tag{8.18}$$

where we took a possible explicit time dependence of the activity packet into account. To get the velocity of the boundaries we have to substitute $x = x_1$ or $x = x_2$ into this equation. We can then substitute eqn 8.6 into this equation to get a formula for the velocity of the boundary, or similarly for the centre of the activity packet,

$$x_\mathrm{c}(t) = \frac{1}{2}(x_1(t) + x_2(t)), \tag{8.19}$$

given by

$$\frac{\mathrm{d}x_\mathrm{c}}{\mathrm{d}t} = -\frac{1}{2\tau\Delta x_1}\int_{x_1}^{x_2} w(x_1, y)\mathrm{d}y - \frac{1}{2\tau\Delta x_2}\int_{x_1}^{x_2} w(x_2, y)\mathrm{d}y. \tag{8.20}$$

The expression on the right-hand side of the equation is zero when the weighting function is symmetrical and shift-invariant, and the gradients of the activity packet at the boundaries are the same except for their sign. These conditions are illustrated in Fig. 8.15. For the Gaussian weighting function, which is symmetrical and shift-invariant, we see that the integral from x_1 to x_2 of the Gaussian centred around x_1 is the same as that for the Gaussian centred around x_2. Also, once we have a symmetrical activity packet, it is clear that the gradients at the boundaries are equal except for their sign, as illustrated in Fig. 8.15B. The velocity of the centre of the activity packet for a symmetrical weighting function is therefore zero ($dx_c/dt = 0$), and the activity packet stays centred around the location where it was initialized.

We have formally derived that the activity packet in models with shift-invariant and symmetrical weight matrices is stable. Eqn 8.20 also tells us when the activity packet is not stable and can hence drift. For example, the velocity of the centre of the activity packet is not equal to zero when the shift invariance of the weight matrix is broken. The weight matrix generated by Hebbian learning on random patterns, as will be discussed in Chapter 9, is not shift-invariant. Such associative memory networks therefore drift away from initial conditions toward a point attractor, as will be discussed in the next chapter.

Another important factor is noise in the system, which we have always to take into account when discussing brain mechanisms. Noise breaks the symmetry as well as the shift invariance of the weighting functions when the noise is independent for each component of the weight. The activity packet in such networks therefore drifts to some points where the shifting forces compensate each other. This leads to a clustering of end states. An example is shown in Fig. 8.16A. Each curve in the plot corresponds to the time evolution of the centre of gravity of the activity packet after the network was initialized with an activity packet centred around a different node in the network. This drift caused by noise has some interesting consequences for operations in the brain. For example, the drift makes an accurate representation of locations over a long time impossible. Indeed, experiments show that the sense of direction in the dark diminishes after some period of time. Note that the drift of the activity packet due to noise decreases with the size of the system because the noise components can average out when the weighting function is the result of the interaction of many noisy nodes.

Another source of asymmetries in the weighting function is irregular or partial training of the network. In the previous examples, we always trained the networks for the same amount of time, with activity packets centred at each node in the network. This not only requires long training sessions, but is also unrealistic in biological terms as the subject would have to explore a new environment in a very regular manner. The effects of partial training are illustrated with the simulations shown in Fig. 8.16B–D. There, we have trained the network with activity packets centred around only 10 different nodes in the network. A partial view of the resulting weight matrix is shown in Fig. 8.16B. The values of the weight matrix are largest at the locations that were used for training. The centre of the activity packet with the resulting weight matrix, not including any noise, also shows a drift for initial states around the trained locations (Fig. 8.16C). This is a point attractor network, discussed more in the next chapter. Note that the locations precisely in-between the trained locations are also stable, but only marginally so. A small deviation would result in a drift to the trained locations.

The drift in the activity packet can be stabilized by a small increase in the excitability of neurons once they have been recently activated. This corresponds to a voltage-dependent non-linearity in the postsynaptic neuron that can help to maintain the firing in a recurrent network. Such voltage-dependent non-linearities could, for example, be implemented by NMDA receptors. We have already mentioned in Chapter 4 that

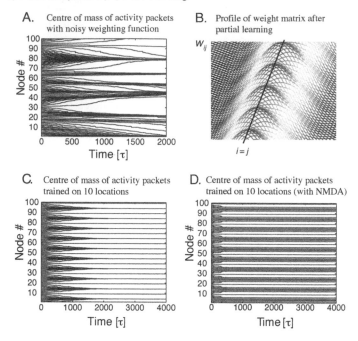

Fig. 8.16 (A) Simulations with noisy weight matrix: time evolution of the centre of gravity of activity packets in a DNF model with 100 nodes. The model was trained with activity packets on all possible locations. Each component of the resulting weight matrix was then convoluted with some noise.
(B) Irregular or partial learning: partial view of the weight matrix resulting from training the network with activity packets on only a few locations.
(C) Time evolution of the centre of gravity of activity packets in DNF model with 100 nodes after training the network on only 10 different locations.
(D) 'NMDA'-stabilization. The network trained on the 10 locations was augmented with a stabiliza- tion mechanism that reduces the firing threshold of active neurons.

NMDA receptors are blocked by magnesium ions when neurons are at rest. This blockade is removed after an increase in the membrane potential. Thus, we can excite the neuron the next time much more easily, if the time necessary to block the channel again is long relative to the time of the next incoming spike.

We can simulate such a voltage-dependent non-linearity with a relatively long time constant by altering the threshold in the activation function of the model neurons. In the simulations shown in Fig. 8.16D we have changed the threshold value α from the value $\alpha = 0$ used in all previous simulations to a lower value of $\alpha = 10$ for neurons that exceeded 50% of their maximal firing rates. The value was reset to $\alpha = 0$ when the neurons fell below this 50% threshold. This change in the simulations was sufficient to increase the number of attractors (see Fig. 8.16D), with most of the states close to the trained locations being stable. Only states far from the trained location drifted initially to the closest attractor state. An increase of the voltage-dependent non-linearity would make more states stable. However, we do not want to make this mechanism too dominant, as we would otherwise lose the competitive nature of the network, which is relevant for most applications of these network models. There is, so

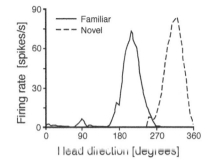

Fig. 8.17 Experimental response of a neuron in the subiculum of a rodent when the rodent is heading in different directions [redrawn from Golob and Taube, *Journal of Neuroscience* 19: 7198–211 (1999)].

far, no direct experimental verification of this proposal, but a direct verification might be possible with well-directed blocking of NMDA receptors. The model predicts that drift in the activity packets should increase, corresponding to a quick confusion in the sense of direction.

8.4   'Path' integration and the Hebbian trace rule ◇

Humans usually have to a certain degree a sense of direction. This suggests that we must have some form of spatial representation in our brain. The sense of direction can be tested with a simple experiment. If a subject is placed in a rotating chair with closed eyes while someone rotates the subject a certain amount, it can be shown that the subject's guess of the new direction is quite accurate. This demonstrates two important issues: first, we have to have a representation of body, or head, direction and, second, we have to have a mechanism to update this information without visual cues.

We already saw that special information is represented with place fields in the hippocampus of rats, and other spacial information, such as head-directions, can also be found there and in other proximate areas. For example, in the subiculum of rodents it was found that firing of neurons represents the direction in which the rodent was heading. An example is shown in Fig. 8.17 from recording activities of a cell when the rodent was rotated in different directions. The solid line represents the response property of this neuron in a familiar maze. The neuron fires maximally for one particular direction and fires with lower firing rates to directions around the preferred direction of this neuron. The shown curve is a tuning curve of head-direction representations in the subiculum. The dashed line represents the new head properties of the same neuron when the rodent is placed in a new, unfamiliar, maze. The new response properties will normally be similar to the previous one, that is, head-direction cells try to maintain approximately their response properties to specific head-directions. However, the results shown were produced in experiments with a rodent that had cortical lesions that weakened the ability to maintain the response properties after the rodent was transferred into a new environment. It was shown that the head-direction neurons continue to fire in the dark, which is another example of physiological working memory through ongoing neural activity after removal of the stimulus. We discuss, in this section, how the representation of the current head-direction can be updated in DNF models.

8.4.1 Path integration with asymmetrical weight kernels

One way of updating the state represented by a DNF layer is to apply an external stimulus to a new location. This is, of course, only possible if we know the absolute value for the new location, which should be represented explicitly so that we can apply an external stimulus at the corresponding location in the network. However, a subject might not have such an absolute value available, for example, when rotating a subject with closed eyes. This is like driving a blindfolded person around in a city and, after some time, asking where we are. To solve this problem we have to 'calculate' the new position from the old position and the changes we made (velocity information including rotation and forward speed) over this time period. This 'calculation' is called path integration, and we will adopt this terminology for the generic situation of calculating a new state representation from an initial state representation plus signals that indicate the change of the state.

We saw in the last section that asymmetries in the weight kernel in DNF models lead to a movement of the activity packet. A proposal for solving the path integration problem involves using such asymmetries in a systematic way. To do this we have to find a way to relate the strength of the asymmetry to the velocity of the movement. A velocity signal can be generated by the subject itself, and we call such information idiothetic cues, where 'idiothetic' means self-generated. Examples are inputs from the vestibular system in mammals, which can generate signals indicating the rotation of the head and proprioceptive feedback from muscles that signal the change in their position. Such signals will be the input to our following models, where we will again concentrate on head-direction as an example.

A proposal as to how idiothetic velocity signals can be used in DNF models of head-direction representations to update the system is shown in Fig. 8.18. For simplicity, we have only shown three nodes of the recurrent network representing the head-direction of a subject, and have only included collateral connections to the neighbouring nodes. In addition to these head direction nodes we included two other nodes (which can also represent a collection of neurons), which we call rotation nodes. We assume for simplicity that the firing rate of these nodes is directly proportional to the velocity of the head movement. The principal idea behind the model is that these rotation nodes can modulate the strength of the collateral connections between DNF nodes. This modulatory influence makes the effective weight kernel within the attractor network in one direction stronger than in the other direction, thus enabling the activity packet to move in a particular direction with a speed that is determined by the firing rate of the rotation nodes.

The effect of rotation node activity on the attractor network has to be modulatory (that is, multiplicative) as opposed to additive because the latter case would produce only an equal external input to all nodes that could not shift the activity packet. The modulatory effect can, for example, be implemented with sigma–pi nodes as introduced in Section 5.6. This, in turn, has several possible implementations on the neuronal level. For the following discussion, it is sufficient to think about two physically close synaptic

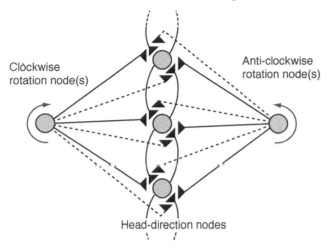

Clockwise
rotation node(s)

Anti-clockwise
rotation node(s)

Head-direction nodes

Fig. 8.18 Model for path integration which shows a few head-direction cells with collateral connections. The rotation nodes represent collections of neurons that signal rotation velocities proportional to their activity. The afferents of the rotation cells can modulate the collateral connections within the head-direction network, which is symbolized with synapses close to the synapses of the collateral connections. Each rotation cell can synapse on to each synapse in the head-direction network. The separation of the connections, as indicated by the solid and dashed lines, is self-organized during learning.

terminals that can interact to produce such non-linear modulation affects.

8.4.2 Self-organization of a rotation network

The major problem we have to solve to make this model biologically realistic is to find a way to self-organize the network. If we simply assume that rotation nodes modulate all synapses equally we cannot move the activity packet. Instead, the network has to learn that the firing in a rotation node that indicates, for example, clockwise rotations should modulate only the appropriate 'clockwise synapses' in the network. Thus, the network has to learn that synapses have strong weights only in response to the appropriate weights in the recurrent network, as indicated by solid lines in Fig. 8.18. The influence of the opposite synapses, indicated by dashed lines, has to at least be weaker. To achieve this, we need a learning rule that can associate the recent movement of the activity packet with the firing of the appropriate rotation node. We therefore need to have a trace, or 'short-term memory', in the nodes, which is related to the recent movement of the activity packet. An example of such a trace term (indicated by a bar over the firing rate) is,

$$\bar{r}_i(t+1) = (1 - \eta)\bar{r}_i(t) + \eta r_i(t). \tag{8.21}$$

This is a discrete version of a leaky integrator and can also be written in a differential form. This trace term represents the sliding average of recent firing, with an exponential sliding window of width characterized by the parameter η. The precise form of this trace term is not essential for the following mechanisms, and other trace terms can be used. With this trace in the firing of the nodes in the recurrent network, we can associate the co-firing of rotation cells with the movement of the activity packet in the recurrent network. The weights between rotation nodes (which have a superscript 'rot') and the synapses in the recurrent network (which have no superscript) can be formed with a Hebbian rule,

$$\delta w_{ijk}^{\text{rot}} = \epsilon r_i \bar{r}_j r_k^{\text{rot}}. \tag{8.22}$$

The parameter ϵ is, as usual, a learning rate. The rule strengthens the weights between the rotation node and the appropriate synapses in the recurrent network. As before, we can form these weights during the learning phase where the firing of the nodes is determined by the firing of external input. This learning phase corresponds to the exploration of an environment by a subject using visual cues and is hetero-associative in the sense that it associates consecutive states during learning.

8.4.3 Updating the network after learning

After the weights have been learned, we can update head-directions of a subject without external input. The dynamic of the model is specified with

$$\tau \frac{\partial h(x,t)}{\partial t} = -h(x,t) + \int_y w^{\text{eff}}(x,y,r^{\text{rot}})r(y,t)r_i^{\text{rot}}(t)\mathrm{d}y, \tag{8.23}$$

where the index i labels the group of nodes of either clockwise or anti-clockwise rotation cells. The weight matrix $\mathbf{w}^{\text{eff}}$ depends on the activity of the rotation nodes, and describes the effective weight kernel within the recurrent network from the collateral connections and the modulatory influence of the idiothetic cues. The modulatory nature of these influences can, for example, be expressed by

$$w_{ij}^{\text{eff}} = (w_{ij} - c)(1 + w_{ijk}^{\text{rot}} r_k^{\text{rot}}), \tag{8.24}$$

though other forms of modulatory functions are possible and generally lead to results similar to the ones outlined below.

The behaviour of the model when trained on examples of one clockwise and one anti-clockwise rotation, with only one rotation speed, is demonstrated in Fig. 8.19. An external position stimulus was applied initially for 10τ to initiate an activity packet, and this activity packet is stable after the removal of the external stimulus when the rotation nodes are inactive. Between $20\tau \le t \le 40\tau$ we applied a clockwise rotation activity corresponding to the activity used during learning. The activity packet then moved in the clockwise direction linearly within this time. The movement stops immediately after the rotation cell firing is abolished at $t = 40\tau$. During $50\tau \le t \le 70\tau$ we applied an anti-clockwise firing rate of the anti-clockwise node that was twice the value used during learning. The activity packet moved at nearly twice the speed in the anti-clockwise direction, demonstrating that the network can generalize to other rotation speeds.

Examples of the weighting functions after learning are shown in Fig. 8.20. The solid line represents symmetrical collateral weighting values $w_{50,i}$ between node 50 and the other nodes in the network. The clockwise rotation weights $w_{50,i,1}^{\text{rot}}$ are shown as a dashed line in the figure. Their functional form is not symmetrical as expected.

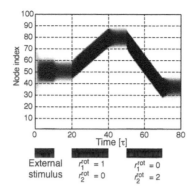

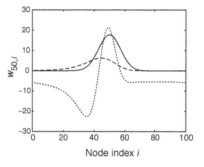

Fig. 8.19 Simulation of a DNF model with idiothetic updating mechanisms. The activity packet can be moved with idiothetic inputs in either clockwise or anti-clockwise directions, depending on the firing rates of the corresponding rotation cells. The experimental stimuli are indicated at the bottom.

Fig. 8.20 The different weighting functions from node 50 to the other nodes in the network after learning. w, solid line; w^{rot}, dashed line; w^{eff}, dotted line.

The corresponding anti-clockwise rotation weights $w_{50,i,2}^{\text{rot}}$, not shown in the figure, are a mirror-image of the dashed line. The resulting effective weighting function (eqn 8.24) is shown as a dotted line in the figure. All the examples are within a feature space with an intrinsic one-dimensional topography. However, path integration can be achieved in analogous ways with feature spaces in higher dimensions as the network self-organizes.

8.5 Distributed representation and population coding

We have discussed in this chapter how information is represented in cortical and some subcortical maps, and we will end this chapter with a more general discussion of distributed coding. We consider here that a stimulus is represented by a vector with components that have values given by the responses (such as firing rates) of neurons in a brain area. We then want to know how many components are actively used to represent a stimulus in the brain. We can distinguish roughly three classes of representation:

1. **Local representation:** In a local representation only one node represents a stimulus in that only one node is active when a particular stimulus is presented. A single node (or neuron) would be sufficient to indicate that a particular stimulus was present. Neurons with such characteristics have been termed cardinal cells, pontifical cells, or grandmother cells. A vector of length N could represent N different features with such a local representation. The number of stimuli that can be encoded by such a vector increases linearly with the number of components (nodes). Reading out which stimulus is represented is very easy with a local representation. In the case of representations with binary nodes that are either 'on' or 'off', which we will consider frequently later, only one node would be 'on' for each possible stimulus.

2. **Fully distributed representation:** The fully distributed representation can be seen as the other extreme, compared to the local representation. A stimulus is encoded by the combination of the activities of all the components in the vector representing a stimulus. In the case of binary nodes we can think of the case where the probability of each node being *on* or *off* is equal (that is, 50%), so that the number of active nodes is 50% on average. The number of different stimuli that can be encoded with such vectors scales exponentially with the number of nodes and is therefore much larger than in the case of local representations. The information stored in a node vector is, however, the same, as they always specify a stimulus uniquely. An advantage of such a representation is that we can define similarities of stimuli by counting how many components of the vector have similar values. This is important for building associations.

3. **Sparsely distributed representation:** Somewhat of a compromise between the above two representations is a sparsely distributed representation. In this scheme only a fraction of the components (nodes) of a vector are involved in representing a certain stimulus. The number of stimuli that can be represented by a vector of length N is then somewhere in-between the cases above. Note that the information content has to be the same in all cases because the information cannot change with the internal representation as long as the representation is information-preserving; only the information content of each node will be different. In the case of binary vectors, we would have a larger probability for a node to be 'off' compared to the probability for the nodes to be 'on'.

8.5.1 Sparseness

To specify more quantitatively how many (or what percentage of) neurons are involved in the neural processing of individual stimuli, we define here a measure of sparseness of a representation. A definition is obvious in the case of binary nodes. If we consider neurons (or population nodes) that are either active ($r = 1$) or not ($r = 0$), then the average number of nodes that are active for a set of stimuli is

$$a = \frac{1}{S} \sum_s \frac{1}{N} \sum_i r_i^s, \tag{8.25}$$

where S is the number of stimuli over which the sparseness is evaluated, and N is the number of neurons in the considered population. In other words, if we consider relative firing rates r that are either 0 if the neuron is not responding or 1 if it is responding, then the sparseness of the representation with binary nodes is defined by the average relative firing rate,

$$a = \langle r_i^s \rangle_{i,s}, \tag{8.26}$$

where the average is taken over the number of neurons in the population and the number of stimuli in the test set. A fully distributed binary representation has in this definition a sparseness of $a = 0.5$, and the sparseness of sparsely distributed representations is less if we restrict ourselves to the case where the number of nodes that are *on* is less than $N/2$. Note that the other case of having more *on*-nodes than *off*-nodes can be mapped to the previous case by redefining the values for the representation of *on* and *off*.

The definition of sparseness in the case of vectors with continuous (real-valued) components is not that obvious. We have then to decide how much weight we put on the contribution of small versus large firing rates. What we would like to do is to take the information in the firing rate as a weighting factor, which means that we should take the firing rate relative to the variance of the firing rate into account. We thus define the sparseness of a representation, again defined as average over a set of stimuli, as

$$a = \frac{\langle r_i^s \rangle_{i,s}^2}{\langle (r_i^s)^2 \rangle_{i,s}}. \tag{8.27}$$

For example, we can measure the firing rate of N neurons in response to a set of S stimuli and estimate the sparseness as

$$a = \frac{\left(\frac{1}{S} \sum_s \frac{1}{N} \sum_i r_i^s \right)^2}{\frac{1}{S} \sum_s \frac{1}{N} \sum_i (r_i^s)^2}. \tag{8.28}$$

The definitions 8.25 and 8.27 are equivalent in the case of binary vectors with components of value 0 and 1. The sparseness of coding with tuning curves, as modelled by DNF models, can be calculated from the size of the activity packet. For example, the sparseness of the end states in the simulation of Fig. 8.9 is $a = 0.56$. Thus, orientation tuning curves in V1 indicate a strongly distributed representation in a hypercolumn. However, we will see that some brain areas, in particular the hippocampus, which is discussed more in the next chapter, are though to have much sparser representations.

8.5.2 Probabilistic population coding

We expect that information about the external world and the processing of information is distributed in the brain, but this representation can be very noisy given the stochastic nature of neuronal activities, as discussed in Chapter 5. Here we discuss probabilistic encoding, the specific way in which a stimulus is coded in a neuron or a population of neurons, and decoding, how a message can be read from the responses of a neuron or a population of neurons. We can express the encoding of a stimulus pattern in terms of the response probability of neurons in a population with a joined probability distribution of neuronal responses conditional on a stimulus s,

$$P(\mathbf{r}|s) = P(r_1^s, r_2^s, r_3^s, ...|s), \tag{8.29}$$

where r_i^s is the stimulus-specific response of neuron i in the population. We will here mainly consider stimulus-specific firing rates as the response, although other response quantities such as the latencies of firings can be treated in the same framework. We are using the symbol P as either meaning the probability for discrete random variables or the probability densities in the case of continuous random variables.

Decoding is the inverse of encoding, that is, we want to deduce what stimulus was presented from the neuronal responses of a neuron or a population of neurons. Decoding brain activity has recently become of much interest in brain–computer interfaces, and the brain may have to perform such computations at some stages. The probability that a stimulus was present, given a certain response pattern of the neurons in the population, is expressed by the conditional probability

$$P(s|\mathbf{r}) = P(s|r_1^s, r_2^s, r_3^s, ...). \tag{8.30}$$

If we know this conditional probability, we can say which stimulus was most likely present given a certain response of the neuron population. It is obvious to choose the most likely stimulus as an answer to the decoding problem,

$$\hat{s} = \arg\max_s P(s|\mathbf{r}), \tag{8.31}$$

where $\hat{s}$ is our estimation of the stimulus and $\arg\max f(x)$ is a function that selects the argument x that maximizes the expression $f(x)$. We can estimate the conditional probabilities $P(\mathbf{r}|s)$ from recordings of cells as stated above, but we need the conditional probability $P(s|\mathbf{r})$. However, these two conditional probabilities are related through the identity called Bayes's theorem.

$$P(s|\mathbf{r}) = \frac{P(\mathbf{r}|s)P(s)}{P(\mathbf{r})}. \tag{8.32}$$

This theorem is important because it tells us how to combine prior knowledge, such as the expected distribution of stimuli, $P(s)$, with some evidence as measured by $P(\mathbf{r}|s)$, to get the posterior distribution $P(s|\mathbf{r})$ from which the optimal estimate (in a statistical sense) of the stimulus can be calculated with eqn 8.31. Note that in the literature there are sometimes discussions and critiques on the 'Bayesian view'. This refers to a more philosophical discussion on the use of probability theory to describe experiments with underlying mechanisms that are thought to be deterministic in nature. In contrast, Bayes's theorem is an identity within probability (or set) theory and is not questioned by statisticians.

$P(r)$ is the proper normalization so that the left-hand side is again a probability. To use the theorem we need to have an estimate of the prior $P(s)$ and the evidence $P(\mathbf{r}|s)$. The normalization is not necessary if we are only interested in finding the most likely stimulus. Let us consider the case of equally likely stimuli. We then need to estimate the probability $P(\mathbf{r}|s)$. However, this is what is given by the tuning curves.

Indeed, we can view this as a function of the stimulus. When treating the probability function as a function of the stimulus, which is usually done by building a concrete model (hypothesis) of the response, this function is then called the likelihood function. Thus, we can ask which sensory stimulus provides the maximum likelihood of the data,

$$\hat{s}_{\mathrm{ML}} = \arg\max_s P(\mathbf{r}|s),\qquad(8.33)$$

which is called the maximum likelihood estimate. In practice we mostly maximize the logarithm of the likelihood because a joined probability of independent variables can be expressed as the product of their marginal probabilities. The logarithm of a product is the sum of the logarithm of the individual terms. Such a sum is often more easy to calculate. Also, note that when we have to take the prior into account we need to use Bayes's theorem to calculate the maximum posterior distribution (MAP; eqn 8.31) to estimate the most likely stimulus causing the neural response.

The importance of the maximum likelihood estimate in statistics is that it is an unbiased estimate, which is an estimate for which the expectation value (mean) of the estimate is equal to the correct parameter, $E(\hat{s}_{\mathrm{ML}} = s)$. Furthermore, the variance of this estimate is optimal in the sense that it approaches the minimum possible variance given by the Cramér–Rao bound,

$$E\left((\hat{s}_{\mathrm{ML}} - s)^2\right) = \frac{1}{I_{\mathrm{F}}},\qquad(8.34)$$

where I_{F} is the Fisher information

$$I_{\mathrm{F}} = -\int p(\mathbf{r}|s)(\frac{\mathrm{d}}{\mathrm{d}s}\ln p(\mathbf{r}|s))^2\mathrm{d}s.\qquad(8.35)$$

The maximum likelihood estimate can therefore provide some reasonable estimates with limited data sets.

8.5.3 Optimal decoding with tuning curves

Tuning curves are commonly deduced from average responses of neurons to many different stimuli, and these curves provide some estimate of the likelihood function. We use again Gaussian tuning curves $f_i(s)$,

$$r_i = f_i(s) = \mathrm{e}^{-(s-s_i^{\mathrm{pref}})^2/2\sigma_{\mathrm{tc}}^2},\qquad(8.36)$$

with width σ_{tc}, and where s_i^{pref} is the preferred stimulus of this node. An example is provided in Fig. 8.21A. Note that we cannot determine the feature value of the stimulus from the firing rate of one neuron unambiguously because a certain firing rate can be the result of two different stimuli. This ambiguity is, however, removed in a population code. A second neuron with a shifted tuning curve, illustrated in Fig. 8.21B, can resolve the ambiguity. In the illustrated example the firing rate of the neuron is higher in the case of the true stimulus corresponding to the right solution compared to the alternative. Note also that the accuracy of the decoding can be different for different values of the stimulus feature value s. A good resolution can be achieved where the tuning curve changes most with respect to the stimulus feature value s, around the

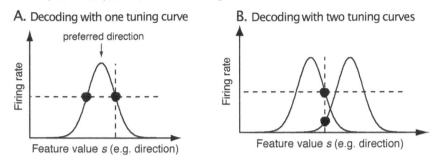

A. Decoding with one tuning curve   **B.** Decoding with two tuning curves

Fig. 8.21 Gaussian tuning curves representing the firing rate of a neuron as a function of a stimulus feature. (A) A single neuron cannot unambiguously decode the stimulus feature from the firing rate. (B) A second neuron with shifted tuning curve can resolve the ambiguity.

largest slope of the tuning curve, $\max(f'(s))$, not at the maximum. However, with noisy data we also have to take the signal to noise ratio into account, which might be highest at the centre of the tuning curves.

In the following we will assume that the response fluctuations of the neurons around this average response profile are independent, so that the conditional probability $P(\mathbf{r}|s)$ can be written as the product of the conditional probabilities of the individual neurons,

$$P(\mathbf{r}|s) = \prod_i P(r_i|s). \tag{8.37}$$

This is called a naive Bayes assumption. We still do not know the individual probability densities and have to guess this. Since we estimated the tuning curves from average responses, and since the average of random numbers tends to be Gaussian distributed (according to the central limit theorem), we use

$$P(r_i|s) = \frac{1}{\sqrt{2\pi}\sigma_i}\mathrm{e}^{-(r_i - f_i(s))^2/2\sigma_i^2}, \tag{8.38}$$

we can calculate the log-likelihood function by taking the logarithm of this expression and viewing it as a function of s. The maximum likelihood estimator can thus be extracted in this situation by minimizing the expression,

$$\hat{s} = \mathrm{argmin} \sum_i \left(\frac{r_i - f_i(s)}{\sigma_i}\right)^2, \tag{8.39}$$

which is a least square fit of the data points r_i (measured firing rates) to the expected firing rates $f_i(s)$ of stimulus s.

8.5.4 Implementations of decoding mechanisms

We can now outline some practical methods for population decoding, which have been suggested as implementations of decoding mechanisms in the brain. The most commonly used method is simply called population vector decoding, which we will use to demonstrate some general properties of decoding with different widths of tuning curves. For this demonstration, we consider a set of neurons with Gaussian tuning curves, as illustrated in Fig. 8.22 for eight neurons. These nodes have equally distributed preferred directions with centres s_i^{pref} every 45 degrees. We will compare a system with two different widths of the receptive fields, $\sigma_t = 10$ degrees shown in Fig. 8.22A, and $\sigma_t = 20$ degrees shown in Fig. 8.22B. We might intuitively think that sharper tuning curves lead to more accurate decoding. This is, however, not the case. The principal reason for this can be seen in the firing rate pattern of the eight nodes in response to a specific stimulus pattern shown in the second row of Fig. 8.22. There, we plotted the noiseless response of the neurons to a stimulus at 130 degrees, indicated by the vertical dashed line. The neurons with preferred direction close to this stimulus value respond heavily. However, we also see a response from some of the neurons in the population with wide receptive fields, which helps in the decoding process.

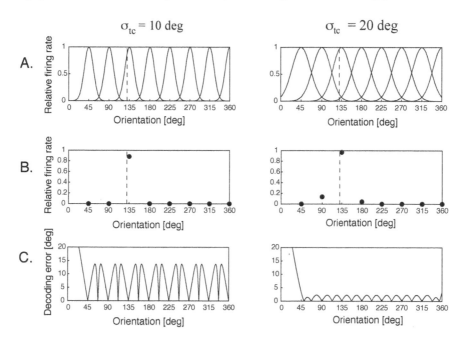

Fig. 8.22 (A) Gaussian tuning curves representing the firing rate of a neuron as a function of a stimulus feature. (B) Example of the firing rates of the eight neurons in response to a stimulus with direction 130 degrees. (C) Decoding error when the stimulus is estimated with a population code.

To decode the stimulus value for the firing pattern of the population we multiply the firing rate of each neuron by its preferred direction and sum the contributions of all the neurons,

$$\hat{s}_{\text{dir}} = \sum_i r_i s_i^{\text{pref}}. \tag{8.40}$$

For a stimulus that coincides with a preferred direction for one neuron, and with small sizes of the receptive fields so that the firing rates of the other neurons can be neglected, we get an estimate that is r_i times the preferred direction of the node that is firing. We will therefore have to apply some further normalization.

In our example, the stimulus values are real values for the direction of the moving object. However, we can apply this method to higher-dimensional stimulus presentations, so that the preferred stimulus of a neuron is a feature vector s_i^{pref}. The estimate (eqn 8.40) is then a vector that is an estimate of the direction of the feature vector, but has a length that depends on the sum of the firing rates. If we are interested in the precise values of the stimulus features, and the nodes have different dynamical ranges r_i^{min}–r_i^{max}, we have to normalize the firing rates to the relative values, and the sum in eqn 8.40 to the total firing rates,

$$\hat{r}_i = \frac{r_i - r_i^{\text{min}}}{r_i^{\text{max}}} \tag{8.41}$$

$$\hat{s}_{\text{pop}} = \sum_i \frac{\hat{r}_i}{\sum_j \hat{r}_j} s_i^{\text{pref}}. \tag{8.42}$$

This is the normalized population vector that can be used as an estimate of the stimulus. The absolute error of decoding orientation stimuli with this scheme in our example of eight neurons is shown in the last row of Fig. 8.22. The decoding error is very large for small orientations because this part of the feature space is not well covered by the population of neurons. Reasonable estimates are, however, achieved for the areas of the feature space that are covered reasonably well by the receptive fields of the neurons. The error is not uniform and depends on the feature values. The average error is much less for the larger receptive fields compared to the average errors of the population of neurons with smaller receptive fields.

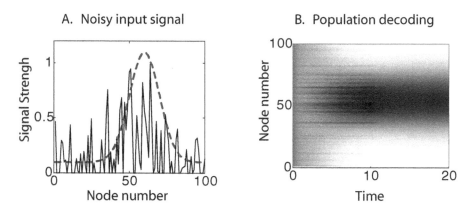

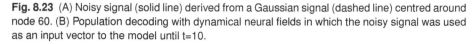

Fig. 8.23 (A) Noisy signal (solid line) derived from a Gaussian signal (dashed line) centred around node 60. (B) Population decoding with dynamical neural fields in which the noisy signal was used as an input vector to the model until t=10.

We have only shown results for the noiseless case. The real test is the performance of estimates with noisy data, which we leave as an exercise. It is well known that other estimation methods can easily outperform the population vector decoding-procedure outlined here. In particular, DNF models can be used for this purpose. These have the advantage of being computationally efficient and biologically plausible. To use DNFs for noisy population decoding we can simply apply a noisy population vector as input to the model. An example is shown in Fig. 8.23. In this example we used a very noisy signal, shown as a solid line in Fig. 8.23A. This was derived from the noiseless Gaussian signal around node 60, shown as a dashed line in the same graph. The noisy input is then applied as input to the DNF model with the program used before (dnf.py). The time evolution for this simulation is shown in Fig. 8.23B. The competition within the model cleans up the signal and finds a winning node that corresponds to the direction of the noiseless signal. There is already some advantage in decoding before the signal is removed at time $t = 10$. This example demonstrates that simple decoding using the maximal value would produce large errors with the noisy signal. However, the maximum decoding can easily be applied to the clean signals after some updates in the DNF model.

9 Recurrent associative networks and episodic memory

This chapter continues the discussion on the dynamics of recurrent networks. However, instead of using the characteristic recurrent weight profile of the last chapter, we now train the networks on random patterns. We show that such networks can function as auto-associative memories, which can rapidly store items and are able to recall stored items from partial information. In contrast to DNF models, which have a continuous manifold of point attractors (continuous attractors for short), the models here have isolated point attractors of their dynamics. We discuss the storage capacity of point attractor networks and their extraordinary robustness to noise and lesions. But memories can also break down rapidly when overloading the network or when lesions become to severe, and we will study the physics of such sharp transitions to amnesic phases. We also review gated recurrent networks such as long short-term memory.

9.1 The auto-associative network and the hippocampus

9.1.1 Different memory types

The words 'learning' and 'memory' can be applied to many different domains. We have already discussed several types of learning and memory, and it is time to conceptualize the different types in some form. In the last chapter, we encountered a type of short-term memory, often called working memory by physiologists, in which representations of concepts seem to be held active by sustained firing of neurons. This type of short-term storage is essential for many mental abilities and thus relates to what psychologists call working memory. We also discussed, in the last chapter, the formation of cortical maps, which is a form of learning and memory on a developmental scales. This type of memory is long term, since these learned organizations can be stable for a long time. However, there are other aspects of learning and memory we would like to comprehend, such as learning concepts, remembering specific events, or learning motor skills.

Fig. 9.1 shows a classification of memory adopted from a review by Larry Squire. In this scheme, memory is distinguished by either being declarative or non-declarative. Declarative memories are explicit memories such as recalling specific events or facts. Recalling specific events, such as remembering what you did this morning, is called episodic memory. Remembering facts, such as the name of the capital of France, is called semantic memory. Non-declarative memory is more implicit, which includes concepts such as procedural and perceptual learning and memory, classical conditioning, and non-associative learning. Procedural learning includes learning motor skills, such as how to ride a bike, or social skills, like learning to function in a group. Perceptual learning includes the formation of cortical maps, which is related to priming in the

Fundamentals of Computational Neuroscience. Third edition. Thomas P. Trappenberg, Oxford University Press. © Oxford University Press 2023. DOI: 10.1093/oso/9780192869364.003.0009

psychology literature. Classical conditioning, such as responding to a bell with an eye blink when the bell was previously combined with an air puff, is another widespread adaptation mechanism in the brain. We will discuss this topic together with reward learning in Chapter 10. All these forms of memory can be related to Hebbian type associative mechanisms. The last category includes non-associative memories, such as reflexes.

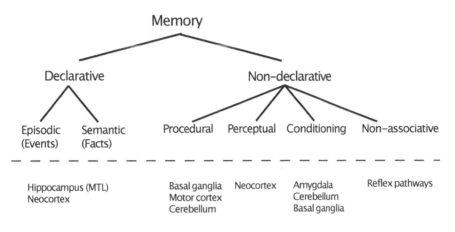

Fig. 9.1 Outline of a memory classification scheme [adapted from Squire, *Neurobiology of Learning and Memory* 82: 171–7 (2004)].

Fig. 9.1 includes, at the bottom, some examples of brain areas in the nervous system that have been associated with such memory concepts. Conditioning has been associated with several brain areas. For example, implicit emotional responses, such as fear have been associated with the amygdala, and the cerebellum has been shown to be involved in eye blink conditioning. We will specifically discuss reward learning in the basal ganglia in the next chapter. The formation or reorganization of cortical maps is an example of perceptual learning, and procedural learning has been associated with the motor cortex, the basal ganglia, and the cerebellum, to name a few. Interestingly, a very specific area called the hippocampus, together with adjacent areas in the medial temporal lobe (MTL), are frequently associated with declarative memory. This area is of particular interest to the discussion in this chapter. While we will discuss the hippocampus as an example, it is important to keep in mind that the models in this chapter are more general and that this area alone is certainly not the only brain area involved in declarative memory. Declarative memory relies heavily on cortical processes, and the precise contribution of the hippocampus in various forms of declarative memory is still under considerable debate.

Before getting more specifically into models of declarative memories, we will contrast this with Chapter 7, where we discussed object recognition in a statistical learning context. Networks in that chapter were aimed at learning to extract central tendencies to allow generalizations to unseen data. The memorization of single instances was destructive, since they cause overfitting. While such types of learning are important in the brain and are likely present in some form of semantic memory, we concentrate

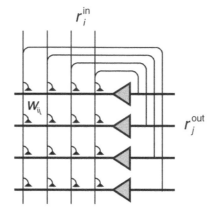

Fig. 9.2 An auto-associative network which consists of associative nodes that not only receive external input from other neural layers but, in addition, have many recurrent collateral connections between the nodes in the neural layer.

here on the learning of specific instances and associative mechanisms, as discussed in Chapter 6.

The principle network considered in this chapter is shown in Fig. 9.2 which is the same type of recurrent network structure as the ones in the last chapter. The only difference between the auto-associative memory discussed in this chapter and the DNF model discussed in Chapter 8 is that the network is trained on a different pattern set. While the DNF models were systematically trained on all possible features to be represented in the map, the networks in this chapter will be trained on distinct patterns, mostly random patterns to demonstrate their ability. We will see that this leads to well-separated point-attractors in these networks, whereas the DNF model had a continuous manifold of point attractors. The models here are therefore called point attractor neural networks (PANNs), or simply attractor neural networks (ANNs), in contrast to the continuous attractor neural networks (CANNs) of Chapter 8.

The model in Fig. 9.2 is similar to the associator network shown Fig. 6.2, except that the input of each node is fed back to all of the other nodes in the network. In this way we can associate a pattern with itself. Such networks are therefore also called auto-associator, although it is possible to realize an auto-associative memory as feedforward architecture called auto-encoders. In this chapter, we are specifically interested in recurrent networks, and we will use the auto-associative network synonymously with the specific form of a recurrent network.

The back-projections in this associative network introduce attractive features into the model. As has already been seen, associators are able to perform some form of pattern completion. After an external input pattern is presented to the network, the network will respond with an output pattern more similar to a trained pattern when Hebbian learning is applied. This response is then fed back as input to the same network, so that the network will respond with a pattern that is again made closer to a learned pattern. We therefore expect that the cycling in a recurrent network can enhance the pattern completion ability of simple one-step associative nodes. The dynamic process of changing responses in the recurrent network will stop when a learned output pattern

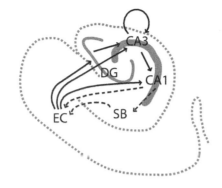

Fig. 9.3 A schematic outline of the medial temporal lobe with some connections mentioned in the text. Some areas are indicated by acronyms including the entorhinal cortex (EC), dentate gyrus (DG), hippocampal subfield cornus ammonis (CA), and subiculum (SB).

is reached.

As we have already seen in Chapter 8, such an attractor state keeps active until another pattern is applied to the network. However, working memory will not be the main focus of the discussions here. Also, while we will talk about asymptotic and stationary states in this chapter which seems contrary to ongoing mental activity, this should not be taken as an argument to dismiss such models since this is only a convenient way describe the system mathematically. Such states are meant to describe some forces in the system within the larger picture of a system with ongoing iterations. We will see that some systems can come close to asymptotic states within a few iterations.

9.1.2 The hippocampus and episodic memory

The models discussed in this chapter have been implicated with hippocampal functions since a theory of the archicortex was proposed by David Marr in 1976. This phylogenetically older part of the cortex is part of the medial temporal lobe and is illustrated in Fig. 9.3 with a coronal section. This structure is called hippocampus for its shape resembling a seahorse, and some of its subfields are labelled CA for cornus ammonis after the Egyptian ram god. This is the same structure in which Bliss and Lomø discovered LTP and which is a primary area examined in plasticity research as mentioned in Chapter 6. Also, we mentioned place fields in Chapter 8, which are often recorded in the hippocampus of rodents, as well as head-direction cells, which are often recorded from the neighbouring subiculum.

The hippocampus has been implicated with the acquisition of episodic memories since the famous case of patient HM. In this patient, large parts of both medial temporal lobes were removed to treat his epileptic condition. Subsequently, he suffered from a form of amnesia marked by the inability to form new long-term memories of episodic events. In contrast, long-term memory that was acquired before the removal of this structure was not impaired. However, he still could learn new motor skills and even acquire some new semantic memories. This condition is called retrograde amnesia. The precise involvement of the hippocampus in memory acquisition and recall is still under intense debate, but it seems that the hippocampus can rapidly store memories of events which may later be consolidated with neocortical information storage.

The hippocampus seems extraordinarily adapted to the rapid storage of complex events. The input to the hippocampus comes primarily from the entorhinal cortex (EC), which receives input from many cortical areas. The coding within these areas, in particular in the dentate gyrus (DG), is very sparse, and we will discuss later how this helps to minimize interference with other memories. The DG is also an area where neurogenesis, the creation of new neuronal cells throughout the lifetime of an organism, has been established. There are two major pathways to subfield CA3, one that first projects to DG, and another which passes through DG, called the perforant pathway. The CA3 region has many collateral connections which contact other cells in CA3 and CA1. These abandoned collaterals, in particular within CA3, have largely inspired the study of recurrent networks of the form shown in Fig. 9.2. CA1 projects back to the EC, but EC also has direct projections to CA1. It is possible that some of the pathways are preferentially active in either a storage or retrieval phase, as discussed further below.

The basic models discussed further in this section only capture some aspects of hippocampal processing, most notably the storage abilities of specific events in auto-associative networks. While such models are capture an important ability of networks, that of forming associative memory in recurrent networks, there are now much more detailed proposals of hippocampal functions with respect to sequence processing, novelty detection, memory consolidation, and other functions. But the basic model was an important milestone in the computational neuroscience.

9.1.3 Learning and retrieval phase

Before we outline the memory abilities of recurrent associative networks in more detail, we must mention a difficulty that occurs when combining associative Hebbian mechanisms with recurrences in the networks. Associative learning depends crucially on relating presynaptic activity to postsynaptic activity that is imposed by an unconditioned stimulus. The recurrent network will, however, drive this postsynaptic activity rapidly away from the activity pattern we want to imprint if the dynamic of the recurrent network is dominant. A solution to the problem is to divide the operation of the networks into two phases, a training phase and a retrieval phase. These phases can be interleaved.

There are several proposals as to how the switching between the learning and retrieval phase could be accomplished in the hippocampus. For example, mossy fibres from granule cells in the DG provide strong inputs to CA3 neurons with the largest synapses found in the mammalian brain, which David Marr termed detonator synapses. Thus, CA3 firing patterns could be dominated by this pathway during a learning phase. In contrast, the perforant pathway could stimulate the CA3 neurons in the retrieval phase, where the CA3 collateral and CA3–CA1 projections could help to complete patterns from partial inputs. This ability could also be supported by different types of synapses and their proximity to the cell body.

Another proposal, investigated by Michael Hasselmo, is that chemical agents, such as acetylcholine (ACh) and noradrenaline (also called norepinephrine), could modulate learning and thereby enable the switching between a retrieval and learning phase.

It has been shown that such neuromodulators facilitate synaptic plasticity and that their presence enhances the firing of the neurons. At the same time, neuromodulators suppress excitatory synaptic transmission, which can then suppress the effects of the recurrent collaterals. The neurons are therefore mainly responsive to external input to the system, which mirrors the proposal of the learning phase that we will generally apply in the following models.

Even if ACh is not directly responsible for switching between learning and retrieval phases in the hippocampus, it is well known that this chemical is important as a modulator of plasticity throughout the cortex. The switching between learning and retrieval phases might also be necessary for the transfer of intermediate-term memories stored in the hippocampus to long-term memory stores in other cortical areas. This might happen during sleep, and fluctuations of ACh during sleep have been detected. There are many further interesting questions, such as the control of the neuromodulation and the time scale of the switching between learning and retrieval, which need further investigation.

9.2 Point-attractor neural networks (ANN)

Many researchers have speculated about the importance of feedback connections within brain networks. Grossberg was among the first to propose, analyse, and popularize such networks in connection with brain processes, since the late 1950s. Other important pioneers include Caianiello, Longuet-Higgins, Willshaw, Edelman, Amari, and Kohonen, among others. For a nice collection of early papers see Shaw and Palm, *Brain theory*, preprint edition, World Scientific (1988). John Hopfield popularized these networks among physicists in the early 1980s. Much of the following is based on work by Amit, Gutfreund, and Sompolinsky. We will now discuss attractor states, since they dominate the time evolution of the dynamic systems discussed here, at least asymptotically. Since it may take a considerably long time for the system to come close to such states, the relevance of such states for brain processes has been questioned. However, we will see that attractor states are reached fairly rapidly in most of the situations discussed here. Also, there is no need for the brain to settle into attractor states. Rather, the rapid path towards attractor states may be sufficient to use them as associative memories. While this suits the real-time processing demands of brain functions much better, we discuss attractor states to analyse the dynamic regimes of the networks.

9.2.1 Network dynamics and training

The dynamic rule of ANNs is the same as the one covered in Chapter 8, although a description with individual nodes is more appropriate to use here. We therefore use the discrete version (eqn 8.1) with external inputs as in eqn 8.6,

$$\tau \frac{\mathrm{d}u_i(t)}{\mathrm{d}t} = -u_i(t) + \frac{1}{N}\sum_j w_{ij}r_j(t) + I_i^{\mathrm{ext}}(t) \tag{9.1}$$

$$r_i = g(u_i), \tag{9.2}$$

and the Hebbian covariance rule for learning N_p patterns with components r_i^μ for pattern μ. When starting this rule with an initial weight matrix of zeros, and using a learning rate of ϵ (see also Section 6.4.2, eqn 6.23), we can write the resulting weight matrix as

$$w_{ij} = \epsilon \sum_{\mu=1}^{N_p} (r_i^\mu - \langle r_i \rangle)(r_j^\mu - \langle r_j \rangle) - c_i. \tag{9.3}$$

We included thereby an inhibition constant, c_i for each receiving node, analogous to the additional inhibition used in Chapter 8. The angular brackets stand for the expected values as used before. This chapter primarily considers training binary patterns. To keep notations consistent with the last chapter, we start with representations $r_i^\mu \in \{0, 1\}$, for which a threshold activation function,

$$r_i = \Theta(u_i; \theta) = \begin{cases} 1 & \text{if } u_i > \theta \\ 0 & \text{otherwise} \end{cases}, \tag{9.4}$$

is appropriate. Note that pattern values, in contrast to state values of the network, are denoted with a superscript for the different pattern numbers.

The literature on ANNs often uses patterns with representation $s_i^\mu \in \{-1, 1\}$, where the letter s is used to allude to an analogy with spin models, discussed more below. This representation is used for most of the discussions in this chapter. Of course, the arguments derived here should not depend on the representation, so some care must be given to the correct translation between the notations. To translate rates $r \in \{0, 1\}$ to spins $s \in \{-1, 1\}$ we can simply multiply the rate values by 2 and subtract a 1, $s = 2r - 1$. Hence, to transform eqns 9.1–9.3 to the s-representation, one can simply use the substitutions

$$r_i = \frac{1}{2}(s_i + 1), u_i = \frac{1}{2}(u_i^s + 1). \tag{9.5}$$

Substituting the rate variables with the spin variables yields

$$\tau \frac{du_i^s(t)}{dt} = -u_i^s(t) + \frac{1}{N} \sum_j w_{ij} s_j + \sum_j w_{ij} + 2I_i^{\text{ext}}(t) - 1, \tag{9.6}$$

$$s_i = g^s(u_i^s) = \text{sign}(u_i^s - 2\theta + 1), \tag{9.7}$$

where the activation function is now appropriately the sign function with some adjusted threshold. The weight values, when expressed with patterns in the s-representations, are

$$w_{ij} = \epsilon \frac{1}{4} \sum_{\mu=1}^{N_p} (s_i^\mu - \langle s_i \rangle)(s_j^\mu - \langle s_j \rangle) - c_i, \tag{9.8}$$

which has the same form as in the r-representation, but with an adjustment in the learning rate.

In contrast to the previous chapter, we are here primarily interested in stationary states as memory states. Stationary states are the states that do not change under the dynamics of the system which are hence marked by $du_i^s/dt = 0$. The dynamic equations are simple in the case of $\sum_j w_{ij} + 2I_i^{\text{ext}}(t) = 1$ using a threshold of $\theta = 0.5$. The stationary states are then fixpoints of the discrete system,

$$s_i(t+1) = \text{sign}\left(\sum_j w_{ij} s_j(t)\right) \tag{9.9}$$

where we have applied the activation function to both sides of the stationary state equation. We first discuss the case $c_i = 0$. Both, the continuous time model (eqns 9.6 and 9.7), and the discrete fixpoint model (eqn 9.9) can illustrate the asymptotic features of the system with weight matrix eqn 9.8. It is only when we are interested in the transient response dynamics of the model, for example when modelling the reaction times of the system, that we have to use the continuous equations.

The attractor models can be considered in a probabilistic context, either with stochastic background input, noisy weights, or probabilistic transmissions. We often speak simply of noise in this context, although it should be clear that this probabilistic description can be more than just unwanted environmental effects. A common noise model used for results shown later is a probabilistic updating rule, which replaces the deterministic activation function (eqn 9.9)

$$s_i(t) = \text{sign}\left(\sum_j w_{ij} s_j(t-1)\right) \tag{9.10}$$

with a probabilistic version

$$P(s_i(t) = +1) = \frac{1}{1 + \exp(-2\sum_j w_{ij} s_j(t-1)/T)}. \tag{9.11}$$

This noise model corresponds to the Boltzmann statistics in thermodynamic systems, and the noise parameter T is therefore sometimes called temperature. The sign function is recovered in the limit $T \to 0$ (see exercise).

The main conclusion of this chapter is that dynamic networks, as introduced in this section, can function as an auto-associative memory devise. This is demonstrated for the fixpoint model and the continuous time model in Fig. 9.4. Both networks were first trained on 10 random patterns. The fixpoint model (Fig. 9.4A) was then initialized with a random pattern, and a noisy version of one pattern was used as external input until $t = 10\tau$ for the continuous time model. Both plots show the normalized dot product, called overlap in these plots, between the network states with each stored pattern while updating the networks. The normalized dot product measures the cosine of the angle between two vectors and is hence equal to one if the vectors are pointing in the same direction and zero when they are perpendicular. In the figure, one of the lines becomes one, which shows that one pattern was retrieved. The simulation with the continuous model demonstrates recovery of a (noisy) memory since we used such a noisy state as input pattern until $t = 10\tau$. We show in this figure a particularly interesting case in which two patterns competed for some time before the correct stored pattern was retrieved. The simulations in the discrete case were started with a random pattern and demonstrate that one of the stored patterns was retrieved. Both simulations also demonstrate working memory with sustained firing after removal of the external input.

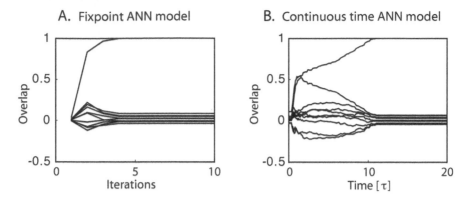

A. Fixpoint ANN model

B. Continuous time ANN model

Fig. 9.4 Examples of results from simulations of ANN models. (A) Simulation of the fixpoint model with program `ann_fixpoint.m`. The overlap here is the normalized dot product of the network states during an update with all of the 10 patterns that were imprinted with Hebbian learning into the network. The network was initialized randomly, and one of the stored patterns was retrieved. (B) Simulation of the continuous time version of an attractor network with program `ann_cont.m`. A noisy version of one stored pattern was applied as external input until $t = 10\tau$.

To demonstrate associative memory, we run a small experiment with binary neurons. We choose to represent these two states as -1 and 1. We can easily transform the network to other state representations, but it turns out that this representation helps with the compactness of the following program. We use hard threshold units in this example with the 'update rule'

$$\mathbf{s}(t+1) = \text{sign}(\mathbf{w}\mathbf{s}(t-1)). \qquad (9.12)$$

The sign function returns -1 if the argument is less than and otherwise 1. This is just another version of a threshold perceptron. We now want to store some patterns $\mathbf{x}^\mu$ in this network. The new part is now how we train this network. We use here the

$$\text{Hebb rule:} \quad \mathbf{w} = \sum_\mu \mathbf{x}\mathbf{x}' \qquad (9.13)$$

This rule has a long history. It was verbally suggested by Donald O. Hebb in the 1940s and formalized by Eduardo R. Caianiello in 1961. This rule basically specifies that the connection between two neurons increases if both neurons are active (s=1) and decreases otherwise. A simulation program of a network with 500 nodes that stores 10 random patterns is given in program `Hopfield.py`.

Programs/Hopfield.py

```
1 import numpy as np
2 import matplotlib.pyplot as plt
3
4 pat=2*np.random.randint(2,size=(500,10))-1#Rand binary pattern
5 w=pat@pat.T                               #Hebbian learning
6 s = pat+10*np.random.randn(500,10)        #Initialize network
7 for t in range(10): s[:,t]=np.sign(w@s[:,t-1]) #Update network
8 plt.plot(s.T@pat/500)                      #plot overlaps
```

Fig. 9.4 shows the results of this simulation by showing the overlap between the network states and the vectors representing the ten random patterns. The value of this overlap is 1 if the two vectors are the same, it is -1 if all the features are inverted, and 0 on average for random relations. After training, the network was started on a random input. While the overlap between the network and the stored pattern is therefore not good initially, we can see that one patterns gets perfectly recalled (overlap = 1). Sometimes the program will result in an overlap of -1 or some other configuration, at it will become clear later why this can happen. The important point here is that we showed that the stored patterns are fix-points under the network dynamics. Interestingly, an overlap of -1 shows that the inverse of the pattern is also a fix-point under the network dynamics.

9.2.2 Signal-to-noise analysis ◇

It is possible to study the recall abilities of fixpoint networks more formally. The state of the network at each consecutive time step is given by the discrete dynamics, eqn 9.9, in which a Hebbian-trained weight matrix can be inserted,

$$s_i(t+1) = \text{sign}[\frac{1}{N}\sum_j\sum_\mu s_i^\mu s_j^\mu s_j(t)]. \tag{9.14}$$

Let us test the network when initialized with one of the trained patterns. Without loss of generality, we can choose $\mu = 1$ for the demonstration. It is then useful to split the terms in the sum over μ into a term for the first training pattern and a second term with the rest of the training patterns,

$$s_i(t+1) = \text{sign}[\frac{1}{N}s_i^1\sum_j s_j^1 s_j(t) + \frac{1}{N}\sum_j\sum_{\mu=2}^{N^{\text{pat}}} s_i^\mu s_j^\mu s_j(t)]. \tag{9.15}$$

The expression $s_j^1 s_j(t)$ in the first term simplifies for the initial condition $s_j(t) = s_j^1$. This product is always one with this choice of training patterns (either 1^2 or $(-1)^2$), and the sum of these ones just cancels the normalization factor N. We then get the expression

$$s_i(t+1) = \text{sign}[s_i(t) + \frac{1}{N}\sum_j\sum_{\mu=2}^{N^{\text{pat}}} s_i^\mu s_j^\mu s_j(t)]. \tag{9.16}$$

We want the network to be stationary for the trained pattern, and the first term does indeed point in the right direction. We call this term the 'signal' part, since it is this part that we want to recover after the updates of the network. The term $\frac{1}{N}\sum_j\sum_{\mu=2}^{N^{\text{pat}}} s_i^\mu s_j^\mu s_j^1$ describes the influence of the other stored patterns on the state of the network, and is called the cross-talk term. This cross-talk term is thought to be analogous to interference between similar memories in a biological memory system. The cross-talk in our formal analysis is a random variable because we used independent random variables s_i^μ as training patterns (see Appendix 3.5). The cross-talk term can thus be considered as 'noise'. The activity of the node i remains unchanged in the next time step as long as the cross-talk term is larger than -1 for $s_i^1 = 1$ or smaller than 1 for $s_i^1 = -1$. The probability of the node changing sign depends on the relative strength of that signal and noise, hence the name of the analysis.

The special case of a network with only one imprinted pattern ($N^{\text{pat}} = 1$) is particularly easy to analyse. In this case, we do not have a cross-talk term so the network stays in the initial state when started with the imprinted pattern. The imprinted pattern is thus a fixpoint of the dynamics of this network,

$$s_i(t+1) = \text{sign}[s_i] = s_i(t). \tag{9.17}$$

What happens if we do not start the network with the trained pattern, but instead start the network simulation with a noisy version of this pattern where some of the components are randomly flipped? In this case, we have to go back to eqn 9.15 and to notice that the sum $\sum_j s_j^\mu s_j(t)$ is always positive as long as we change fewer than half of the signs of the initial pattern. We therefore retrieve the learned pattern even when we initialize the network with a moderately noisy version of the trained pattern. The retrieval is also very fast, as it takes only one time step. The pattern will remain stable for all following time steps. The trained pattern is therefore a point attractor of the network dynamics, because initial states close to the trained pattern are attracted by this point in the state space of the network. As an interesting side note, if the number of flipped states is more than half of the number of nodes in the network, then the inverse pattern $s_i = -s_i^1$ is retrieved. Thus, the inverse of a trained pattern is also an attractor of such networks.

Now let us turn to the situation when we train the network on more than one pattern, ($N^{\text{pat}} > 1$). Let us further discuss the case of a pattern component $s_i^1 = 1$. The state of the corresponding node is preserved when the network is initialized with the first pattern, only if the contribution from the cross-talk (noise) term is larger than -1. The cross-talk term is a random variable because we used random variables s_i^μ as training patterns, as mentioned before. The mean of the random term is zero because the individual components are independent and the mean of the individual components is zero. Thus, we can expect some cases in which some of the many trained patterns are stable. However, the probability of the cross-talk term reversing the state of the node depends on the variance of the noise term. We therefore have to estimate the variance of the cross-talk term.

In our example, we used a training pattern with components that were equally distributed between values -1 and 1. Each part of the sum in the cross-talk term is therefore an equally distributed number with values -1 or 1. The sum of such binary random numbers over the training patterns (except the pattern that we used as the initial condition for the network) is a binomial distributed random number with mean zero and standard deviation $\sqrt{N^{\text{pat}} - 1}$. The large sum of such random numbers over the number of nodes in the network is then well approximated by a Gaussian distribution with mean zero and standard deviation $\sqrt{(N^{\text{pat}} - 1)N}$ (see Appendix 3.5). We finally have to take the normalization factor, N, in the cross-talk term into account, and the standard deviation of this 'noise' term is therefore,

$$\sigma = \sqrt{\frac{(N^{\text{pat}} - 1)}{N}} \approx \sqrt{\frac{N^{\text{pat}}}{N}} = \sqrt{\alpha}. \tag{9.18}$$

In this equation we have introduced the load parameter, $\alpha = N^{\text{pat}}/N$, which specifies the number of trained patterns, relative to the number of nodes in the network.

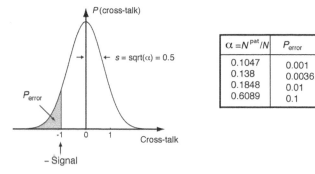

Fig. 9.5 The probability distribution of the cross-talk term is well approximated by a Gaussian with mean zero and variance $\sigma = \sqrt{\alpha}$. The value of the shaded area marked P_{error} is the probability that the cross-talk term changes the state of the node. The table lists examples of this probability for different values of the load parameter α.

With knowledge of the probability distribution of the cross-talk term, we can specify the probabilities of the cross-talk term changing the activity value of the node. The probability of the cross-talk term producing values less than -1 is illustrated in Fig. 9.5. Such an integral of a Gaussian is given by the error function (see eqn 3.54),

$$P_{error} = \frac{1}{2}[1 - \mathrm{erf}(\frac{S}{\sqrt{2}\sigma})], \tag{9.19}$$

where S is the strength of the signal, which is equal to one in our case, and σ is the variance of the cross-talk term, as estimated above. To ensure that the probability of the cross-talk term changing sign is less than a certain value, that is, $P_{error} < P_{bound}$, we need a load parameter less than

$$\alpha < \frac{1}{2[\mathrm{erf}^{-1}(1 - 2P_{bound})]^2}. \tag{9.20}$$

The expression for the cross-talk term distribution tells us that the probability of the component flipping sign is small when the load parameter of the network is small ($\alpha \ll 1$), that is, if the number of patterns in the training set is much smaller than the number of connections per node in the network ($P \ll N$). In particular, if we train the network on a number of patterns that is equal to 10% of the number of nodes in the network, that is, $P = 0.1N$, then the probability that the component will flip signs is less than 0.001. Some other examples are listed in the table in Fig. 9.5.

9.2.3 The phase diagram

The signal-to-noise analysis shows that it is likely for a moderate number of trained patterns to be still fixpoints of the network dynamics. However, an increasing number of training patterns will increase the probability of flipping signs in the activities of nodes. The flipped states can cause further nodes to flip signs in the next time step, and even cause an avalanche effect which leads the network state away from the trained pattern. Quantitative values for the parameters at which the memory breaks down can

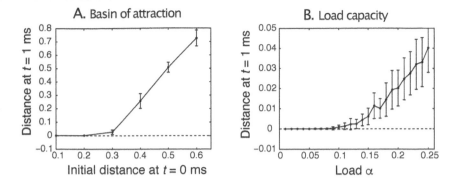

Fig. 9.6 Simulation results for an auto-associative network with continuous time, leaky-integrator dynamics, $N = 1000$ nodes, and a time constant of $\tau = 10$ ms. (A) Robustness to noise pattern recall. Average distance between network state and memory state at $t = 1$ ms as a function of the distance at time $t = 0$ ms, for a fixed number of training patterns ($N_p = 100$). (B) Average distance with different loads for a fixed distance of initial states ($d_0 = 0.01$).

only be derived from a more detailed analysis of the dynamics. One way to do this is to use simulations as outlined in Fig. 9.4.

The pattern completion ability of the associative nodes makes the trained patterns point attractors of the network dynamics in networks with small load parameters, as demonstrated in Fig. 9.4. Fig. 9.6 demonstrates the memory breakdown more systematically. These simulations were done with a larger network of $N = 1000$ nodes with a continuous time ANN with time constant $\tau = 10$ ms and a larger weight amplitude to allow faster convergence. We monitored the state of the network by calculating the distance, defined by

$$d(\mathbf{a}, \mathbf{b}) = \frac{1}{2}\left(1 - \frac{\mathbf{a}'\mathbf{b}}{||\mathbf{a}||\ ||\mathbf{b}||}\right), \tag{9.21}$$

between the training vector $\mathbf{a} = \mathbf{s}^1$ and the state of the system $\mathbf{b} = \mathbf{s}$. In contrast to the overlap measure used in Fig. 9.4, we here normalized the dot product so that the value is equal to the percentage of changed signs as compared to the training vectors.

In Fig. 9.6A, the network was started with a specific number of reversed components (flipped bits) of one training vector, and the distance of the network to this training vector was measured at $t = 1$ ms (0.1τ). The results demonstrate that the network converges, on average, to a trained pattern if the initial distance is less than a certain value around $d_{BA} \approx 0.3$. The trained pattern is therefore a point attractor under the dynamics of the network with a basin of attraction of size d_{BA}.

In Fig. 9.6B we show the results where the number of training patterns was changed and the network was initialized with a fixed small number (1%) of flipped bits of one training pattern. An analysis of networks with sparse connectivity shows that the relevant load parameter is the number of training patterns relative to the number of connections per node, C,

$$\alpha = \frac{N^{\mathrm{pat}}}{C}. \tag{9.22}$$

Of course, the number of connections per node is equal to the number of nodes in a fully connected network. The relatively sharp transitions between the domain in which the network can restore a noisy version of a training pattern to its original state, and the domain where the network is not able to retrieve the pattern has the signature of a phase transition, which is a transition between domains of a system with different properties. The transition point when the memory breaks down as the load is increased is called the load capacity, α_c, of the network.

The load capacity of auto-associative networks can be analysed in much more depth by realizing a useful correspondence of ANN models to so-called spin models developed in statistical physics. The binary states of the nodes are interpreted as spins, or little magnets, that can have two orientations, up or down. These 'magnets' interact with all the other magnets in the network. Two neighbouring magnets try to align each other in the same direction if the interaction between two magnets is positive (positive weight value). However, thermal noise is another force which tends to randomize the direction of the magnets (spins of the nodes). This randomizing force gets stronger with increasing temperature, T. The competition between the magnetic force, which tends to align the magnets, and the thermal force, which tends to randomize the directions, results in a sharp transition between a paramagnetic phase, in which there is no dominant direction of the magnets, and a ferromagnetic phase, in which there is a dominating direction of the elementary magnets. These phases have very different physical properties, and the transition is therefore called a phase transition.

Powerful analytical methods have been developed to describe systems of interacting spins. The situation in auto-associative networks is, however, further complicated by the fact that the force between the nodes is not consistently positive, but is instead somewhat random with a Gaussian distribution with positive and negative weights. The resulting conflicting forces can result in complicated spin states of the system. Such systems are known as frustrated systems or spin glasses; the latter alludes to the correspondence with glasses that have similar properties. Spin glasses are complicated systems and only partially tractable with standard methods of statistical mechanics, such as mean field theory. However, a breakthrough mathematical trick called the replica method was able to generalize the methods so that these can be applied to spin glasses. Physicists such as Daniel Amit have considerably advanced our understanding of attractor neural networks using such methods.

The phase diagram of the ANN model is summarized schematically in Fig. 9.7. This phase diagram outlines the phase boundaries as a function of two parameters, the load parameter, α, on the abscissa and the temperature, T (specifying the noise in the network), on the ordinate. A detailed analysis of such noisy network models shows that the shaded region in the phase diagram is where point attractors exist that correspond to trained patterns. The network in this phase is therefore useful as an associative memory. For vanishing noise, $T = 0$, a transition point to another phase occurs at around $\alpha_c(T = 0) \approx 0.138$. For load parameters larger than this value, the network is in a frustrated phase (spin glass phase), in which point attractors of trained memories become unstable. This frustrated phase is reached for smaller values of the load parameter if we include noise in the network. For strong noise the behaviour of the system is mainly random. Simulations have confirmed the validity of the analytical results.

The formal analysis of the network in this section describes the average behaviour of infinitely large networks. This is a good assumption in the sense that networks in the

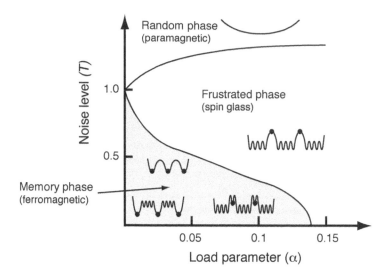

Fig. 9.7 Phase diagram of the attractor network trained on a binary pattern with Hebbian imprinting. The abscissa represents the values of the load parameter $\alpha = N^{\mathrm{pat}}/C$, where N^{pat} is the number of trained patterns and C is the number of connections per node. The ordinate represents the amount of noise in the system. The shaded region is where point attractors proportional to the trained pattern exist. The behaviour of the different phases is indicated with various cartoons of the energy landscape, where the states of training patterns is indicated with dots (see text) [adapted from Amit, Gutfreund and Sompolinsky, *Physical Review Letters* 55: 1530–3 (1995), and Hertz, Krogh, and Palmer, *Introduction to the theory of neural computation*, Addison-Wesley (1991)].

nervous system are comprised of many thousands of highly interconnected neurons. The transitions are less sharp in finite systems of networks with a finite number of nodes. Also, the behaviour of a particular network depends strongly on the specific realization of the training pattern. The phase diagram is therefore specific to the choice of training pattern, which we chose to be random binary numbers. Nevertheless, the example outlines the general picture that attractor states can be expected in recurrent networks, and that phase transitions to a phase in which the memory system breaks down (an amnesic phase) is possible under various circumstances. Breakdowns occur only after the network is brought to its limits. A load capacity of $\alpha_c \approx 0.138$ means that over 1000 memories can be stored in a system with nodes receiving 10,000 inputs, as is typical for neurons in the brain. This provides plenty of states that a small patch of cortex could store.

9.2.4 Spurious states and the advantage of noise ◇

It seems that noise would only be destructive for the memory abilities of the associative network. However, this is not entirely the case. To see how noise can help the memory performance of ANN, let us study how a mixture of some trained patterns behaves under the dynamics of the network. For example, let us start the network with a pattern that has the sign of the majority of the first three patterns,

Table 9.1 The possible states of three binary nodes and their summed value

s^1	s^2	s^3	$s^1 + s^2 + s^3$
1	1	1	3
1	1	-1	1
1	-1	1	1
1	-1	-1	-1
-1	1	1	1
-1	1	-1	-1
-1	-1	1	-1
-1	-1	-1	-3

$$s_i(t = 0) = s_i^{mix} = \text{sign}(s_i^1 + s_i^2 + s_i^3). \tag{9.23}$$

The state of the node after one update of this node with the discrete dynamics (eqn 8.1) is then

$$s_i(t = 1) = \text{sign}(\frac{1}{N} \sum_j \sum_{\mu=1}^{N^{\text{pat}}} s_i^\mu s_j^\mu \text{sign}(s_j^1 + s_j^2 + s_j^3))$$

$$= \text{sign}(\frac{1}{N} \sum_j (s_i^1 s_j^1 + s_i^2 s_j^2 + s_i^3 s_j^3)\text{sign}(s_j^1 + s_j^2 + s_j^3)$$

$$+ \frac{1}{N} \sum_j \sum_{\mu=4}^{N^{\text{pat}}} s_i^\mu s_j^\mu \text{sign}(s_j^1 + s_j^2 + s_j^3)) \tag{9.24}$$

The last term is again a cross-talk term, which can be shown to be of the same magnitude as the cross-talk term in the case of a trained pattern. The magnitude of the signal term itself can have different values. For example, if the components s_i^1, s_i^2, and s_i^3 all have the same value, which happens with a probability of 1/4, then we can pull out this value from the sum in the signal term,

$$\frac{1}{N} \sum_j (s_i^1 s_j^1 + s_i^2 s_j^2 + s_i^3 s_j^3)\text{sign}(s_j^1 + s_j^2 + s_j^3)$$

$$= s_i^1 \frac{1}{N} \sum_j (s_j^1 + s_j^2 + s_j^3)\text{sign}(s_j^1 + s_j^2 + s_j^3). \tag{9.25}$$

The components in the remaining sum of the signal term can have various values as can be seen from the possible combinations of components as listed in Table 9.1. We get a contribution of 3 if the signs of all three nodes s_j^1, s_j^2, and s_j^3 are the same. This happens again with probability 1/4. The remaining 3/4 of the time we get a contribution of 1. On average we therefore get a signal that is 3/2 of the signal of a trained pattern. However, the signal term is different when one sign of the nodes s_i^1, s_i^2, or s_i^3 is different from that of the other ones, which happens with probability 3/4. For example, if s_i^3 has a different sign from s_i^1 and s_i^2, we can write the signal term as

$$\frac{1}{N} \sum_j (s_i^1 s_j^1 + s_i^2 s_j^2 + s_i^3 s_j^3)\text{sign}(s_j^1 + s_j^2 + s_j^3)$$

$$= s_i^1 \frac{1}{N} \sum_j (s_j^1 + s_j^2 - s_j^3)\text{sign}(s_j^1 + s_j^2 + s_j^3). \qquad (9.26)$$

The average values of the remaining sum can be evaluated as before, showing that this is equal to 1/2. We conclude that we have, on average, a signal that has the strength of

$$\frac{1}{4} * \frac{3}{2} + \frac{3}{4} * \frac{1}{2} = \frac{3}{4}$$

times the signal when updating a trained pattern. This indicates that there can be mixture states of the trained patterns that are also attractors in the system. These are an example of what is called a spurious state in the network; attractors that are different from the pattern used to train the network. Those strange memory states have been termed schizophrenic states to allude to apparent memory recalls with strange content. The analysis here shows the possibility that under certain conditions some memory recalls are contaminated by other memory states, even more than through the usual cross-talk term analysed above.

We found that the average strength of the signal for the spurious states is less than the average strength for trained patterns. This makes the spurious states, under normal conditions, less stable than attractors related to trained patterns. This can be used to our advantage by forcing the system out of the spurious states should it be attracted by an initial pattern close to them. We can do this by introducing noise into the system. With an appropriate level of noise we can kick the system out of the basin of attraction of some spurious states and into the basin of attraction of another attractor. It is likely that the system will then end up in a basin of attraction belonging to a trained pattern as these basins are often larger for moderate load capacities of the network. Noise can thus help to destabilize undesired memory states.

9.2.5   Noisy weights and diluted attractor networks

Fig. 9.6 shows that ANN memories are remarkably robust to noise, both in terms of recall of noisy patterns (Fig. 9.6A), or to noise (cross-talk) produced by an additional pattern (Fig. 9.6B). The curves show that there is perfect recall for a wide range of noise. However, there is a sudden and extensive breakdown when the noise level passes a critical value. Such sharp transitions are a consequence of the attractor dynamics in such networks.

Also, we can ask how robust the network is to noise in the weight matrix, deletion of synapses, or the loss of whole nodes. Results of corresponding simulations are shown in Fig. 9.8. In these simulations of the fixpoint model, we used 1000 nodes, and the memory of a stored pattern was tested when the ANN was initialized with pattern that had 10 components flipped compared to a stored pattern. The graphs show the mean and standard deviation over 100 runs.

Fig. 9.8a shows the robustness and breakdown of the memory model when adding static Gaussian noise to the weight matrix. The abscissa denotes the strength of this noise and is in units of the variance of the weight matrix. Haim Sompolinsky showed that this model has a similar phase diagram to the one shown in Fig. 9.7 with the temperature replaced by the noise strength. Fig. 9.8b shows how robust the system is to deleting synapses. Indeed, a very high percentage of synapses have to be destroyed

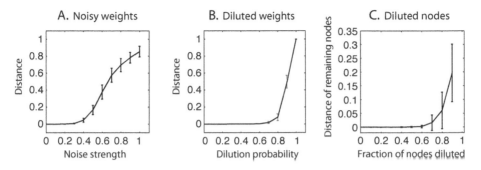

Fig. 9.8 Simulation results for a fixpoint ANN with 1000 nodes, which was trained on 50 patterns and tested on initial states of a stored pattern with 10 flipped bits. Error bars show standard deviations. (A) Mean distance between network state and stored pattern after 10 updates with different levels of static noise in the weight matrix. (B) Mean distance with diluted weight matrices. The abscissa gives the probability that a weight value was set to zero. (C) Mean distance with a fraction of nodes set to zero.

before the system breaks down, although this breakdown is then rapid. Of course, the brain is not fully connected as the model used here as baseline. These simulations demonstrate that attractor networks are possible in much less connected networks. Finally, the large robustness and sudden breakdown also holds true when deleting whole nodes. Of course, the nodes which are removed cannot be compared to the memory states, so the graph depicts the percentage error in the remaining nodes. Again, a very high percentage of nodes have to be removed before the attractor breaks down.

9.3 Sparse attractor networks and correlated patterns

The load capacity for the noiseless ANN model with standard Hebbian learning on random binary patterns is $\alpha_c \approx 0.138$. These training patterns are, on average, uncorrelated. The sensory signals driving the learning in our brains are, on the contrary, often correlated in some way. For example, the visual patterns on the retina are correlated across space, and specific images (for example, a fish) are commonly seen in conjunction with other images (for example, water). Correlations between the training patterns worsens the performance of the network, since the cross-talk term can yield high values in this case. A solution to this problem is to use a preprocessing step in which the representations of the training pattern get modified to yield orthogonal patterns. Orthogonal patterns have the property that the dot product between them is zero,

$$\mathbf{s}^{\mu\prime}\mathbf{s}^{\nu} = \delta^{\mu\nu}. \tag{9.27}$$

We used thereby the Kronecker symbol defined by

$$\delta^{\mu\nu} = \begin{cases} 1 & \text{if } \mu = \nu \\ 0 & \text{otherwise} \end{cases}. \tag{9.28}$$

The cross-talk term for such patterns is exactly zero, so the network can store up to C patterns, that is, $\alpha_c = 1$.

One can use this fact to maximize the storage capacity by minimizing the average overlap between the patterns. A typical engineering approach would be to calculate a matrix with elements representing the dot product between the patterns in the training set,

$$Q_{\mu\nu} = \sum_i s_i^\mu s_i^\nu. \tag{9.29}$$

For linearly independent training vectors, we can invert this matrix and use it in the learning rule to orthogonalize the patterns. This learning rule is known as the pseudo-inverse method,

$$w_{ij} = \frac{1}{N} \sum_{\mu\nu} s_i^\mu (\mathbf{Q}^{-1})_{\mu\nu} s_j^\nu, \tag{9.30}$$

which results in a storage capacity of $\alpha_c = 1$. However, calculating the inverse of such a matrix is biologically not very plausible, although we can still use this learning rule in simulations as long as we can argue that the orthogonalization can be implemented by biological means.

Reaching the optimal storage capacity is not necessarily what is needed in biological systems. Using a random remapping of correlated patterns is thus a possible mechanism to handle correlated patterns in attractor networks. This can be combined with remapping to a sparser representation which will further reduce overlaps between patterns.

9.3.1 Sparse patterns and expansion recoding

Decreasing the cross-talk between stored patterns, such as by using sparse patterns, increases the storage capacity of associative networks. Indeed, the brain seems to use this strategy with the help of expansion recoding. An example illustrating the principle of expansion recoding using a single-layer perceptron is shown in Fig. 9.9. The system has two input channels that can have four different combinations of input values if we restrict ourselves to binary patterns, namely $(0,0), (0,1), (1,0)$, and $(1,1)$. The perceptron has four output nodes, and we have included a variable firing threshold with a bias in the activation function implemented by an additional input node with constant activation value (see Chapter 7). In the figure, we specified an example of the weight values for which a network with threshold output nodes transforms the initial pattern representation into an orthogonal representation. All four patterns can therefore be stored in a subsequent auto-associative memory network with only four nodes.

Expansion recoding can also be realized with competitive networks. Common to the expansion schemes is that the number of nodes representing a pattern is expanded, while at the same time the representation is made more sparse. We mentioned already that sparse codes are thought to be used in the hippocampus, and these codes might be produced by expansion recoding in the dentate gyrus which has a large number of granule cells. Expansion coding might also be at work in the cerebellum, where mossy fibres contact a large number of granule cells, which exceed, by far, the number of mossy fibres.

Expansion recoding indicates that the load capacities of attractor networks can be larger for patterns with sparse representations. Alessandro Treves and Edmund Rolls analysed the storage capacity of attractor networks with such sparsely distributed

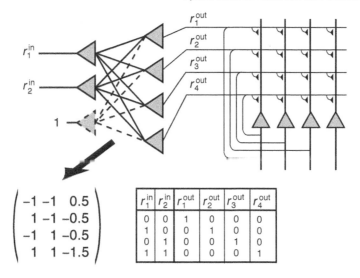

$$\begin{pmatrix} -1 & -1 & 0.5 \\ 1 & -1 & -0.5 \\ -1 & 1 & -0.5 \\ 1 & 1 & -1.5 \end{pmatrix}$$

r_1^{in}	r_2^{in}	r_1^{out}	r_2^{out}	r_3^{out}	r_4^{out}
0	0	1	0	0	0
1	0	0	1	0	0
0	1	0	0	1	0
1	1	0	0	0	1

Fig. 9.9 Example of expansion recoding that can orthogonalize a pattern representation with a single-layer perceptron. The nodes in the perceptron are threshold units, and we have included a bias as a separate node with constant input. The orthogonal output can be fed into a recurrent attractor network where all inputs are fixpoints of the attractor dynamics.

random patterns and found, in the limit of small a and large networks, a storage capacity of

$$\alpha_c \approx \frac{k}{a \ln(1/a)}, \tag{9.31}$$

where k is a constant that depends weakly on some details of the network and the pattern representations, but is roughly on the order of 0.2–0.3. The number of patterns in a pattern set with sparseness $a = 0.1$ that can be stored in an attractor network with nodes that have 10,000 synapses can therefore exceed 20,000, more than enough for many memory requirements in small brain areas. Note, however, that the information content does not change. The enhanced storage capacity of the network has to be compared with the reduction of the amount of information that can be stored in a sparse representation compared to that in a representation with more active components. The information is proportional to $a \ln(1/a)$, the denominator in eqn 9.31. The amount of information that can be stored in the network stays approximately constant.

We have only analysed weight matrices produced with basic Hebbian correlation rules. There are many other possible learning algorithms which can produce different weight matrices. It is interesting to ask what would be the best possible solution for a weight matrix. To be more precise, if we have a certain training set, we can ask what the load capacity of the network is, with a weight matrix that was produced with the optimal learning rule. To answer this question, we have to try out all the possible weight matrices, which is, of course, a daunting task. However, methods from statistical physics can help us to get the answer to this question, as shown by Elizabeth Gardner. She found that the maximal storage capacity of auto-associative networks with binary patterns and sparse representations is:

Table 9.2 The contributions of the four possible firing patterns of pre- and postsynaptic firing rates to the Hebbian covariance matrix, and the probability of the occurrence of these patterns for training sets with patterns of sparseness a

r_i	r_j	$\tilde{w}$	$P(\tilde{w})$
0	0	a^2	$(1-a)^2$
0	1	$-a(1-a)$	$a(1-a)$
1	0	$-a(1-a)$	$a(1-a)$
1	1	$(1-a)^2$	a^2

$$\alpha_c = \frac{1}{a\ln(1/a)}. \tag{9.32}$$

Comparing this result with sparse Hebbian networks (eqn 9.31) shows that the simplest Hebbian rule comes close to giving the maximum value.

9.3.2 Control of sparseness in attractor networks

The investigation of the properties of attractor networks with sparse patterns is important when studying brain functions. Indeed, the ANN models used so far will not work with sparse patterns since the network dynamics try to make half of the nodes active, as shown below. The important question is how one can ensure that the sparseness of retrieved states, a^{ret}, has the sparseness of training patterns, a. There are several possible solutions to the problem of achieving the right retrieval sparseness. One is to adjust the firing thresholds of the nodes appropriately so that only a nodes can fire in the retrieval process. However, adjusting the thresholds of neurons with respect to the firing of all the nodes in the networks is a non-local operation that has to be carefully implemented to be biologically plausible.

Another possibility, already illustrated in Chapter 8, is to include additional inhibition, on top of that produced by the Hebbian covariance rule, to control the overall activity in the network. Let us demonstrate this with binary patterns that have components 0 and 1, where 0 indicates no firing and 1 indicates firing of the node. The sparseness of the pattern is then given by the number of nodes that are active. The patterns are imprinted with a Hebbian rule

$$w_{ij} = \frac{1}{\sqrt{N^{\text{pat}}}} \sum_{\mu} (r_i^{\mu} - a)(r_j^{\mu} - a) - C. \tag{9.33}$$

Each pattern contributes four possible combinations of pre- and postsynaptic firing to the weight values. To shorten the presentation, let us use the short form $\tilde{w} = (r_i^{\mu} - a)(r_j^{\mu} - a)$. The four possible values for $\tilde{w}$ are listed in Table 9.2, together with their respective probabilities. The mean of each contribution is

$$\langle \tilde{w} \rangle = \sum \tilde{w} P(\tilde{w}) \tag{9.34}$$

$$= a^2 - (1-a)^2 - 2a^2(1-a)^2 + a^2(1-a)^2 = 0, \tag{9.35}$$

and the variance is

$$\langle \tilde{w}^2 \rangle = \sum \tilde{w}^2 P(\tilde{w}) = a^2(1-a)^2. \tag{9.36}$$

The mean and the variance of the weight distribution after imprinting a large number N^{pat} of patterns, using the central limit theorem and taking the normalization and inhibition into account, is

$$\langle w \rangle = -C \tag{9.37}$$

$$\langle w^2 \rangle = a^2(1-a)^2. \tag{9.38}$$

If this weight matrix is used with an iterative rule for updating the states of the system,

$$r_i - \Theta(h_i) = \Theta(\sum_j w_{ij}r_j - \theta), \tag{9.39}$$

where Θ is the step gain function and θ is the firing threshold, the stationary state must obey the self-consistent condition,

$$\frac{P(h_i > 0)}{P(h_i < 0)} = \frac{a^{\text{ret}}}{1 - a^{\text{ret}}}. \tag{9.40}$$

Since a^{ret} nodes are active, the probability density of the net input, $P(h)$ is a Gaussian with mean $-Ca^{\text{ret}}$ and variance $\sigma^2 = a^2(1-a)^2 a^{\text{ret}}$, as illustrated in Fig. 9.10. Thus,

$$P(h_i > 0) = \frac{1}{2} - erf(\frac{Ca^{\text{ret}} + \theta}{\sqrt{2}\sigma}), \tag{9.41}$$

$$P(h_i < 0) = \frac{1}{2} + erf(\frac{Ca^{\text{ret}} + \theta}{\sqrt{2}\sigma}), \tag{9.42}$$

and the appropriate inhibition constant, or threshold, can be calculated from

$$a^{ret} = \frac{1}{2} - erf(\frac{Ca^{\text{ret}} + \theta}{\sqrt{2}\sigma}). \tag{9.43}$$

The equation seems to indicate that a fine tuning of parameters is necessary. However, we have not taken the attractor dynamics of the stored patterns into account. These will bias the networks to the desired sparseness once the inhibition (or threshold) brings the network activity into the right range. Simulation results for a network of 500 nodes, trained on 40 patterns with sparseness $a = 0.1$, are shown in Fig. 9.11. The two curves show the average retrieval sparsness and the average Hamming distance, respectively, and standard deviations within 10 runs are indicated with error-bars. The threshold was thereby set to $\theta = 0$, and the curves show results for different values of the inhibition constant C.

The curves in Fig. 9.11 were produced with the program annSparse.py. First, we set the network parameters such as the number of nodes nn, the sparseness of the training patterns a, and the number of patterns to be learned (npat). We then average over 10 runs. The sparse patterns are produced by setting, at first, all pattern values to zero and then set a components to zero with a trick using a random permutation of the indices. These patterns are then trained with the Hebbian rule and tested against different values of the inhibitory shift. Note that we start the network with a disturbed version of the first pattern to test the attractor ability.

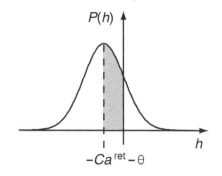

Fig. 9.10 A Gaussian function centred at a value $-Ca^{\text{ret}}$. Such a curve describes the distribution of Hebbian weight values trained on random patterns and includes some global inhibition with strength value C. The shaded area is given by the Gaussian error function described in Appendix 3.5.

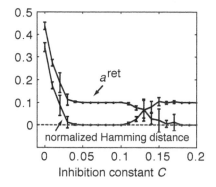

Fig. 9.11 Simulation of fixpoint ANN for pattern with sparseness $a = 0.1$.

Programs/annSparse.py

```
1  # Sparse auto-associative network
2  import numpy as np
3  import matplotlib.pyplot as plt
4
5  nn=500; a=0.1; npat=40
6  aret=np.zeros((20,10))
7  hd=np.zeros((20,10))
8
9  for irun in range(10):
10     pat=np.zeros((nn,npat));
11     for i in range(npat):
12         idx=np.random.permutation(nn)
13         pat[idx[:int(a*nn)],i]=1
14     w=(pat-a)@(pat-a).T; w=w/np.sqrt(npat); ic=-1
15     sparsity=np.arange(0,0.2,0.01)
16     for c in sparsity:
17         ic=ic+1
```

```
18      s=pat[:,0]; s[:10]=1−s[:10]
19      for t in range(10): s=((w−c)@s)>0
20      aret[ic,irun]=np.sum(s)/nn
21      hd[ic,irun]=((1−s).T@pat[:,0]+s.T@(1−pat[:,0]))/nn
22 plt.errorbar(sparsity,np.mean(aret,axis=1),yerr=np.std(aret,axis=1))
23 plt.errorbar(sparsity,np.mean(hd,axis=1),yerr=np.std(hd,axis=1))
```

9.4 Chaotic networks: a dynamic systems view ◠

This section contains a short excursion into the theory of dynamic systems which
will show us why we have called the memory states of auto-associative memories
'point attractors', and which will give us further insight into the possible behaviour
of recurrent networks. In particular, we will outline the conditions under which a
recurrent network has point attractors. We will also show that recurrent networks
with biologically more plausible, non-symmetric weight matrices, in comparison to
the symmetric weight matrices resulting from simplified Hebbian learning, frequently
have properties similar to those of the Hebbian counterpart.

We have already stressed the dynamic nature of the models when recurrences
are involved. In general, models with continuous dynamics are described in dynamic
systems theory by a set of coupled, ordinary, first-order differential equations, the
so-called equations of motion. Note that higher-order ordinary differentials can be cast
into a set of coupled first-order differential equations.

$$\frac{d\mathbf{x}}{dt} = \mathbf{f}(\mathbf{x}). \tag{9.44}$$

This is a coupled set of equations that only appears to be a single equation since we have
used a compact vector notation. The dynamics of a recurrent network with continuous
dynamics (eqn 9.1) is a special form of eqn 9.44, and an auto-associative network is
therefore formally a dynamic system. Recurrent networks with discrete dynamics, for
example the systems specified by eqn 8.1, are still dynamic systems, but with discrete
dynamics.

It is useful to know some of the basic terminology of dynamic systems theory. The
number of equations, that is, the number of nodes in the network, define the dimensionality of the systems, and recurrent neural networks must therefore be considered
as high-dimensional dynamic systems. The vector $\mathbf{x}$ in eqn 9.44 is called a state vector,
and a set of values for all components is called a state. A state describes a point within
the high-dimensional state space, the space of all possible state values. The evolution
of the state, defined by the equations of motion, describes a trajectory, a path in state
space.

9.4.1 Attractors

Dynamic systems can display a variety of different dynamic behaviour. We have
already seen some examples of recurrent networks in which the networks converged
to a fixpoint of the dynamic equations. This is a point in the state space, and it is for
this reason that we called this point a point attractor. Other forms of attractors are also

possible in dynamic systems. For example, the attractor can be a loop within the state space, a so-called limit cycle, in which the system cycles through a continuous set of points. Such movements in state space would appear in the components as oscillations, and oscillations in the brain may well be described by such types of attractors of neural networks. We can also define the dimensionality of an attractor. For example, a line attractor has a dimensionality of one, and a point in the state space has a dimensionality of zero. Higher-dimensional attractors are also possible in dynamic systems, although it is often difficult to find corresponding regularities in the movements of the system.

So far, we have only considered regular movements of dynamic systems. However, we know of examples of dynamic systems that display movements that are not completely regular, but yet are also not completely stochastic (like noise). For example, a system can be attracted by two points in the phase space with irregular domination of these two attractor points. A popular example of a chaotic system is the Lorenz system defined by the equations of motion

$$\frac{dx_1}{dt} = a(x_2 - x_1) \tag{9.45}$$

$$\frac{dx_2}{dt} = x_1(b - x_3) - x_2 \tag{9.46}$$

$$\frac{dx_3}{dt} = x_1 x_2 - cx_3. \tag{9.47}$$

Note that we can write this system as a recurrent network of three nodes with sigma and sigma–pi couplings such as

$$\frac{dx_i}{dt} = \sum_j w^1_{ij} x_i + \sum_{jk} w^2_{ijk} x_j x_k \tag{9.48}$$

with

$$\mathbf{w}^1 = \begin{pmatrix} -1 & a & 0 \\ b & -1 & 0 \\ 0 & 0 & -c \end{pmatrix} \quad \text{and} \quad \mathbf{w}^2 = \begin{cases} w^2_{213} = -1 \\ w^2_{312} = -1 \\ 0 \quad \text{otherwise} \end{cases}. \tag{9.49}$$

An example of a trajectory of the Lorenz system, showing the famous Lorenz attractor, is plotted in Fig. 9.12. With the above-mentioned definition of the dimensionality of an attractor, we must consider two points to have a dimensionality larger than zero and less than one. It then becomes a question of how to define such fractional dimensionalities, although we will not go into these discussions here. For our purposes it is enough to realize that there can be fractional dimensional attractors, from which the term fractals, often mentioned in the dynamic systems literature, is derived.

Fig. 9.12 was produced with the program `Lorenz.py`. The point to note here is that this is very similar to the previous recurrent network simulations except the slightly modified network equation.

Programs/Lorenz.py

```
1  # Plot trajectory of Lorenz system
2  import numpy as np
3  import matplotlib.pyplot as plt
4  from scipy.integrate import solve_ivp
```

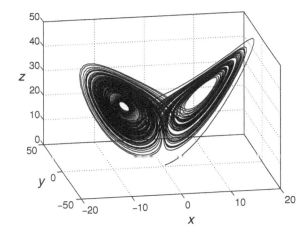

Fig. 9.12 Example of a trajectory of the Lorenz system from a numerical integration within the time interval $0 \le t \le 100$. The parameters used were $a = 10$, $b = 28$, and $c = 8/3$.

```
5
6  def udot(t,u):
7      a=10.; b=28.; c=8/3.
8      return a*(u[1] − u[0]), u[0]*(b−u[2])−u[1], u[0]*u[1]−c*u[2]
9
10 u0 = [1.0, 1.0, 1.0]  # Initial state
11 t_span = (0.0, 30.0)
12 t = np.arange(0.0, 30.0, 0.01)
13 u = solve_ivp(udot, t_span, u0, method='LSODA', t_eval=t)
14 fig = plt.figure(); ax = plt.axes(projection='3d')
15 ax.plot(u.y[0, :], u.y[1, :], u.y[2, :])
```

The movement around fractal attractors is very irregular, yet there is still some order. Such movements are therefore very different from random movements, as such movements are dominated by noise. We call such behaviour deterministic chaos. It is deterministic because there is no noise in the equations and the future states of the system are uniquely defined by the initial conditions. In contrast, stochastic systems include noise, so that systems that start with identical initial conditions can evolve in different ways.

9.4.2 Lyapunov functions

In this chapter, we have outlined that point attractors of recurrent networks are useful as memories, and chaotic fluctuations in such systems are not normally desirable. While chaotic fluctuations are not desirable within the basic ANN models discussed here, chaotic networks may have useful properties that are employed by the brain. For example, EEG measurements of normal brain activity indicate a chaotic brain dynamic on a system level, while synchronized modes seem to occur in epileptic seizures. It is hence of considerable interest to examine under which conditions recurrent networks have point attractors, and under which conditions dynamic, chaotic behaviour is expected.

From dynamic systems theory, we know that a system has a point attractor if a

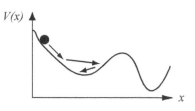

Fig. 9.13 A ball in an 'energy' landscape.

Lyapunov function exists. The idea behind this statement can be illustrated with the help of Fig. 9.13. We illustrate there a 'landscape' in which a ball, driven by gravity and influenced by friction, can roll down a hill into a valley. The ball will ultimately come to a halt at the minimum (the valley) of the function describing the landscape. More formally, if there is a function $V(\mathbf{x})$ that never increases under the dynamics of the system,

$$\frac{\mathrm{d}V(\mathbf{x})}{\mathrm{d}t} \leq 0, \tag{9.50}$$

where the $\mathbf{x}$ is governed by the dynamic equations of the system (eqn 9.44), then there has to be a point attractor in the system (as long as the state space is bounded), corresponding to the minimum of the function V. If such a function exists with the required properties, then this function is called a Lyapunov function in dynamic systems theory and an energy function in physics. Indeed, we encountered this view of the network dynamics in predictive coding in Chapter 7.

Can we find such a function for the recurrent networks? The answer is that we know of a function that fulfils the conditions under certain circumstances. Let us illustrate this for the special case of the discrete dynamics, eqn 8.1,

$$h_i(t+1) = \sum_j w_{ij} r_j(t) + I_i^{\mathrm{ext}}(t). \tag{9.51}$$

For this system, we propose to study the following function,

$$V(r_1, ..., r_N) = -\frac{1}{2} \sum_i \sum_j w_{ij} r_i r_j - \sum_i I_i^{\mathrm{ext}} r_i. \tag{9.52}$$

The change of this function in one time step is given by

$$
\begin{aligned}
\Delta V &= V(t+1) - V(t) \\
&= -\frac{1}{2} \sum_k \sum_j w_{kj} r_k(t+1) r_j(t+1) + \frac{1}{2} \sum_k \sum_j w_{kj} r_k(t) r_j(t) \\
&\quad - \sum_k I^{\mathrm{ext}} [r_k(t+1) - r_k(t)].
\end{aligned}
\tag{9.53}
$$

It is easiest to consider this model with sequential updates. In this case, when the ith node is updated, the other nodes stay constant, that is, $r_k(t+1) = r_k(t)$ for $k \neq i$.

Only terms from node i contribute to the change of the function V, and the change of this function at this time is given by

$$\Delta V = -\frac{1}{2}r_i(t+1)\sum_{j\neq i}w_{ij}r_j(t) - \frac{1}{2}r_i(t+1)\sum_{k\neq i}w_{ki}r_k(t)$$

$$+\frac{1}{2}r_i(t)\sum_{j\neq i}w_{ij}r_j(t) + \frac{1}{2}r_i(t)\sum_{k\neq i}w_{ki}r_k(t) - I_i^{\text{ext}}[r_i(t+1) - r_i(t)]$$

$$= [r_i(t+1) - r_i(t)][\sum_{j\neq i}\{\frac{1}{2}(w_{ij}+w_{ji})r_j(t)\} + I_i^{\text{ext}}]. \tag{9.54}$$

This difference is zero if $r_i(t+1) = r_i(t)$, but this would mean that we have already reached a stationary state. The most interesting case occurs when $r_i(t+1) \neq r_i(t)$. Then we have to inspect the second term more carefully, and we notice that the result depends on the weight matrix. Let us first examine the case of Hebbian learning that results in a symmetrical weight matrix, $w_{ij} = w_{ji}$. In this case, we have $(w_{ij} + w_{ji})/2 = w_{ij}$, and the second factor in the last equation equals $h_i(t)$ according to eqn 9.51. We can therefore write eqn 9.54 as

$$\Delta V = -[r_i(t+1) - r_i(t)]h_i(t). \tag{9.55}$$

Let us consider again a system with binary states. If $r_i(t) = 1$, then it must be true that $h_i(t) < 0$ in order to have $r_i(t+1) = -1$. If $r_i(t) = -1$ then it must be true that $h_i(t) > 0$ in order to have $r_i(t+1) = 1$. In both cases we have $\Delta V < 0$ and hence a Lyapunov function. The system therefore always converges to a stable state, each of which corresponds to the trained patterns, as we saw in the last section.

9.4.3 The Cohen–Grossberg theorem

Michael Cohen and Stephen Grossberg studied more general systems with continuous dynamics of the form

$$\frac{dx_i}{dt} = -a_i(x_i)\left(b_i(x_i) - \sum_{j=1}^{N}(w_{ij}g_j(x_j))\right) \tag{9.56}$$

with functions a_i and b_i. This dynamic equation corresponds to the leaky integrator dynamics (eqn 9.1) with generalizations such that the time constants and the activation functions can be different for each individual node in the network. Cohen and Grossberg found a Lyapunov function under the conditions that

1. **Positivity** $a_i \geq 0$: The dynamics must be a leaky integrator rather than an amplifying integrator.
2. **Symmetry** $w_{ij} = w_{ji}$: The influence of one node on another has to be the same as the reverse influence.
3. **Monotonicity** $\text{sign}(dg(x)/dx) = \text{const}$: The activation function has to be a monotonic function.

The statement that under these conditions a Lyapunov function exists has come to be known as the Cohen–Grossberg theorem. This theorem proves the existence of point attractors of the noiseless recurrent networks under the conditions just outlined.

9.4.4 Asymmetrical networks

Synaptic weights between neurons in the nervous system cannot be expected to fulfil the condition of weight matrix symmetry required to guarantee stable attractors in these networks. Also, we have studied so far weight matrices that have arbitrary negative and positive values. Positive weight values represent excitatory synapses, while negative values represent negative synapses. Neurons receive a mixture of input from excitatory and inhibitory presynaptic neurons, but each class of neurons often makes only one type of synaptic contact which defines the neuron type as either excitatory or inhibitory. Note that this is called Dale's principle, though this is also not always observed. For example, there are two types of dopamine receptors, D1 and D2, in spiny neurons of the caudate nucleus, which have opposite effects on EPSPs. However, if we observe this rule here, this corresponds to a weight matrix in which the signs within each column have to be consistent (all the elements in a column, corresponding to the synaptic efficiencies of one presynaptic neuron, are either positive or negative). This violates the symmetry condition of the weight matrix in the Cohen–Grossberg theorem, since an inhibitory node could then only receive inhibitory connections and vice versa. However, the Cohen–Grossberg theorem only describes the special case in which we can prove that networks have point attractors, while it is still possible that networks have point attractors, even if the conditions for the Cohen–Grossberg theorem are not fulfilled. We will now test how networks that violate some of the conditions of the Cohen–Grossberg theorem behave.

Let us start by studying a particularly simple case of non-symmetrical weight matrices. Each matrix can be decomposed into a symmetrical and an antisymmetrical part,

$$\mathbf{w} = g^{\mathrm{s}}\mathbf{w}^{\mathrm{s}} + g^{\mathrm{a}}\mathbf{w}^{\mathrm{a}}, \tag{9.57}$$

where

$$w^{\mathrm{s}}_{ij} = w^{\mathrm{s}}_{ji} \tag{9.58}$$

$$w^{\mathrm{a}}_{ij} = -w^{\mathrm{a}}_{ji}, \tag{9.59}$$

and g^{s} and g^{a} are parameters. These parameters allow us to study network conditions while varying the strength of the symmetrical and antisymmetrical parts of the weight matrix. A simple example of symmetrical and antisymmetrical matrices is to set the magnitude of all components of $\mathbf{w}^{\mathrm{s}}$ and $\mathbf{w}^{\mathrm{a}}$ equal to one,

$$w_{ij} = \begin{cases} g^{\mathrm{s}} + g^{\mathrm{a}} & \text{for} \quad i > j \\ 0 & \text{for} \quad i = j \\ g^{\mathrm{s}} - g^{\mathrm{a}} & \text{for} \quad i < j \end{cases} \tag{9.60}$$

Let us study by simulations how networks with such matrices behave. We will use a network with dynamics specified by eqn 8.1 using a sigmoidal activation function. To get an indication as to whether the networks have reached a steady state (point attractor) we measure the square difference of the states of two consecutive time steps of the network,

$$d(t) = (|\mathbf{r}(t)| - |\mathbf{r}(t-1)|)^2. \tag{9.61}$$

This distance is zero if the network has converged to a point attractor, and positive otherwise. The values of this convergence indicator are plotted on a grey scale for different values of strength values, g^s and g^a, in Fig. 9.14A. The value is zero for symmetrical weight matrices, as predicted by the Cohen–Grossberg theorem (horizontal line at $g^a = 0$). What is especially interesting is that a stationary state is reached as long as the strength of the asymmetrical part of the weight matrix is smaller than the strength of the symmetrical part of the weight matrix. This indicates that only strong asymmetries destroy point attractors in the network.

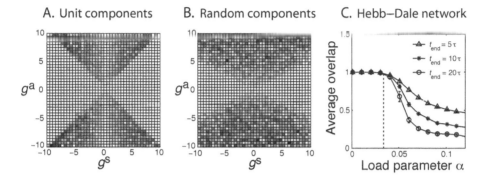

Fig. 9.14 (A) Convergence indicator for networks with asymmetrical weight matrices where the individual components of the symmetrical and antisymmetrical matrix are of unit strength. (B) Similar to (A) except that the individual components of the weight matrix are chosen from a Gaussian distribution. (C) Overlap of the network state with a trained pattern in a Hebbian auto-associative network that satisfies Dale's principle.

Of course, weight matrices with components of unit strength are a drastic simplification of biological systems. In Fig. 9.14B we show another example where the components in the symmetrical and antisymmetrical matrices were chosen from a Gaussian distribution, which is typical for weight matrices trained with Hebbian rules (see Section 6.4.2). The results are similar to the previous experiment in that the asymmetry has to be quite strong before the network displays signs of the onset of chaos. Strong asymmetries are only achieved if an excitatory connection from one neuron to another is countered by strong inhibition of the other neuron, or vice versa.

The next experiment was performed to test networks with separate excitatory and inhibitory nodes, which comply with Dale's principle and still utilize basic Hebbian imprinting. We simulated networks with weight matrices chosen by the following procedure. We first generated a symmetrical weight matrix through Hebbian learning. We also generated another matrix of the same size, in which we randomly assigned excitatory and inhibitory nodes. We then deleted (set to zero) all the entries in the weight matrix that were either inconsistent with the nature of the node (to be inhibitory or excitatory), or which would result in a direct feedback between the nodes. This procedure generated a highly diluted weight matrix that is consistent with biological constraints (while still being Hebbian). The overlap of the network state with a stored pattern after different durations of network cycles is shown in Fig. 9.14C. The results indicate that the storage capacity of this network coincides with the storage capacity of the ANN network with equivalent dilution, indicated by the vertical dashed line. This demonstrates that the theoretical results about the behaviour of recurrent networks that we discussed in the first part of this chapter and that were obtained in highly idealized networks are likely to carry over to networks with more biologically realistic constraints.

Programs/annChaos.py

```
1  import numpy as np
2  import matplotlib.pyplot as plt
3
4  # Assymetric network model
5  nn = 251; dt = 0.1
6
7  wa = np.random.normal(size=(nn,nn))
8  ws = np.random.normal(size=(nn,nn))
9  for i in range(nn):
10     wa[i,i] = 0; ws[i,i] = 0
11     for j in range(i):
12         wa[i,j] = -wa[j,i]
13         ws[i,j] = ws[j,i]
14
15 u_dif = np.zeros((41,41))
16 for a in range(41):
17     print(a)
18     gs = (a-21)*0.5
19     for b in range(41):
20         ga = (b-21)*.5
21         w = gs*ws+ga*wa
22         u = 2*np.random.random(size=(nn,1))-1
23         for t in np.arange(0,50,dt):
24             s = np.tanh(u); u = (1-dt)*u+dt*w@s
25         norm1 = u.T@u
26         for t in np.arange(0,10,dt):
27             s = np.tanh(u); u = (1-dt)*u+dt*w@s
28         u_dif[a,b]=np.sqrt(abs(u.T@u-norm1))
29
30 plt.imshow(u_dif)
```

The program `annChaos.py` was used to generate Fig. 9.14A and B. We thereby create weight matrices with components that are either all 1 (Line 3) or all random following a normal distribution (Line 4). The version chosen in this example is the random weight matrices as used in Fig. 9.14B . While we choose values for all components, half of them are overwritten later to enforce the symmetry and antisymmetry by appropriate copying of the values from the lower triangular part of the matrix into the upper part. Self-connections are set to zero, which is commonly done in attractor networks. We then loops over different contributions of the symmetric and antisymmetric weights stored in `ws` and `wa`. The network is then initialized with a random state, and we use the Euler method to update the quasi-continuous network. The norm of the network states u at $t = 50$ is then stored in variable `norm1` so that it can be compared to the network stated after some more interations. The difference between the networks states indicates if the network is still moving around. Note that this program runs for a relatively long time compared to the other programs in this book.

9.4.5 Non-monotonic networks

We have so far only violated the condition of the Cohen–Grossberg theorem regarding the symmetry of the weight matrix. However, the theorem indicates that networks can also behave chaotically when violating other constraints. Masahiko Morita and others have studied models of Hebbian-trained networks with non-monotonic activation functions. They found that point attractors still exist in such networks and demonstrated the profoundly enhanced storage capacities of those networks. Their results also indicate that the point attractors in these networks have basins of attraction that seem to be surrounded by chaotic regimes. The basins of attraction are like islands in a chaotic ocean. These chaotic regimes can have important functions. For example, they can indicate when a pattern is not recognized because it is too far from any trained pattern in the network. Non-monotonic activation functions seem, on first inspection, biologically unrealistic. However, we have to keep in mind that nodes in these networks can represent collections of nodes, and a combination of neurons can produce non-monotonic responses. An effective non-monotonicity can also be the result of appropriate activation of excitatory and inhibitory connections, although such possibilities are largely unexplored.

9.5 The Boltzmann Machine

9.5.1 ANN with hidden nodes

A much more general form of recurrent network was introduced by Geoffrey Hinton and Terrance Sejnowski in the mid-1980s which they called the Boltzmann machine. These recurrent networks with symmetric weights incorporate an important aspects over the basic ANN discussed before. That is, these networks have hidden nodes that are not connected to the outside world directly. As with perceptrons, hidden nodes allow an unlimited internal structure that allows in principle an unbounded complexity of internal computations. Such networks can then also be used to build deep networks, and they plaid an important way in the development of deep learning. Also of note is that Geoff and Terry introduced these networks as stochastic generalizations of the basic noiseless attractor model discussed by Hopfield, although we discussed the stochastic version already above.

While it has long been recognized that a system with enough hidden nodes can approximate any dynamical system, finding practical training rules for such systems has been a major challenge for which there was only recently major progress. These machines use unsupervised learning to learn hierarchical representations based on the statistics of the world. Such representations are key to more advanced applications of machine learning and to human abilities.

The basic building block is a single-layer network with one visible layer and one hidden layer. An example of such a network is shown in Fig. 9.15. The nodes represent a random variable similar to the Bayesian networks discussed earlier. We will specifically consider binary nodes that mimic neuronal states which are either firing or not. The connections between the weights w_{ij} specify how much they influence the on-state of connected nodes. Such systems can be described by an energy function. The energy between two nodes that are symmetrically connected with strength w_{ij} is

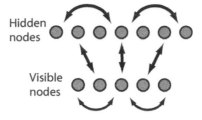

Hidden nodes

Visible nodes

Fig. 9.15 A Boltzmann machine with one visible and one hidden layer.

$$H^{nm} = -\frac{1}{2}\sum_{ij} w_{ij}s_i^n s_j^m. \tag{9.62}$$

The state variables, s, have superscripts n or m which can have values v or h to indicate visible and hidden nodes. We consider the probabilistic update rule,

$$p(s_i^n = +1) = \frac{1}{1 + \exp(-\beta\sum_j w_{ij}s_j^n)}, \tag{9.63}$$

with inverse temperature, β, which is called the Glauber dynamics in physics, and describes the competitive interaction between minimizing the energy and the randomizing thermal force. The probability distribution for such a stochastic system is called the Boltzmann–Gibbs distribution. Following this distribution, the distribution of visible states, in thermal equilibrium, is given by

$$p(\mathbf{s}^v; \mathbf{w}) = \frac{1}{Z}\sum_{m \in h} \exp(-\beta H^{vm}), \tag{9.64}$$

where we summed over all hidden states. In other words, this function describes the distribution of visible states of a Boltzmann machine with specific parameters, $\mathbf{w}$, representing the weights of the recurrent network. The normalization term, $Z = \sum_{n,m} \exp(-\beta H^{nm})$, is again the partition function, which provides the correct normalization so that the sum of the probabilities of all states sums to 1.

Let us consider the case where we have chosen enough hidden nodes so that the system can, given the right weight values, implement a generative model of a given world. Thus, by choosing the right weight values, we want this dynamical system to approximate the probability function, $p(\mathbf{s}^v)$, of the sensory states (states of visible nodes) caused by the environment. To derive a learning rule, we need to define an objective function. In this case, we want to minimize the difference between two density functions. A common measure for the difference between two probabilistic distributions is the Kulbach–Leibler divergence,

$$\text{KL}(p(\mathbf{s}^v), p(\mathbf{s}^v; \mathbf{w})) = \sum_{\mathbf{s}}^v p(\mathbf{s}^v) \log \frac{p(\mathbf{s}^v)}{p(\mathbf{s}^v; \mathbf{w})} \tag{9.65}$$

$$= \sum_{\mathbf{s}}^v p(\mathbf{s}^v) \log p(\mathbf{s}^v) - \sum_{\mathbf{s}}^v p(\mathbf{s}^v) \log p(\mathbf{s}^v; \mathbf{w}). \tag{9.66}$$

To minimize this divergence with a gradient method, we need to calculate the derivative of this 'distance measure' with respect to the weights. The first term in the difference in eqn 9.66 is the entropy of sensory states, which does not depend on the weights of the Boltzmann machine. Minimizing the Kulbach–Leibler divergence is therefore equivalent to maximizing the average log-likelihood function,

$$l(\mathbf{w}) = \sum_{\mathbf{s}}^{v} p(\mathbf{s}^v) \log p(\mathbf{s}^v; \mathbf{w}) = \langle \log p(\mathbf{s}^v; \mathbf{w}) \rangle. \tag{9.67}$$

Of course, we have seen the argument for maximizing the log-likelihood function several times before, although we now put this into the context of a recurrent model. In other words, we treat the probability distribution produced by the Boltzmann machine used as a generative model as a function of the parameters, w_{ij}, and choose the parameters which maximize the likelihood of the training data (the actual world states). Therefore, the averages of the model are evaluated over actual visible states generated by the environment. The log-likelihood of the model increases the better the model approximates the world. A standard method of maximizing this function is gradient ascent, for which we need to calculate the derivative of $l(\mathbf{w})$ with respect to the weights. We omit the detailed derivation here, but we note that the resulting learning rule can be written in the form

$$\Delta w_{ij} = \eta \frac{\partial l}{\partial w_{ij}} = \eta \frac{\beta}{2} \left(\langle s_i s_j \rangle_{\text{clamped}} - \langle s_i s_j \rangle_{\text{free}} \right). \tag{9.68}$$

The meaning of the terms on the right-hand side is as follows. The term labelled 'clamped' is the thermal average of the correlation between two nodes when the states of the visible nodes are fixed. The termed labelled 'free' is the thermal average when the recurrent system is running freely. The Boltzmann machine can thus be trained, in principle, to represent any arbitrary density functions, given that the network has a sufficient number of hidden nodes.

This result is encouraging as it gives as an exact algorithm to train general recurrent networks to approximate arbitrary density functions. The learning rule looks interesting since the clamped phase could be associated with a sensory-driven agent during an awake state, whereas the freely running state could be associated with a sleep phase. Unfortunately, it turns out that this learning rule is too demanding in practice. The reason for this is that the averages, indicated by the angular brackets in eqn 9.68, have to be evaluated at thermal equilibrium. Thus, after applying each sensory state, the system has to run for a long time to minimize the initial transient response of the system. The same has to be done for the freely running phase. Even when the system reaches equilibrium, it has to be sampled for a long time to allow sufficient accuracy of the averages so that the difference of the two terms is meaningful. Further, the applicability of the gradient method can be questioned since such methods are even problematic in recurrent systems without hidden states since small changes of system parameters (weights) can trigger large changes in the dynamics of the dynamical systems. These problems prevented, until recently, more practical progress in this area. Hinton and colleagues developed more practical systems which are described next.

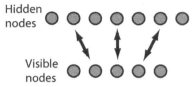

Fig. 9.16 Restricted Boltzmann machine in which recurrences within each layer are removed.

9.5.2 The restricted Boltzmann machine and contrastive Hebbian learning

Training of the Boltzmann machine with the above rule is challenging because the states of the nodes are always changing. Even with the visible states clamped, the states of the hidden nodes are continuously changing for two reasons. First, the update rule is probabilistic, which means that even with constant activity of the visible nodes, hidden nodes receive variable input. Second, the recurrent connections between hidden nodes can change the states of the hidden nodes rapidly and generate rich dynamics in the system. We certainly want to keep the probabilistic update rule since we need to generate different responses of the system in response to sensory data. However, we can simplify the system by eliminating recurrent connections within each layer, although connections between the layers are still bi-directional. While the simplification of omitting collateral connections is potentially severe, any of the abilities of general recurrent networks with hidden nodes can be recovered through the use of many layers, which bring back indirect recurrencies. A restricted Boltzmann machine (RBM) is shown in Fig. 9.16.

When applying the learning rule of eqn 9.68 to one layer of an RBM, we can expect faster convergence of the rule due to the restricted dynamics in the hidden layer. We can also write the learning rule in a slightly different form by using the following procedure. A sensory input state is applied to the input layer, which triggers some probabilistic recognition in the hidden layer. The states of the visible and hidden nodes can then be used to update the expectation value of the correlation between these nodes, $\langle s_i^v s_j^h \rangle^0$, at the initial time step. The pattern in the hidden layer can then be used to reconstruct approximately the pattern of visible nodes. This alternating Gibbs sampling is illustrated in Fig. 9.17 for a connection between one visible node and one hidden node, although this learning can be done in parallel for all connections. The learning rule can then be written in the form,

$$\Delta w_{ij} \propto \langle s_i^v s_j^h \rangle^0 - \langle s_i^v s_j^h \rangle^\infty. \tag{9.69}$$

Alternating Gibbs sampling becomes equivalent to the Boltzmann machine learning rule (eqn 9.68) when repeating this procedure for an infinite number of time steps, at which point it produces pure fantasies. However, this procedure still requires averaging over long sequences of simulated network activities, and sufficient evaluations of thermal averages can still take a long time. Also, the learning rule of eqn 9.69 does not seem to correspond to biological learning. While developmental learning also takes some time, it does not seems reasonable that the brain produces and evaluates long sequences of responses to individual sensory stimulations. Instead, it seems more reasonable to allow some finite number of alternations between hidden responses and

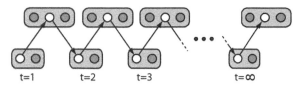

Fig. 9.17 Alternating Gibbs sampling.

the reconstruction of sensory states. While this does not formally correspond to the mathematically derived gradient leaning rule, it is an important step in solving the learning problem for practical problems, which is a form of contrastive divergence introduced by Geoffrey Hinton. It is heuristically clear that such a restricted training procedure can work. In each step we create only a rough approximation of ideal average fantasies, but the system learns the environment from many examples, so that it continuously improves its expectations. While it might be reasonable to use initially longer sequences, as infants might do, Hinton and colleagues showed that learning with only a few reconstructions is able to self-organize the system. The self-organization, which is based on input from the environment, is able to form internal representations that can be used to generate reasonable sensory expectations and which can also be used to recognize learned and novel sensory patterns.

The basic Bolzmann machine with a visible and hidden layer can easily be combined into hierarchical networks by using the activities of hidden nodes in one layer as inputs to the next layer. Hinton and colleagues have demonstrated the power of restricted Boltzmann machines for a number of examples. For example, they applied layered RBMs as auto-encoders where restricted alternating Gibbs sampling was used as pre-training to find appropriate initial internal representations that could be fine-tuned with backpropagation techniques.

9.5.3 Example of basic RMB on MNIST data

While the principles behind RBMs are mathematically advanced, their implementation is straight forward, at least in its basic form. This is implemented in program RBM.py. We can illustrate the principle with a simplified one layer model and training this on some examples from the MNIST data set. The network consists of $784 = 28 \times 28$ nodes as this is the size of the input. We chose 100 hidden nodes. We then selected single examples for each number from the training set.

Programs/RBM.py

```
 1  import numpy as np
 2  import matplotlib.pyplot as plt
 3  import pandas as pd
 4
 5  #sigmoid activation fcn
 6  sig = lambda x: 1 / (1 + np.exp(-x))
 7
 8  #data selection
 9  df = pd.read_csv('mnist_784.csv')
10  X = df.iloc[:,0:784].values/255
11
```

```
12  ndata=10;  nhidden=100;   nvisible=28*28;   nepochs=200
13  e=0.01;   noise=0.05;   ngibbs=3;   T=1/4
14  w= 0.1*np.random.randn(nvisible,nhidden)
15  vbias= np.zeros(nvisible);   hbias= np.zeros(nhidden)
16
17  X = np.array([X[34,:],X[8,:],X[5,:],X[7,:],X[9,:],
18                X[0,:],X[32,:],X[15,:],X[17,:],X[22,:]])
19
20  # RBM training
21  err = np.zeros(nepochs)
22  for epoch in range(nepochs):
23    for v in X:
24      h  = sig(v @ w + hbias)
25      hsample = h > np.random.rand(nhidden)
26      vrecon = sig(w @ hsample + vbias)
27      hrecon = sig(vrecon @ w + hbias)
28      w += e*(np.outer(v,h) - np.outer(vrecon,hrecon))
29      hbias+= e*(h-hrecon);   vbias+= e*(v-vrecon)
30      err[epoch] = ((v-vrecon)**2).sum()
31  plt.plot(err,'.');  plt.xlabel('epoch');  plt.ylabel('error')
32
33  # Plot interations of noisy patterns
34  r = np.random.rand(ndata,nvisible) < noise
35  flipped = (1-r)*X + r*(1.-X)   #flip random bits in input
36  plt.figure()
37  for g in range(ngibbs):
38    for i in range(10):
39      plt.subplot(ngibbs,10,g*10+i+1);   plt.axis('off')
40      plt.imshow(flipped[i].reshape(28,28),'gray');  plt.draw()
41      h = sig(1./T*(flipped[i] @ w+ hbias)) > np.random.rand(nhidden)
42      flipped[i] = sig(1./T*(w @ h + vbias)) > np.random.rand(nvisible)
```

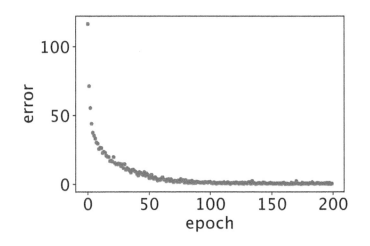

Fig. 9.18 Reconstruction error during training of MNIST examples.

We then train the network by applying a pattern, calculating the hidden activation that represents the probability, sampling the activation of the hidden state with this probability, using this activation to calculate the reconstruction activity for the input nodes, and then using the corresponding terms to modify the weight values.

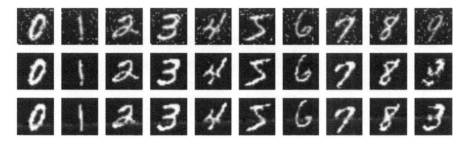

Fig. 9.19 Reconstruction of noisy version of the learned patterns. Each row is one iteration of Gibbs sampling.

For the reconstruction, we initialize the visible nodes with a noisy version of the image by flipping a certain percentage of pixels. The results shown in Fig. 9.18 show that most of the noise is easily removed in basically one iteration of recall through reconstruction. In the example shown, the only error was made in for the last digit. Of course, results will change with different noise examples.

To illustrate the Boltzmann machine in a deeper-layered structure, we briefly outline a demonstration by the Hinton group. The online demonstration can be run in a browser from https://www.cs.toronto.edu/ hinton/digits.html, and a stand alone version of this demonstration is available at this book's resource page. An image of the demonstration program is shown in Fig. 9.20. The model consists of a stacked layer of restricted Boltzmann machines. We called the first layer the model retina in the figure. The system also contains a recognition-readout-and-stimulation layer. The model retina is used to apply images of handwritten characters to the system. The recognition-readout-and-stimulation layer is a brain-imaging and stimulation device from and to the uppermost RBM layer. This device is trained by providing labels as inputs to the RBM for the purpose of 'reading the mind' or response of the brain. This layer learns to give patterns in the uppermost layer a name by mapping them to their meaning, as supplied during supervised learning of this device. This is somewhat analogous to brain–computer interfaces developed with different brain-imaging devices such as EEG, fMRI, or implanted electrodes. The advantage of the simulated device is that it can read the activity of every neuron in the upper RBM layer. The device can also be used with the learned connections in the opposite direction to stimulate the upper RBM layer with typical patterns for certain image categories. This can also represent sensory input such as auditory instructions.

The model for this demonstration was also trained on the MNIST data. All layers of this model were first treated as RBMs with symmetrical weights. Specifically, these were trained by applying images of handwritten characters to the model retina and using three steps of alternating Gibbs sampling for training the different layers. The evolving representations in each layer are thus purely unsupervised. After this basic training, the model was allowed, for fine-tuning purposes, to develop different weight values for the recognition and generative models.

The simulations provided by Hinton demonstrate the ability of the system after training. The system can be tested in two ways, either by supplying a handwritten

Concept input   Recognition readout and stimulation

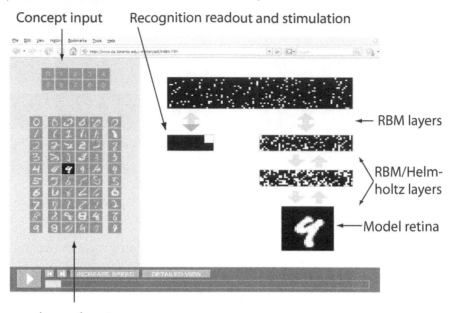

Image input

Fig. 9.20 Simulation of restricted Boltzmann machine by Geoffrey Hinton and colleagues, available at https://www.cs.toronto.edu/ hinton/digits.html.

image and asking for recognition, or by asking the system to produce images of a certain letter. These two modes can be initiated by selecting either an image or by selecting a letter category on the left-hand side. In the example shown in Fig. 9.20, we selected an example of an image of the number 4. When running the simulation, this image triggers response patterns in the layers. These patterns change in every time step, due to the probabilistic nature of the updating rule. The recognition read-out of the uppermost layer does, therefore, also fluctuate. In the shown example, the response of the system is 4, but the letter 9 is also frequently reported. This makes sense, as this image does also look somewhat like the letter 9. A histogram of responses can be constructed when counting the responses over time, which, when properly normalized, corresponds to an estimate of the probability over high-level concepts generated by this sensory state. Thus, this mode tests the recognition ability of the model.

The stimulation device connected to the upper **RBM** layer allows us to instruct the system to 'visualize' specific letters, which corresponds to testing the generative ability of the model. For example, if we ask the system to visualize a letter 4 by evoking corresponding patterns in the upper layer, the system responds with varying images on the model retina. There is not a single right answer, and the answers of the system change with time. In this way, the system produces examples of possible images of letter 4, proportional to some likelihood that these images are encountered in the sensory world on which the system was trained. The probabilistic nature of the system much better resembles human abilities to produce a variety of responses, in contrast to the mapping networks discussed in Chapter 7 which were only able to produce single answers for each input.

9.6 Re-entry and gated recurrent networks

We have so far discussed recurrent networks with symmetric weights as shown on the left in Fig. 9.21. While symmetric connections between neurons seems at first unrealistic, it might be good to remind ourselves that the discussion has been mainly on the level of population nodes, and that many connections between brain areas are often reciprocal. Thus, while a strict symmetry should not be expected in the brain, the importance of such models lies in their ability to shed light on some dynamical properties of neural networks.

Nevertheless, we now consider the important class of more general recurrent networks with directed models that can build loops in the networks as shown on the left in Fig. 9.21. We consider such recurrent neural networks in their common setting with deterministic neurons, although it is possible to generalize the architectures to the stochastic case. Even though the neurons in the following discussions are deterministic, such architectures can change neuron activation in an ongoing way even with constant input. Thus, such networks are still dynamical systems and they represent some form of universal approximators for temporal modelling. It is hence useful to revisit temporal modelling with such networks.

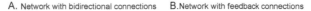

A. Network with bidirectional connections   B. Network with feedback connections

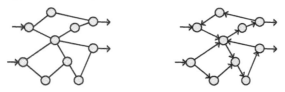

Fig. 9.21 Illustration of two principle cyclic networks with (A) graphs with bi-directional links and (B) directed graphs.

9.6.1 Sequence processing

Our examples of neural network applications have focused on perception tasks where an output (label) should be predicted from one input vector. An extension of such basic static object recognition is that of processing sequences. There are many types of sequence task applications such as predicting the weather from past observations, or the processing of language. While it is common to have naturally sequential data, there are even reasons to process static data in a sequential form such as searching large images in patches to look for specific objects. Doing this is more memory-efficient. The human visual system uses sequence processing as scenes are commonly explored by a series of eye movements called saccades. We will start discussing such sequence processing with the basic tasks of temporal predictions where a value of a sequence at position t is to be predicted from previous data points,

$$x(t) = f(x(t-1), x(t-2), ...).\tag{9.70}$$

In general, we should talk about a sequence position, though we commonly view a sequence as a time series. It is hence common to use the symbol t for the index of a sequence position.

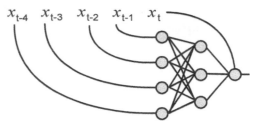

x_{t-4} x_{t-3} x_{t-2} x_{t-1} x_t

Fig. 9.22 Example of a tabbed delay line to represent temporal sequences to a neural network.

We will now consider several architectures of systems for such temporal processing. The first one we should consider is to use a regular feed-forward network to do sequence prediction from a finite number of previous sequence data. For example, we can place sequence values of n previous values of the sequence into an input vector

$$\mathbf{x} = \begin{pmatrix} x(t-1) \\ \dots \\ x(t-1-n) \end{pmatrix}, \tag{9.71}$$

and then do a one-step-ahead prediction of the value $s(t)$ as the output,

$$y = x(t). \tag{9.72}$$

In Fig. 9.22, we visualized the generation of the input vector by tabbing the input sequence with delay lines of different lengths. Representing a finite portion of a sequence in this spatial way is thus sometimes called a tabbed delay line. With such a representation of a time sequence we can immediately apply a deep neural networks for the sequence forecasting. An example of such a simple network with one hidden layer is also shown in Fig. 9.22.

For the following discussion, let's simplify this network with only one hidden node as shown in Fig. 9.23A. We can generalize this easily again to more hidden nodes and many layers of hidden nodes; we have just chosen this simple version for the illustration purposes. With this reduced figure it becomes clear that we assume that the values of the inputs at different times can have different influences on the sequence prediction as we allow the weights to the hidden node to have different values that of course must be learned. This is the most general case, at least for a fixed length of the input sequence. However, if we are looking for a specific pattern in the input sequence which could occur at any position, then we can again use a convolution over the input vector to search for this pattern. For example, in text processing of the sentence 'You should take an umbrella because it is raining', the word 'umbrella' is highly predictive of the word 'raining', although the relative position is variable. Convolutional neural networks have smaller filters compared to dense networks. This will save us parameters as we already discussed for position invariant feature detection in images. The one-dimensional convolutional solution is illustrated in Fig. 9.23B. A model with fewer parameters will usually require less training examples to learn, and convolution makes sense in many cases.

We can reduce the network complexity even further if we assume that the previous time steps only influence the current time point in a transient or diminishing way. This

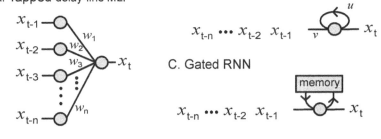

A. Tapped-delay-line MLP

B. Recurrent Neural Network (RNN)

C. Gated RNN

Fig. 9.23 Different ways of sequence processing with neural networks. The illustrations just show one example hidden note, but these networks should be considered with multiple nodes and commonly more layers. (A) A standard feed-forward network (MLP) where the input represents a vector of previous sequence data. (B) A basic recurrent neural network (RNN). (C) A gated recurrent neural network (gRNN) with explicit memory.

is often a good assumption. For example, it is well known that the probability of a sunny day is higher following a sunny day than a rainy day. We can describe a situation where the current value influences future time points at $t + u\delta t$ of the activation of the hidden nodes with

$$\mathbf{h}(t) = \mathbf{vx}(t) + \mathbf{uvx}(t-1) + \mathbf{u}^2\mathbf{vx}(t-2) + ..., \tag{9.73}$$

where u are weights with value less then 1. We can then simplify this network with the architecture shown in Fig. 9.23C where we represent the exponentially decaying memory of the input by a delayed input to the hidden node of its previous value. Mathematically, we are only replacing a diminishing sum with a recursive form,

$$\mathbf{h}(t) = \mathbf{vx}(t) + \mathbf{u}\left(\mathbf{vx}(t-1) + \mathbf{uvx}(t-2) + ...\right) \tag{9.74}$$
$$= \mathbf{vx}(t) + \mathbf{uh}(t-1), \tag{9.75}$$

which is illustrated in Fig. 9.23C. In this way we are not longer restricted in building networks for a finite sequence with the tabbed delay line approach. Compared to separate weights for inputs at different times, we introduced here a form of weight sharing in the sense that only the relative times of the sequence is important. This assumption is similar to the position invariance assumption in convolutional networks, and building in this assumption in our architecture reduces parameters. Note that this form represents the recurrent networks for an autoassociator as discussed before. We introduce this hear again in this form to discuss important generalizations. The assumption of a diminishing influence from previous time steps has the form of an exponential decay, which is not always appropriate. For example in natural language processing it is common that a given word has relations to other distant words. We can overcome this problem with explicit memory, as illustrated in Fig. 9.23C. We will shortly explore how we can implement such a memory in neural networks, for example with gated networks.

To finalize this simplest form of a recurrent neural network, we include a non-linearity in the layer. For example, the equations for a recurrent layer with a $\tanh(x)$ activation function is,

$$\mathbf{h}(t) = \tanh\left(\mathbf{w}\{\mathbf{x}(t), \mathbf{h}(t-1)\}\right). \tag{9.76}$$

We have thereby used a concatenation notation in the second line, $\{\mathbf{x}, \mathbf{h}\}$ for the vectors $\mathbf{x}$ and $\mathbf{h}$, and we have also concatenated the weight vectors $\mathbf{v}$ and $\mathbf{u}$ into the vector $\mathbf{w}$.

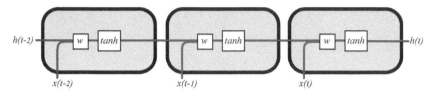

Fig. 9.24 Illustration of a basic RNN unrolled in time (adapted from Chris Olah's blog).

A useful way to visualize this simple RNN is shown in Fig. 9.24, which is an adaptation from the popular blog by Chris Olah. This way of representing the recurrent network will help us to discuss some advanced forms of RNNs later. The illustration shows the computational graph for three time steps, so it shows the unrolling the network in time. This solves a big question you might have about how to train such networks, given that the values of the activation of nodes depend on the activations at previous time steps. With the unfolding in time for a certain number of time steps we see that the networks is basically equivalent to a deep feed-forward network, albeit with shared weights in the different (time)-layers. It is therefore possible to use backpropagation learning on these networks, which is called backpropagation-through-time.

So, by the end, what have we gained? We simplified the graph of a feed-forward network and replaced it with a recursive version, only to unfold it in time again in order to train it. However, note that we have to do the unrolling only during training. Also, we a form of weight sharing that makes sense similar to convolutional layers when we look for similar operations at different times in a sequence. Models with shared weights are somewhat easier to train than the ones with more independent weights and do not tend to overfit as easily. The exponential form of the memory limits the usefulness of such networks. The next section addresses this issue.

9.6.2 Basic sequence processing with multilayer perceptrons and recurrent neural networks in Keras

In the following we demonstrate the implementation of sequence processing with a very simple example. The sequence data are thereby generated from a sine wave at ten discrete equidistant time points within one period

$$x(t) = \sin(\frac{2\pi}{10}t) \quad \text{for} \quad t = 0, ..., 9. \tag{9.77}$$

These data points are shown in Fig. 9.25A with crosses that have been generated using the following program.

Listing 9.1 sinSequence.ipynb (part 1)

```
1  import numpy as np
2  import matplotlib.pyplot as plt
3  from keras import models,layers,optimizers,datasets,utils,losses
4
5  # Sine data with 10 steps/cycle
6  seq = np.array([np.sin(2*np.pi*i/10) for i in range(10)])
7  print(seq)
```

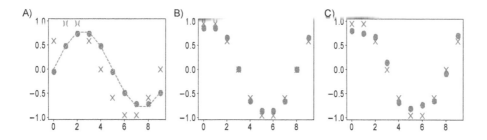

Fig. 9.25 Results of sequence predictions from a sequence that is produced by a sine function. (A) Prediction of the consecutive value in the sequence. The blue crosses show the true value and the orange dots show the results of a simple MLP. The dashed line shows the average of data points with the same value of the preceding data point. (B) Prediction of the consecutive value in the sequence from the two previous values where the predictions are from a simple MLP. (C) Same as (B) except that the predictions are made by a simple RNN.

We then prepare a data set for the specific learning tasks. The first learning tasks will be the one to predict the values of $y = x(t + 1)$ from the value at the previous time step, $x(t)$. Thus, the training set is created by choosing a random example of the sequence points as feature value for the input and uses the next point in the sequence as the target.

Listing 9.2 sinSequence.ipynb (part 2)

```
1  Num_sequences=200
2  x_train=np.array([])
3  y_train=np.array([])
4  for i in range(Num_sequences):
5    ran=np.random.randint(10)
6    x_train = np.append(x_train,seq[ran])
7    y_train = np.append(y_train,seq[np.mod(ran+1,10)])
8
9  x_test=np.array(seq)
10 y_test=np.array(np.roll(seq,-1))
```

Here we used the modulo function to code the periodic conditions of this time series. We then set up a MLP as we did in Chapter 7 to predict the labels after training.

Listing 9.3 sinSequence.ipynb (part 3)

```
1  #MLP1
2  inputs = layers.Input(shape=(1,))
3  h = layers.Dense(10, activation='relu')(inputs)
4  outputs= layers.Dense(1, activation='tanh')(h)
5  model = models.Model(inputs, outputs)
6
```

```
 7  model.compile(loss='mean_squared_error', optimizer='adam')
 8  print(model.summary())
 9  model.fit(x_train, y_train, epochs=1000, batch_size=100, verbose=0)
10
11  # evaluate
12  y_pred = model.predict(x_test, batch_size=10, verbose=1)
13  plt.plot(y_test,'x')
14  plt.plot(y_pred,'o')
15  a = np.array([i for i in range(10)])
16  b = np.roll( np.flip(a,0),-4)
17  plt.plot(((y_test[a]+y_test[b])/2),'—')
```

Here we used a single hidden layer with ten nodes. The plot is shown in Fig. 9.25A. This function to be learned is of course ill-defined as there are always two places in one period with the same function values that are either followed by a larger or a smaller value. This is reflected in the results of this experiment. For example, take the first point for which the input is $x = 0$. The correct next value in the sequence should be around $y \approx 0.6$. The next time the input value is around 0, at the sixth point in the sequence, the corresponding next value in the sequence is around $y \approx -0.6$. Hence, the network seems to learn to average over these responses and comes up with a predicted response around 0. The predictions of the other points can also be derived from the average. The average is shown in Fig. 9.25A with a dashed line which shows that this is indeed what the network seems to learn.

Of course, the prediction of consecutive the y value can be made with the knowledge of the previous two points in a sequence. We can set this up in a similar way as earlier and test an MLP for the prediction.

Listing 9.4 sinSequence.ipynb (part 4)

```
 1  #MLP2
 2  inputs = layers.Input(shape=(2,))
 3  h = layers.Dense(2, activation='relu')(inputs)
 4  outputs= layers.Dense(1, activation='tanh')(h)
 5  model = models.Model(inputs, outputs)
 6
 7  model.compile(loss='mean_squared_error', optimizer='adam')
 8  print(model.summary())
 9  model.fit(x_train,y_train,epochs=1000,batch_size=100,verbose=0)
10
11  # evaluate
12  y_pred = model.predict(x_test, batch_size=10, verbose=1)
13  plt.plot(y_test,'x')
14  plt.plot(y_pred,'o')
```

The results shown in Fig. 9.25B and C are much better and the predictions are quite good and can even be made better with more training. The main points that deviate from the correct results are the ones close to values $y = 1$ and $y = -1$. These values are a bit harder to reach, given that we used a sigmoidal tanh function where these values represent the extremes. Note that we only used two hidden neurons to keep the model even smaller than the previous one. While we used 10 hidden neurons for a total of 31 parameters in the previous experiment, here we are only using a model with 9 parameters.

Finally, we can implement this sequence prediction with a simple recurrent network. This is achieved with the Keras code in part 5 `sinSequence.ipynb`. Key to using the Keras RNN layer is that the input shape is expected to have the form

$$(\text{batch\_size, sequence\_length, feature\_dimension}).$$

We thus included the reshaping at the beginning of this code. We are only using one node for the simple RNN node, and this model therefore has only five parameters (a weight and bias for the input connection, a weight and bias of the recurrent connection, and a weight for the output). Again, we can make the fit even better with more nodes or with more training, but the purpose here is to demonstrate the ability of the minimal networks. We could even remove the output node and use the output of the recurrent node as the prediction of the sequence with reasonable results. Such a model has only three parameters.

Listing 9.5 sinSequence.ipynb (part 5)

```
1  # RNN
2  x_train=np.reshape(x_train ,(200,2,1))
3  x_test=np.reshape(x_test ,(10,2,1))
4
5  inputs = layers.Input(batch_shape=(None,2,1))
6  x = layers.SimpleRNN(1, activation='tanh')(inputs)
7  outputs= layers.Dense(1, activation='tanh')(x)
8  model = models.Model(inputs, outputs)
9
10 model.compile(loss='mean_squared_error', optimizer='adam')
11 print(model.summary())
12
13 model.fit(x_train ,y_train ,epochs=1000,batch_size=100,verbose=0)
14 # evaluate
15 y_pred = model.predict(x_test, batch_size=10, verbose=1)
16 plt.plot(y_test ,'x')
17 plt.plot(y_pred ,'o')
```

9.6.3 Long short-term memory (LSTM) and sentiment analysis

As outlined earlier, the basic recurrent network has the form of a memory that takes earlier states into account. However, the influence of these states fades exponentially when the weight values are smaller than 1, which they have to be as otherwise the recurrent influence would exponentially overwhelm the input. The basic RNN is hence a form of short-term memory. Such a short-term memory is usually not sufficient for many applications. For example, in natural language processing it is necessary to take some context into account that might be remote relative to words at the current sequence position. Hence, some memories should only 'kick in' at some appropriate time which itself might be triggered by another word. It is thus important to gate some of these memories until they are useful at a later state of processing.

The first network which has taken longer-term memory into consideration is called LSTM which stands for 'long short-term memory'. This network is illustrated in Fig. 9.26.

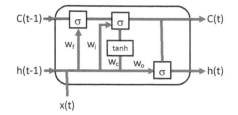

Fig. 9.26 Long short-term memory (LSTM) [adapted from colah's blog at https://colah.github.io/posts/2015-08-Understanding-LSTMs].

This gated network introduces another cell state $c(t)$ which represents an intrinsic memory state. Its value is forwarded to the next time step and can be modified in each time step with two separate operations, a forgetting gate f_t and a input (write) gate i_t,

$$\mathbf{c}(t) = \mathbf{f}(t)\,\mathbf{c}(t-1) + \mathbf{i}(t)\,\tilde{\mathbf{c}}(t). \tag{9.78}$$

The new memory addition depends on the new input and is calculated as

$$\tilde{\mathbf{c}}(t) = \tanh(\mathbf{w}_c\{\mathbf{x}(t), \mathbf{h}(t-1)\} + \mathbf{b}_c) \tag{9.79}$$

As a reminder, the curly brackets signify here a concatenation operation. This is like a usual hidden layer equation used in the basic RNN. The gating functions themselves are learned with corresponding weight values and a sigmoid gain function of the logistic variety to scale these terms to the range between 0 (total forgetting, no memory update) and 1 (keep memory state, add new input fully),

$$\mathbf{f}(t) = \sigma(\mathbf{w}_f\{\mathbf{x}(t), \mathbf{h}(t-1)\} + \mathbf{b}_f) \tag{9.80}$$
$$\mathbf{i}(t) = \sigma(\mathbf{w}_i\{\mathbf{x}(t), \mathbf{h}(t-1)\} + \mathbf{b}_i). \tag{9.81}$$

Finally, we produce an output for the recurrent node from this new memory state

$$\mathbf{h}(t) = o(t)\tanh(\mathbf{c}(t)) \tag{9.82}$$

which itself is gated by the learned influences of the inputs, namely

$$\mathbf{o}(t) = \sigma(\mathbf{w}_o\{\mathbf{x}(t), \mathbf{h}(t-1)\} + \mathbf{b}_o). \tag{9.83}$$

In order to demonstrate an LSTM in Keras we follow the common example of a sentiment analysis. Sentiment analysis is here just another example of classification in the context of giving documents some labels representing sentiments like good or bad. We use here the Large Movie Review Dataset (IMDB), which contains 50,000 movie reviews which are either positive or negative. The task is to use half the documents for training and test the other half if the sentiment of the test reviews can be predicted. Such a program is included in the Keras examples of which we provide here IN a simplified version.

This example gives us the opportunity to discuss some text representations. The representation called a bag of words consists of a large vector the size of the vocabulary with each component of this vector indicating the number of times this word occurs in the text. We now want to represent the text itself as a sequence of words, which is a much better way to approach natural language processing (NLP). With a one-hot representation of a vocabulary letter, we would then have a high-dimensional yet very sparse representation. A sequence would then be a sequence of such high-dimensional sparse vectors. Another way of word representations would be to give every word a unique integer. While this helps with the dimensionality of the representation, this representation does not capture relations between words. A common first step in NLP is therefore to learn an embedding. An embedding, more specifically a word embedding here, transforms an arbitrary representation to a dense vector space representation in which words that are commonly related within a task are close in embedding space. In Keras, we can realize this with an embedding layer. Keras datasets include the IMBD data set as a list of unique words as integers. The following code reads in the data, restricts the vocabulary size to 20,000 unique words, and then represents each document as a string of eight unique words (maxlen = 8) to reduce the size of this example so we can execute it on a simple laptop. If the document has less than eight words, then the Keras function pad_sequences() would using some 0 padding to make sure each document is of length maxlen here.

Listing 9.6 LSTM.ipynb (part 1)

```
1  from keras.preprocessing import sequence
2  from keras import models,layers,optimizers,datasets,utils,losses
3
4  vocabulary_size = 20000
5  maxlen = 8
6  batch_size = 32
7
8  (x_train, y_train), (x_test, y_test) =
9       datasets.imdb.load_data(num_words=vocabulary_size)
10 x_train = sequence.pad_sequences(x_train, maxlen)
11 x_test = sequence.pad_sequences(x_test, maxlen)
```

We can then define the model, where the input is immediately funneled into the embedding layer so that this layer can be trained within the task. The embedding representation is then used in the LSTM layer, and finally we use a single sigmoid node for the classification of the sentiment. We also added dropout to the output of the recurrent layer for some regularization to prevent overfitting. Adding dropout to the recurrent layer is a bit trickier as small perturbations errors can stack up in the recurrent network dynamics and hence lead to problems of correct recall. The recurrent layers in Keras therefore have parameters which include dropout in these layers that are strongly recommended. In this example, we used a high dropout rate. This model is then compiled and trained on the binary cross-entropy as shown in part 2 of LSTM.ipynb.

Listing 9.7 LSTM.ipynb (part 2)

```
1  inputs = layers.Input(shape=(maxlen,))
2  e=layers.Embedding(max_features, 128)(inputs)
3  h=layers.LSTM(128, dropout=0.8, recurrent_dropout=0.8)(e)
4  h=layers.Dropout(0.7)(h)
5  outputs=layers.Dense(1, activation='sigmoid')(h)
6  model = models.Model(inputs, outputs)
```

The evaluation accuracy is around 70 per cent after this short training. However, this is only a small example of a simple language processing task. In general, it is good to learn vector embeddings on better tasks such as a language model that aims to predict the next word in a sequence. Good word embeddings have been achieved with large data sets. Two popular ones are called Word2Vec and GloVe, and it is possible to download these to use for a pre-trained embedding. Using recurrent models with sophisticated word embeddings are among the best current language models.

Listing 9.8 LSTM.ipynb (part 3) with output

```
 1 model.compile(loss='binary_crossentropy',
 2 optimizer='adam',
 3 metrics=['accuracy'])
 4
 5 model.fit(x_train, y_train, batch_size=batch_size, epochs=4,
 6           validation_data=(x_test, y_test))
 7 score, acc = model.evaluate(x_test, y_test, batch_size=batch_size)
 8 print('Test accuracy:', acc)
 9
10 Train on 25000 samples, validate on 25000 samples
11 Epoch 1/4
12 25000/25000 [==============================] - 69s 3ms/step -
13 loss: 0.6255 - acc: 0.6346 - val_loss: 0.5540 - val_acc: 0.7084
14 Epoch 2/4
15 25000/25000 [==============================] - 65s 3ms/step -
16 loss: 0.5342 - acc: 0.7339 - val_loss: 0.5421 - val_acc: 0.7140
17 Epoch 3/4
18 25000/25000 [==============================] - 66s 3ms/step -
19 loss: 0.4938 - acc: 0.7592 - val_loss: 0.5411 - val_acc: 0.7148
20 Epoch 4/4
21 25000/25000 [==============================] - 65s 3ms/step -
22 loss: 0.4633 - acc: 0.7801 - val_loss: 0.5611 - val_acc: 0.7159
23 25000/25000 [==============================] - 4s 160us/step
24 Test accuracy: 0.71588
```

9.6.4 Other gated architectures and attention

A popular slightly simplified variant of LSTM is the gated recurrent unit (GRU) shown in Fig. 9.27A. This model is defined by the following equations

$$\mathbf{z}(t) = \sigma(\mathbf{w}_f\{\mathbf{x}(t), \mathbf{h}(t-1)\}) \tag{9.84}$$

$$\mathbf{r}(t) = \sigma(\mathbf{w}_r\{\mathbf{x}(t), \mathbf{h}(t-1)\}) \tag{9.85}$$

$$\tilde{\mathbf{h}}(t) = \tanh(\mathbf{w}\{x(t), \mathbf{r}_t h(t-1)\}) \tag{9.86}$$

$$\mathbf{h}(t) = (1 - \mathbf{z}_t)\mathbf{h}(t-1) + \mathbf{z}_t\tilde{\mathbf{h}}_t. \tag{9.87}$$

This model has still a read gate r and a write gate z, but it uses the hidden state itself as the memory state. It is therefore a slightly more compact version of the LSTM with fewer parameters. Both the GRU and LSTM usually exhibit similar performance.

There are also a variety of other extensions of the basic gated recurrent units discussed above. A major additional step is to take the idea further in form of an external memory. The first version of such a model was called the neural Turing machine (NTM). The basic idea is to use a separate external memory with reading and writing gates. The

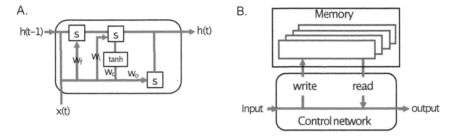

Fig. 9.27 (A) Gated recurrent unit (GRU; see Chris Olah's blog). (B) Differentiable neural computer (DNC; see https://www.deepmind.com/blog/differentiable-neural-computers.)

memory itself is thereby a combination of an location-based memory and a content-addressable memory. It is also important that all such operations are differentiable in order to train such recurrent models with backpropagation through time. The advanced version of NTM is therefore called the differentiable neural computer (DNC). Such an architecture is outlined in Fig. 9.27B.

Instead of going into the details of variations of gated recurrent networks, it is useful to mention one more ingredient in recent models that seems to be crucial in boosting performance: attention. Attention has been considered an important part of human information processing since the release of William James' seminal book *The Principles of Psychology* in 1890. At its heart, attention captures the ability of humans to orient towards important information, or to weight certain information as greater than others and to inhibit others. Different forms of attention have been identified in the brain. One well-known fact is the ability of some networks in the early visual system to emphasize salient features such of having letter 'A' in a sea of letters 'C'. This leads to the common effect that we perceive salient objects as 'popping out', which greatly narrows down the search time for such objects.

This feature-based bottom-up attention is not the only effect. Indeed, our ability to direct attention, either to spatial locations or to objects, shows some form of top-down attention. Some consequences of attention on neuronal firings have been recorded. For example, Fig. 9.28A shows experimental responses of neurons that are sensitive to objects moving in a certain direction in the visual scene. Response curves of neurons are called "tuning curves" in neuroscience. The squares show when the subject attends a 'fixation point' and hence not attending the motion, while the circles show the effect of attending to motion. Interestingly, the modulation of the neuron activity is not additive but better described by multiplication. This is demonstrated in Fig. 9.28B with the program below. We draw a Gaussian which curves down slightly (blue curve). When adding a constant we get shifted dashed blue curve, whereas if we multiply the original curve with 1.5 we get the red curve that represents the experimental results in Fig. 9.28A.

Listing 9.9 attention.ipynb

```
1   import numpy as np
2   import matplotlib.pyplot as plt
3
4   f = lambda x: np.exp(−x**2)−0.2
```

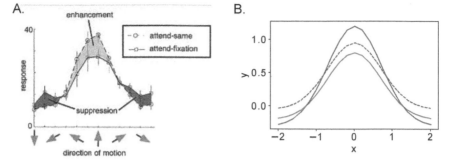

Fig. 9.28 Illustration of the effect of attention on the activation of neurons. (A) Example experimental results. Reprinted from *Current Biology* 14 (9), Julio C. Martinez-Trujillo and Stefan Treue, 'Feature-Based Attention Increases the Selectivity of Population Responses in Primate Visual Cortex', pp. 744–51, Figure 4a, doi.org/10.1016/j.cub.2004.04.028, Copyright ⓒ 2004 Cell Press. Published by Elsevier Ltd. All rights reserved). (B) Illustration of the additive and multiplicative effect on a tuning curve.

```
5   x = np.linspace(-2,2,21)
6
7   plt.plot(x,f(x))
8   plt.plot(x,f(x)+.15,'b--')
9   plt.plot(x,f(x)*1.5,'r')
```

Including information-processing principles of attention has been an important factor in machine learning. For example, attention has strongly influenced sequence-to-sequence processing such as in language translation. Gated memory networks already represent some form of attention since the release of information that is triggered by some context can be seen as attention. In general, attention can be seen mathematically as some form of non-linear processing. The simplest form is thereby a multiplicative gating as shown earlier. For example, we can take the output of a regular layer $f(\mathbf{W}\mathbf{x})$ and multiply this with new parameters $\mathbf{V}$ as in

$$\mathbf{y} = \mathbf{V} * f(\mathbf{W}\mathbf{x}). \tag{9.88}$$

The attention parameters $\mathbf{V}$ can then be learned from supervised learning. It is now common to include such attention modules in modelling sequence-to-sequence processes. A good introductory tutorial of this subject is given by Jason Brownlee at https://machinelearningmastery.com/encoder-decoder-attention-sequence-to-sequence-prediction-keras.

IV

System-level models

10 Modular networks and complementary systems

This chapter explores combinations of basic networks, starting with a discussion of modular mapping networks that can improve the performance of monolithic networks through the strategy of divide-and-conquer. The following discussion of modular recurrent networks explores how coupled dynamical system could balance between the independence of the modules and the cooperation between them. This seems important when considering coupled networks in the brain with drastic consequences of catastrophic synchronization when this balance is disrupted. A system-level example of interacting networks is a model of a complementary memory systems.

10.1 Modular mapping networks

There are a multitude of discussions in the literature about modular architectures and the way in which modules can interact and organize themselves. For example, Marvin Minsky discussed some of his thoughts in his book *The society of mind*. Another example is the committee machine first described by N. J. Nilson in 1965, and the pandemonium suggested by O. G. Selfridge in 1958. To get a deeper understanding of such information-processing architectures within the neural network framework we have to study how neural networks can be combined and interact. We will review some properties of modular networks that are comprised of the basic networks we discussed in previous chapters. The whole system can still be called a neural network, but the fact that we can distinguish subsystems in those networks makes them modular for our purposes.

It is possible to view modular networks as large-scale networks with constraints. An example of a purely physical constraint is the following. Consider a completely interconnected network with a number of elements (nodes) of the order of the neurons in the brain (say conservatively 10^{11}) and with individual interconnecting axons of 0.1 μm radius. Placing the nodes on the surface of a sphere and allowing the interior of the sphere to be densely packed with the axons would result in a sphere with a diameter of more than 20 km. The constraints of the physical extent of interconnecting 'wires' therefore demands some more economic solutions. We will see in this chapter that there are many important advantages of modular structures within large systems.

In light of our earlier discussion of completely connected neural networks as universal function approximators (see Chapter 7), it is obvious to ask why modular specialization is used in the brain. Some suggestions of the functional significance of modular specialization in visual processing have been outlined by the British psychologist Alan Covey. He speculated that, if the cortex uses inhibition to sharpen

Fundamentals of Computational Neuroscience. Third edition. Thomas P. Trappenberg, Oxford University Press. © Oxford University Press 2023. DOI: 10.1093/oso/9780192869364.003.0010

various visual attributes, such as colour, edges, or orientations, then it is possible to use local inhibition, which can be implemented with inhibitory interneurons within retinotopic maps, as long as the different attributes are kept separate. Such a specialization would also allow the separate attentional amplifications of separate features. Other advantages of task decompositions and modular architectures include learning speed, generalization abilities, representation capabilities, and task realizations within hardware limitations.

10.1.1   Mixture of experts

There are many possible architectures for modular networks, and we will concentrate here only on some fundamental examples that can give us a feeling for specific properties of modular networks. In this section we start by combining feedforward mapping networks in various ways. An example of such an architecture, called the mixture of experts, is illustrated in Fig. 10.1. In this architecture we have a column of parallel working modules or experts. Each of these experts receives potentially the same input. Another module, called the gating network, also receives some input from the general input stream. The purpose of the gating network is to weight the outputs of the expert networks appropriately to solve a specific task. The weighted outputs of the expert networks are then combined by the integration network. In the first examples below, this combination is done by summing the weighted outputs of the experts. Since the weighting values are supplied by the outputs of the gating network, the integration network can be viewed as a network with sigma–pi nodes mentioned in Section 5.6.

What are the benefits of using such an approach rather than using a single large mapping network, especially as we know that a large mapping network is a universal function approximator and can thus solve any mapping task (in principle). An example can illustrate some of the benefits of such a modular architecture. In Fig. 10.2A we plotted the absolute function $f(x) = |x|$. It is difficult to approximate this piecewise linear function with a single mapping network due to the sharp discontinuity at $x = 0$. However, a single linear node can represent each branch of the function. By dividing the

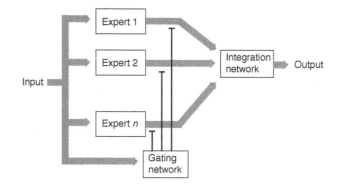

Fig. 10.1 An example of a type of modular mapping network called mixture of experts. Each expert, the gating network, and the integration network are usually mapping networks. The input layer of the integration network is composed of sigma–pi nodes, as the output of the gating network weights (modulates) the output of the expert networks to form the inputs of the integration network.

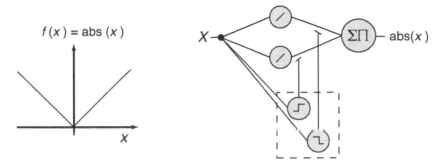

A. Absolute function

$f(x) = \text{abs}(x)$

x

B. Mixture of expert for absolute function

X

$\Sigma\Pi$ — abs(x)

Fig. 10.2 (A) Illustration of the absolute function $f(x) = |x|$ that is difficult to approximate with a single mapping network. (B) A modular mapping network in the form of a mixture of experts that can represent the absolute function accurately.

problem into these subproblems we can employ a simple solution for the subproblems.

This modular network is an example of the divide-and-conquer strategy often used in technical applications. Also, this seems to be a strategy used frequently in our daily lives in order to solve complex problems. By dividing a problem into subproblems it is possible that each subproblem can be solved by simple means. For example, functions that can only be represented by a mapping network with hidden nodes can always be decomposed into linear separable subfunctions. We then still have to solve the problem to combine these subfunctions in the appropriate way, which is sometimes not trivial. In the case of the absolute function illustrated in Fig. 10.2A we can solve this by a simple network of two threshold nodes, one that is active for positive input values and one that is active for negative values, as illustrated in Fig. 10.2B. The outputs of the expert networks are then gated by the outputs of the gating network by simply multiplying the outputs of the experts by the gating values.

Training such networks is a major concern when we want those systems to be able to solve specific tasks in a flexible manner. Training the experts alone now has two components: one is to assign the experts to particular tasks, and the other is to train each expert on the designated task. However, even with trained experts we still have to train the gating network, which is a form of a credit-assignment problem. Note that the division of the training into a task assignment phase and an expert training phase may be useful in solving the training problem, but in biological systems we might not be able to divide the learning into these separate steps. We will see below an example where the different steps are combined. Several training methods have been proposed in the neural network and machine learning literature. We will not discuss these here in detail as their relevance for brain processes is still not clear. Instead we will follow an instructive example.

10.1.2 The 'what-and-where' task

Several studies have shown that the brain has two partly distinguished visual pathways: the ventral visual pathway, which is mainly concerned with the recognition of objects; and the dorsal visual pathway, which is particularly well adapted to selecting objects for action for which the spatial coordinates are important. The two pathways are sometimes simply termed the 'what' and the 'where' pathways, respectively, although this is certainly a drastic simplification of the processing within the brain. Performing object recognition and determining the location of objects in a single network are difficult tasks, and we therefore use this example to illustrate the benefits of a modular network with separate experts for translation-invariant object recognition and object-invariant location recognition.

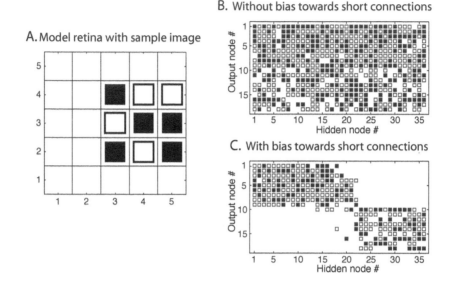

Fig. 10.3 Example of the 'what-and-where' tasks. (A) 5×5 model retina with 3×3 image of an object as an example. (B) Connection weights between hidden and output nodes in a single mapping network. Positive weights are shown by solid squares, while open squares symbolize negative values. (C) Connection weights between hidden and output nodes in a single mapping network when trained with a bias towards short connections [adapted from Jacobs and Jordan, *Journal of Cognitive Neuroscience* 4: 323–36 (1992)].

Robert Jacob, Michael Jordan, and Andrew Barto demonstrated the principal ideas in 1991. They used a simple model retina of 5×5 cells on which different objects represented by different 3×3 patterns can be placed in nine different locations (see the example in Fig. 10.3A). A network that can solve this 'what-and-where' task can be designed to have 26 input channels, consisting of 25 for the retinal input and one for the task specification. The desired output can be represent with 18 nodes, the first nine specify nine objects and the second nine specify the locations. This representation is local in each subtask since only one node for the location and object identity is active at any time. Jacobs and co-workers have demonstrated that a single network with a hidden layer of 36 nodes can solve the task after training the multilayer mapping network with back-propagation learning. However, the authors also demonstrated improved performance with modular networks, for reasons summarized next. Note that the use of back-propagation learning is acceptable in this circumstance since the algorithm is only used to find an example of a network that can solve the problem and no claim of biological plausibility for this step is necessary for the questions asked in this study.

A general problem that diminishes learning in single networks is conflicting training information. Conflicting training information can cause different problems. For example, the network will quickly adapt to reasonable performances of the 'what' task if we train the network first entirely on this task. The representations of the hidden layers will, however, change in a subsequent learning period on the 'where' task, which is likely to conflict with the representation necessary for the 'what' task. This temporal cross-talk is generally a problem in training sets with conflicting training patterns. In addition, there can be conflicting situations within one training example due to the distributed nature of the representations. This is called spatial cross-talk. The division of the tasks into separate networks can abolish both problematic cross-talk conflicts.

The above discussion suggests that modular networks have important merits, though we haven't yet solved the problem of establishing a modular network that can solve the what-and-where task. An important contribution of Jacobs, Jordan, and Barto was to demonstrate that modular networks can learn task decomposition. For this they used a gating network that increased the strength to the expert network that significantly improved the output of the system. An increased dedication of such an expert ensured the increased learning of this expert in response to subsequent training examples of the same tasks because the back-propagated error signal is modulated by the gating weights, and the module that contributed most to the answer will also adapt most to the new example. Another expert can then take on the representation of another task since a training example of another task would probably diminish the performance of the already specialized expert.

It is interesting to note that this is example provides some insight into the nature–nurture debate. In the above example it is obvious that architectural constraints can influence the specific task decomposition found through learning. The 'where' task is linear separable, so that a single-layer network can represent this task and is easier to train compared to a more complicated network. A simple expert without hidden layer therefore tends to be used for the 'where' task. In contrast, the 'what' task requires hidden nodes to achieve shift-invariant object recognition. A simple perceptron-like expert is likely to produce insufficient improvements, so that the gating network would not assign this task to this expert. Thus, architectural constrains influence the acquisition of specific abilities, but these inherent abilities are not necessarily fixed and can still be changed by specific learning.

In the above example, the experts were chosen ad hoc. Another question is how modularity could evolve through learning. An example of this was outlined by Jacobs, and Jordan in a subsequent study. In this study they considered a physical location of the nodes in a single mapping network and used a distance-dependent term in the objective function, which leads to a weight decay favouring short connections. The multilayer network was trained on the objective (or error) function

$$E = \frac{1}{2}\sum_i (r_i^{\text{out}} - y_i)^2 + \lambda \sum_{ij} \frac{d_{ij} w_{ij}^2}{1 + w_{ij}^2}. \tag{10.1}$$

The first term is the common mean square error between the actual and desired output of the network (as in eqn 7.8), which enforces the correct functioning of the network. The second term is yet another weight decay term (see Section 6.3.2) that makes solutions with large weight values between distant nodes unfavourable. Fig. 10.3B and 10.3C indicate the connections between the hidden nodes and the output nodes trained on the what-and-where task, as outlined above, with a single 25–36–18 feedforward mapping network. In Fig. 10.3B the network was trained entirely on the MSE objective function (that is, $\lambda = 0$), whereas Fig. 10.3C shows an example of the results when trained with the bias term that enforces short connections. As can be seen, the connections from the hidden layers to the output nodes, and therefore the hidden nodes themselves, were separated in relation to the two separate tasks. More hidden nodes were thereby allocated to the more difficult 'what' task. A learning procedure with such physical constraints therefore leads to a modularization of the network.

10.1.3 Product of experts

We mentioned in Chapter 7 that the normalized output of a feedforward mapping network with a competitive output layer can be interpreted as the probability that an input vector has a certain feature or belongs to a certain class symbolized by the output node. The previously discussed modular networks can easily be generalized to allow similar interpretations if the summed outputs of the expert networks are normalized. We can thus view the mixture of experts as a collection of experts whose weighted opinion is averaged (added and re-normalized) to determine the probability of the feature value. However, if we are considering probabilities, it is much more natural to consider products of probabilities that would determine the joined probability of independent events. This was pointed out by Geoffrey Hinton, and he proposed an architecture that he named product of experts. He not only stressed some of the advantages of such networks but also alluded to their biological plausibility when compared to empirical data.

To illustrate this further, consider 10 experts that are asked to state their opinion of what the likely increase in sea levels is due to global warming. The answers, expressed as (Gaussian) probability distributions is shown in Fig. 10.4 with dotted lines. If we combine these answers as a sum, and normalizing the sum to get again a probability density function, the answer would be as indicated with the dashed line in the figure. Summing density functions results in wide distribution that do not provide precise answers. The sum of experts only indicates that there is a wide range of answers. However, if we give all experts the same weight (ignoring that the first expert on the left denies global warming), we should also take into account how consistent experts are and how much support the final answer has from the distribution of expert opinions. This is much better described by the product of experts, shown with a solid line in the figure.

A product of experts can produce much sharper probability functions. The reason for this is that even a large probability assigned by one expert can be largely suppressed by low probabilities assigned by other experts. A large probability is only assigned to events for which there is some agreement between the experts. This helps with another problem in density estimation, that of estimating densities with low probabilities. Areas with low densities are more difficult to estimate well, since events in these areas have low probabilities of occurring. Errors in the estimation are therefore larger than areas in which many events can be used to estimate the density functions. An overestimation of rare events is thus common in statistical analysis. Products of experts are less prone

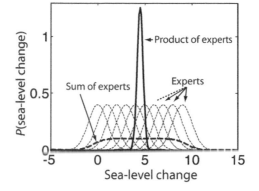

Fig. 10.4 Demonstration of combining expert opinions in different ways. The expert opinions, shown as normal distributions with different centres (dotted lines), are summed and re-normalized in the dashed line. The solid line represents the normalized product of the experts.

to such errors. Or, in other words, opinions of experts outside their domain of expertise have less of an effect when other experts confirm that these areas are of less relevance.

10.2 Coupled attractor networks

In contrast to the combination of feedforward networks in the previous section, this section discusses the combination of basic recurrent networks. Such modular recurrent networks can also be viewed as a subdivided recurrent network. An example is illustrated in Fig. 10.5A where an overall recurrent network is divided into a network with two groups of nodes. It is useful to distinguish between connections (or weights) between nodes in the same group (intra-modular connections) and connections (or weights) between nodes of different groups (inter-modular connections). The whole system is, of course, still a recurrent network and thus basically still one large dynamic system. However, by distinguishing the different types of connections and neuronal groups, we can study more explicitly systems with strongly coupled subsystems and weak interaction between such subsystems. In general, neither the nodes within the groups, nor the nodes between groups, have to be completely connected. However, we will simplify the discussion by considering fully connected attractor networks of the types discussed in Chapter 9.

10.2.1 Imprinted and composite patterns

Similar to the discussions in the last chapter, we now discuss the associative storage abilities of such modular attractor networks, following largely some discussions by Yaneer Bar-Yam. The main purpose is to show that there is a sensitive balance between the strength of connection between subnetworks in order to influence processes in other subnetworks, and the ability of the subnetworks to function semi-autonomously.

Let us first compare the extremes of coupled attractor networks, one single point attractor network as discussed in Chapter 9 versus two single point attractor networks. As an example we want to imprint into this system all objects that can be described

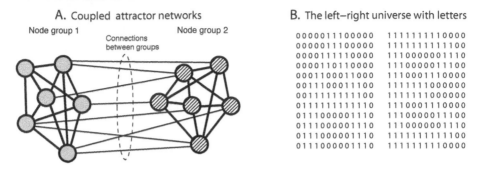

Fig. 10.5 (A) Coupled (or subdivided) recurrent neural networks. The nodes in this example are divided into two groups (the nodes of each group are indicated with different shadings). There are connections within the nodes of each group and between nodes of different groups. (B) The left–right universe that is made up of words with two letters.

by two independent feature vectors representing, for example, shape and colour. We consider therefore three different shapes {*circle, square, triangle*} and three different colours {*red, blue, green*}. The possible training set with this example consists thus of nine possible combinations {*red circle, blue circle, ...*}. Another example, a world with letter images on the left and right visual fields, respectively, is shown in Fig. 10.5B. In general, with m possible feature values (objects), one can build m^2 possible (combined) objects as long as there are no correlations between the features that would make certain combinations more likely than others.

Let us now consider a separate attractor network for each feature. From the discussion in Chapter 9 we know that a network with 1000 nodes can store around 138 patterns (feature values) when random representations of the feature values are trained with the Hebbian rule. A network with two such independent subnetworks, each carrying the information of one feature, could store

$$P = (\alpha_c N/m)^m = 138^2 = 19,044 \tag{10.2}$$

objects represented by all possible feature combinations, where m is the number of features (or the number of modules) with an equal number of nodes N/m. The number of patterns that can be stored in a single network is only

$$P = \alpha_c N. \tag{10.3}$$

To store all the 19,044 possible objects in one attractor network, we need a network with at least $N = 19,044/\alpha_c = 138,000$ nodes. The saving of resources of the modular network in terms of nodes is very impressive (2000 versus 138,000), and the savings are even more impressive if we consider the number of weights we have to use ($1000^2 + 1000^2 = 2 \times 10^6$ versus $138,000^2 \approx 2 \times 10^{10}$).

Why, then, would we ever want to use large single networks? The answer is that we have to use them if we want to represent correlations of features and remember specific objects. For example, if we want to remember a green square and a blue triangle, then we have to imprint these two objects with the specific combination of the features, and not the other possible combinations. If we do this we can recall the objects from partial information; for example, green can trigger the memory of green square. In the case of separate networks the input of green cannot trigger any memory in the 'shape' network, and we would potentially recall all possible combinations of features even if they were not part of the set of objects we used for training.

10.2.2 Signal-to-noise analysis

The previous discussion suggests that a certain intermediate level of coupling between attractor neural networks is likely to be necessary for more complex (and realistic) processing in the brain. We can get some further insight into the behaviour of coupled attractor networks using a signal-to-noise analysis along the lines of that outlined in Chapter 9. We consider an overall network of N nodes that can be divided into

$$m = \frac{N}{N'} \tag{10.4}$$

modules, each having the same number of nodes N'. The weights are trained with the Hebbian rule

$$w_{ij} = \frac{1}{N} \sum_{\mu=1}^{P} \xi_i^\mu \xi_j^\mu. \tag{10.5}$$

However, we modulate the weight values between the modules with a factor g. Formally, we can define a new weight matrix with components

$$\tilde{w}_{ij} = g_{ij} w_{ij}. \tag{10.6}$$

The components of a modulation matrix **g** are given by

$$g_{ij} = \begin{cases} 1 & \text{if nodes } i, j \text{ are within the same module} \\ g & \text{otherwise} \end{cases}. \tag{10.7}$$

To shorten the statement 'if nodes i, j are within the same module', we define a set $m(i)$ that lists all the node numbers that are in the same module as node number i.

The next step in the signal-to-noise analysis is to evaluate the stability of the imprinted pattern. First we will evaluate an imprinted pattern that is made up of the subvectors of each module that were imprinted together. Without loss of generality we can evaluate again the first pattern $\mu = 1$, that is, $s_i(t) = \xi_i^1$. We can then separate the signal terms from the noise terms in the updating rule as outlined in Chapter 9. This gives

$$s_i(t+1) = \text{sign}(\frac{N'}{N}\xi_i^1 + g\frac{N-N'}{N}\xi_i^1 + \dots$$
$$\dots \frac{1}{N} \sum_{j \in m(i)} \sum_{\mu \neq 1} \xi_i^\mu \xi_j^\mu \xi_j^1 + \frac{g}{N} \sum_{j \notin m(i)} \sum_{\mu \neq 1} \xi_i^\mu \xi_j^\mu \xi_j^1). \tag{10.8}$$

From this we can identify the signal and noise terms. The strength S of the signal term is the factor in front of the desired signal ξ_i^1, and the variance of the noise term is determined by the remaining part analogously to the procedure described in Chapter 9. In summary we get

$$\text{signal: } S = \frac{N'}{N} + g\frac{N-N'}{N} = \frac{1}{m} + g\left(1 - \frac{1}{m}\right)$$

$$\text{noise: } \sigma = \sqrt{\frac{P-1}{N}}\sqrt{\frac{1}{m} + g^2\left(1 - \frac{1}{m}\right)} \tag{10.9}$$

$$\approx \sqrt{\frac{P}{N}}\sqrt{\frac{1}{m} + g^2\left(1 - \frac{1}{m}\right)} = \sqrt{\alpha z_1}.$$

We introduced in the last line a shorthand notation z_1 that encapsulates the difference between the modular networks ($m > 1$) and the standard single network ($m = 1$) for which $z_1 = 1$. The parameter α is again the load parameter defined in eqn 9.18. Further discussions on the load capacity depend again on the error bound we impose on the network (see eqn 9.19). To simplify the formulas we introduce the shorthand notation,

$$z_2 = [\text{erf}^{-1}(1 - 2P_{\text{error}})]^2. \tag{10.10}$$

With these terms we can write the capacity bound (eqn 9.20), generalized to modular networks started in a trained pattern, as

$$\alpha < \frac{S^2}{2z_1 z_2}. \tag{10.11}$$

We called the limiting case the critical load parameter or the storage capacity, α_c, which is plotted for $P_{\text{error}} = 0.001$ and different values of g and m in Fig. 10.6A. With only one module, we recover the results of Chapter 9. However, with more than one module ($m > 1$) the results depend on the relative strength of the intramodular weights relative to the intermodular weights, which we parametrized with g. With values of $g < 1$ we get less support from the signals of the other modules, so that the load capacity of the networks diminishes.

In contrast to the previous case we can start the network from states that correspond to different subpatterns in the different modules. We can consider all kinds of combinations of patterns in different modules, but for the following discussion there are two most interesting and limiting cases. The first one occurs when all the subpatterns in the modules are chosen to be the first training pattern except for the module to which the node under consideration belongs. For this module we choose a random initial state and ask how strong the intermodular coupling strength has to be in order for the other modules to trigger the corresponding state in the module with the random initial state. We thus study the network with the starting state

$$s_j(t) = \begin{cases} \eta_j \text{ for } j \in m(i) \\ \xi_j^1 \text{ otherewise} \end{cases}, \tag{10.12}$$

where the variable η_j is a random binary number. The state of the network after one update is then

$$s_i(t+1) = \quad \text{sign}(g\frac{N-N'}{N}\xi_i^1 + \dots$$

$$\dots \frac{1}{N}\xi_i^i \sum_{j \in m(i)} \xi_j^1 \eta_j + \text{other noise-terms for } \mu \neq 1). \tag{10.13}$$

The corresponding strength of the signal is determined by the first factor. The second term is an additional noise term that has to be added to the noise term of the previous

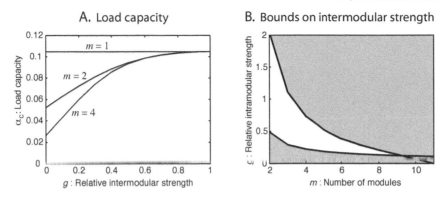

Fig. 10.6 Coupled attractor neural networks: results from signal-to-noise analysis. (A) Dependence of the load capacity of the imprinted pattern on relative intermodule coupling strength g for different numbers of modules m. (B) Bounds on relative intermodule coupling strength g. For g values greater than the upper curve the imprinted patterns are stable. For g less than the lower curve the composite patterns are stable. In the narrow band in-between we can adjust the system to have several composite and some imprinted patterns stable. This band gets narrower as the number of modules m increases and vanishes for networks with many modules.

case (eqn 10.9). However, this noise term contributes only with $1/(mN)$ and, since we consider large networks, we can ignore this small contribution. In summary we get

$$\text{signal: } S = \frac{N-N'}{N}g = (1 - \frac{1}{m})g \ .$$
$$\text{noise: } \sigma \approx \sqrt{\alpha z_1} \tag{10.14}$$

We can insert these expressions into eqn 10.11 from which we can derive a lower bound on the relative intracoupling strength g (for a given number of modules m and load parameter α) that we have to impose if we want to be able to trigger the first pattern in the module that we started in a random state. This is given by

$$g^2 > \frac{2\alpha z_2}{(m-1)(1 - \frac{1}{m} - 2\alpha z_2)}. \tag{10.15}$$

This lower limit on g is plotted in Fig. 10.6B as the line restricting the white area from below (for $P_{\text{error}} = 0.001$ and $\alpha = 0.01$). The curve confirms the intuitive conjecture that the g-factor can be reasonably small if the number of modules increases because an increasing number of modules results in an increasing relative number of nodes that are pointing in the desired direction.

We can also study the reverse case with

$$s_j(t) = \begin{cases} \xi_j^1 \text{ for } j \in m(i) \\ \eta_j \text{ otherwise} \end{cases} \tag{10.16}$$

as starting state. With this starting state we can ask how low the g-factor has to be in order for the substate ξ^1 in one module to be stable while all the other modules are pulling in other directions. The state of the network after one update with this starting state is

$$s_i(t+1) = \text{sign}(\frac{N'}{N}\xi_i^1 + \frac{g}{N}\xi_i^i \sum_{j \notin m(i)} \xi_j^1 \eta_j + \text{other noise-terms for } \mu \neq 1). \quad (10.17)$$

We can again neglect the additional noise term and use

$$\begin{aligned} \text{signal: } S &= \frac{N'}{N} = \frac{1}{m} \\ \text{noise: } \sigma &\approx \sqrt{\alpha z_1} \end{aligned} \qquad (10.18)$$

in the signal-to-noise analysis. Thus, if we want to be able to keep a state of a module stable (free from interferences from the other modules) the g-factor has to obey

$$g^2 < \frac{1 - 2\alpha z_2 m}{2\alpha z_2 m(m-1)}. \qquad (10.19)$$

The upper limit on g from these considerations is plotted in Fig. 10.6B as the line restricting the white area from above. With g-factors somewhere in the white area we could find points where patterns in different modules are relatively stable while still responding to some influence from the other patterns.

The analysis discussed here is only intended to allude to the possible interaction between subnetworks in modular networks, and many simplifying assumptions have been made. For example, we have assumed that intermodular weights have been trained with all patterns. In more realistic circumstances we would train intermodular connections for only specific subpattern combinations and could thus allow the white area to extend to higher values of m. Also, we have seen that the values from the signal-to-noise analysis do not accurately describe the full dynamics in such networks. Nevertheless, what is striking from our analysis is that there is a limit on the number of modules in the system when we want to have a system with a sensible balance of modular independence and modular interactions. This restricts the modularity that can be utilized in complex systems at each level. To be able to utilize many modules to encapsulate certain functionalities we have to combine these many modules within a hierarchical structure where on each level we have a restricted number of branches. We conjecture that the sensible balance of cooperation versus independence between modules is a driving force behind possible structures of complex systems such as the brain.

10.3 Sequence learning

While we have mainly analysed point attractor states to highlight the pattern completion ability of associative networks, the brain is much more dynamic in that some memories can trigger other memories, and the importance of sequential aspects in brain processing is increasingly realized. In this section we briefly discuss sequence learning and show that sequence learning in associative networks can benefit from modular architectures.

The principal idea behind the application of recurrent networks to sequence learning has already been discussed in Section 8.4, where we have seen that hetero-associations between consecutive states can move the system between attractor states. It is useful to distinguish between auto-associative weights

$$w_{ij}^A = \frac{1}{N} \sum_\mu s_i^\mu s_j^\mu, \qquad (10.20)$$

which associate patterns with themselves, and hetero-associative weights

$$w_{ij}^H = \frac{1}{N} \sum_\mu s_i^{\mu+1} s_j^\mu, \qquad (10.21)$$

which are associations between different, in this case consecutive, patterns. Both auto-associative and hetero-associative connections are necessary to achieve robust sequence memory. The principal idea is that the hetero-associations drive the system to a new, possibly noisy version, of a consecutive memory state, and that the auto-association helps to clean up the noisy version of the new state. For example, Hopfield considered a model with asymmetrical weights

$$w_{ij} = w_{ij}^A + \lambda w_{ij}^H \qquad (10.22)$$

in his 1982 paper. However, he also found that this basic model only works for very short sequences. Many variations of this basic model have subsequently been proposed, including refined choices of hetero-associative weights and temporally varying parameters λ. However, here we focus on a solution within a modular network.

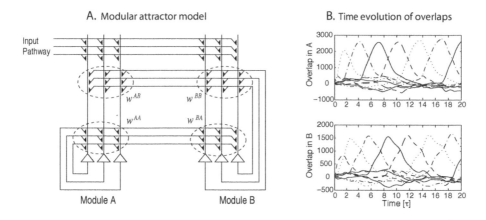

Fig. 10.7 (A) A pair of connected recurrent modules A and B. (B) Overlap of the net activation $\mathbf{u}(t)$ of nodes in each module with the stored patterns in a sequence of length 10 during recall. [Adapted from Lawrence, Trappenberg and Fine, *Neurocomputing* 69: 634–41 (2006); see also Sommer and Wennekers, *Neurocomputing* 65–66: 449–54 (2005).]

We consider a modular network as shown in Fig. 10.7A. This network consists of two auto-associative models labelled A and B, which are coupled through a hetero-associative coupling $\mathbf{w}^{AB}$. The reverse intermodular coupling is auto-associative. Results of the simulations are shown in Fig. 10.7B as overlaps between the internal activation $\mathbf{u}(t)$ of the nodes and the stored patterns. As the activation overlap rises for a particular pattern in module B (Fig. 10.7B, bottom), module A begins moving toward the next pattern in the sequence (Fig. 10.7B, top) due to the B→A hetero-associations. As the activation overlap rises for a particular pattern in A, B follows shortly behind from the A→B auto-associations. Note that only four different line styles where used in Fig. 10.7B, so that some patterns share the same line style.

Further analysis of this network shows that long sequences can be learned by this architecture. Similar architectures have been proposed for hippocampal functions, with suggestions that the CA3 subfield represents one auto-associative subnetwork, and that recurrencies in the hippocampus through the dentate gyrus provide the anatomical substrate for the other auto-associator. Thus architectures could then not only support the rapid learning of sequences within the hippocampus, but these learned sequences could also be used to anticipate sensory states and thus guide behaviour. Modular attractor networks, with auto-associative and/or hetero-associative components, have also been used to model behavioural data such as the influence of mood on memory recall. The characterization of interacting recurrent networks is thus an important area of research within computational neuroscience.

10.4 Complementary memory systems

We will now start to outline some more specific examples of system-level models of brain functions, still with a particular emphasis on modular networks. We start with a specific hypothesis on the implementation of working memory in the brain. We reserve the term 'working memory' for a concept as used by cognitive scientists, although the term is frequently used by physiologists to refer to an apparent memory through ongoing neuronal activity, as discussed in Chapter 8. We use the term short-term memory for this latter concept and discuss here their relation.

Since working memory is a concept derived from behavioural studies, it is not easy to define this construct precisely, and many different views of this concept in terms of definition and functional roles exist in the literature. The reason that it is useful in cognitive science is that it is a very appealing concept when describing possible mechanisms of complex cognitive processes that seem to rely on some form of workspace, which provides the necessary buffer to hold information to solve complex tasks. Examples of such complex cognitive tasks include language comprehension, mental arithmetic, and all forms of reasoning that are necessary for problem-solving and decision making. Working memory is different from the specific form of short-term memory (STM) discussed in Chapter 8 because many complex cognitive tasks also rely on other forms of memory. For example, episodic memory, which is possibly mediated by the hippocampus, and semantic memory, as supported by functions of the neocortex, can be necessary to directly solve complex tasks faced by humans.

10.4.1 Distributed model of working memory

Several models of working memory have been advanced in the literature, and the models by Alan Baddeley have been particularly influential. However, here we out-line a conceptual model of working memory proposed by Randall O'Reilly, Todd Braver, and Jonathan Cohen, which is based on a modular structure as summarized in

Fig. 10.8. Three modules are included in this model, each having some characteristic functionalities.

It is often difficult to distribute specific functionalities in a distributed system as there are interactions within the system and the system properties frequently rely on the whole system. Nevertheless, what we have in mind here is to assign to each module a different memory functionality in terms of short-, intermediate-, and long-term memory.

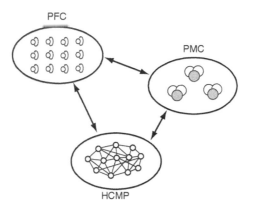

Fig. 10.8 Modular system with short-, intermediate-, and long-term memory, which are associated with functionalities of the prefrontal cortex (PFC), the hippocampus and related areas (HCMP), and the perceptual and motor cortex (PMC), respectively [adapted from O'Reilly, Braver, and Cohen, in *Models of working memory*, Miyake and Shah (eds), Cambridge University Press (1999)].

The module labelled PFC has many (mainly) independent recurrent subsystems represented as single recurrent nodes. Each such node could hold a specific, previously presented, item of information over a short period of time through reverberating neural activity. This module thus mimics basic operations sometimes attributed to the prefrontal cortex (see Chapter 8). The structure labelled HCMP represents structures such as the hippocampus that we identified as suitable for rapid learning of associations as required for episodic memory (see Chapter 9). This form of memory is based on rapid synaptic plasticity, in contrast to the predefined weights of short-term memory in cortical maps. The module labelled PMC, which stands for perceptual and motor cortex, is aimed at describing more slowly learned concepts such as semantic memory or action-repertoires. The interesting scientific question is to study how the different memory models interact and how the brain utilizes the kind of information that is necessary to perform complex mental tasks. O'Reilly and collaborators discussed such complementary systems in more depth, which is highly recommend as further reading. Here we will only focus on a specific issue of working memory which is repeatedly discussed in the literature.

10.4.2 Limited capacity of working memory

It is easy to remember very quickly a small list of numbers such as '31, 27, 4, 18'. However, the ability to recall a list of numbers (without repeated learning) breaks down drastically when the list has a few more items. Try '62, 97, 12, 73, 27, 54, 8'. The memory required to perform such a task depends strongly on short-term memory mechanisms. However, in light of the discussion above we think of them more as limitations of working memory. The limited capacity of working memory was described in 1928 by H. S. Oberley. G. Miller coined the phrase 'magical number 7 ± 2' for this limit. It is now clear that the precise limit depends strongly on the specific task that has to be performed, and the apparent limit can be modified by other processes. For example, a waiter is often highly skilled in quickly remembering long lists of orders. This is made possible by utilizing 'mental tricks' such as grouping items together. However, when more carefully ruling out such mental tricks in experiments, it seems that a limit around four items is more common.

The very limited capacity of working memory is puzzling if we remember that we can easily build systems that can rapidly store many thousand of items. It is also an important issue since there are some indications that the individual capacity of working memory is a good predictor of success in completing courses, indeed some argue even more than classical measurements of IQ. Thus, a larger storage capacity should make us fitter to survive, and we can ask why evolution was not able to increase the working memory capacity considerably. The search for the reasons behind the limited capacity of working memory is therefore prominent in cognitive neuroscience.

There are many hypotheses about the reasons behind the limited capacity of working memory. Donald Broadbent was among the first to point out that this hints to a bottleneck in the information-processing capabilities of the brain. Nelson Cowan advanced this further by investigating more specifically how limits in the attentional system, which is often an essential part of working memory models, could account for the data. Another suggestion is that short-term memory due to reverberating neural activity, which is also a essential ingredient in most working memory models, could hold the key. For example, we outlined in Chapters 8 and 9 how such short-term memory could be realized in an attractor network. Such networks are limited to represent a single item at each time. However, Lisman and Idiart pointed out that different objects could be encoded in different high-frequency subcycles of low-frequency oscillations. In the following we will discuss two further suggestions, mainly as an exercise in applying previous discussions to the quantification of these suggestions. The first example is based on a spike-train representation of objects, whereas the second example brings us back to interacting recurrent modules.

10.4.3 The spurious synchronization hypothesis

Experimental results of human performance in a typical working memory experiment are shown in Fig. 10.9. In these experiments, Steven Luck and Ed Vogel showed images with N^{obj} simple objects, such as objects with different shapes and/or colours, to a subject. After a delay of 900 ms, the subject was presented with a second image, and the subject had to judge if the two images were identical or not. The performance of the subjects, as measured by the average percentage of correct responses, is plotted in Fig. 10.9A with solid squares as a function of the number of objects (squares) in the images. A sharp breakdown of the performance with an increasing number of objects in the image can be seen. With similar experiments the authors demonstrated in addition that: (1) the capacity limit does not depend on the number of features of objects relevant for making the decision; (2) the visual working memory is independent of the load in the verbal working memory; (3) the capacity limit is not due to an increase of the number of decisions that have to be made for an increasing sample set.

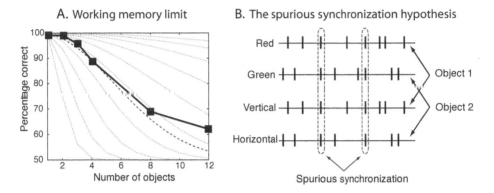

Fig. 10.9 (A) The percentage of correct responses (recall ability) in human subjects in a sequential comparison task of two images with different numbers of objects N^{obj} (solid squares). The dotted lines illustrate examples of the functional form as suggested by the synchronization hypothesis. The dashed line corresponds to the results with $P^{SS}(2) = 0.04$, where P^{SS} is the probability of spurious synchronization. (B) Illustration of the spurious synchronization hypothesis. The features of the object are represented by different spike trains, so that the number of synchronous spikes within a certain resolution increases with an increasing number of objects [adapted from Luck and Vogel, *Trends in Cognitive Science* 2: 78–80 (1998)].

Luck and Vogel also suggested a possible reason for the limited capacity of working memory. Their idea is based on the assumption that a feature is represented by a particular spike train, as illustrated in Fig. 10.9B. We assume that a feature is coded by a spike train with an arbitrary code (that is, a random spike train), and that the decoding of the spike trains is limited by a finite resolution of the spike times. The different features of different objects could be represented by synchronized spike trains. This is a popular way of solving the binding problem, the problem of relating the different features of one object when those features are represented in different brain areas. Of course, we have to assume that different objects are represented by different spike trains. However, it is possible that some spikes in the different spike trains for the different objects fall within the same time window, as illustrated in Fig. 10.9B. As this is based purely on random coincidences, we call this type of synchronization spurious synchronization. The number of coincident spikes between some objects does increase if we increase the number of objects in a set. At some point the level of spurious synchronization would become very large, possibly large enough to destroy the ability to distinguish between the objects. This, as argued by Luck and Vogel, could explain the breakdown of performance in their experiments.

The idea of spurious synchronization as the reason behind the capacity limit of working memory is very appealing. It would, for example, predict that the capacity limit does not depend on the number of features that an object has as found experimentally. The explanation for this within the spurious synchronization hypothesis is that each additional feature of one object would in any case be synchronized with the other features of the object so that only the number of objects with different spike trains would matter.

Computational neuroscience offers some way of testing this hypothesis further, specifically by quantifying the hypothesis so that it can be compared more directly to experimental data. This can be done for the above hypothesis by using only basic combinatorics. The number of pairs N^{PAIRS} in a set of N^{obj} objects is given by

$$N^{\text{pairs}} = \binom{N^{\text{obj}}}{2} = \frac{N^{\text{obj}}!}{2! \, (N^{\text{obj}} - 2)!}. \tag{10.23}$$

With a given neural code, such as that specified by a given probability distribution of the spikes, there will be a given probability of spurious synchronization between two spike trains, which we symbolize as $P^{\text{ss}}(2)$. The probability of not having spurious synchronization between two spike trains is then $1 - P^{\text{ss}}(2)$. The probability of spurious synchronization between at least two spike trains in a set of N^{obj} spike trains (pattern) is then given by

$$P^{SS}(N^{\text{obj}}) = 1 - \left(1 - P^{\text{SS}}(2)\right)^{N^{\text{pairs}}}, \tag{10.24}$$

because the spike trains are independent which means that the probabilities simply multiply. An increasing probability of spurious synchronization decreases the performance in the object comparison task. We can thus quantify the hypothesis of Luck and Vogel with a functional expectation of the percentage of correct recall given by

$$P^{\text{correct}} = \left(1 - P^{\text{SS}}(N^{\text{obj}})\right) + \left(P^{\text{SS}}(N^{\text{obj}})\right) 0.5. \tag{10.25}$$

The second term on the right-hand side is added because a random answer can be expected if objects cannot be correctly separated. The recall performances from eqn 10.25 for various values of the probabilities of spurious synchronization between two spike trains are shown as dotted lines in Fig. 10.9A. The dashed line corresponds to the spurious synchronization hypothesis with $P^{\text{SS}}(2) = 0.04$. We see that we can use the quantification of the hypothesis to extract some parameters that can be further compared to experimental data. For example, the probability of spurious synchronization between two spike trains can be compared to models of spike trains that take realistic values for spike distributions, firing rates, and time precision into account.

The comparison of experimental and theoretical data also indicates some possible discrepancies that should be analysed further. For example, the experimentally observed transition seems a little bit sharper than the one derived from the spurious synchronization hypothesis. Also, there seems to be a strong deviation for large numbers of objects that could indicate a separate effect on working memory. We will not follow this line of research further as the discussion was only intended to illustrate that the quantification of hypotheses is often important and should enable us to develop better models in the future.

10.4.4 The interacting-reverberating-memory hypothesis

The previous discussion on interacting memory modules offers another possible reason behind the limited capacity of working memory. We have seen that we can build separate memory modules in which to store separate items, and storing more items would only require more memory modules. However, we also discussed that interactions in the brain are necessary to solve complex tasks, and we have seen already that there is a sensible balance between the number modules and the interaction strength between them to allow for some flexibility in the operation of the system.

In this section we will quantify this observation in terms of dynamic neural field models, which, as argued in Chapter 8, model some aspects of representations in cortical maps. For example, we can think about reverberating neural activity in the frontal cortex that holds information of high-level concepts and activates lower-level details that make up specific objects. So while the implementation in the brain is likely based on distributed activity in the brain, we will simplify the discussion here by showing the concept with a single feature dimension.

Neural field models with appropriate balance of centre-surround inhibition and local excitation have the ability to store features with ongoing neural activity, as outlined in Section 8.3.2. An example is shown in Fig. 10.10A, which demonstrates that an external stimulus applied until $t = 10\tau$ was memorized with ongoing neural activity after the external stimulus was removed. This short-term memory ability is what we are using in the following simulations. The program used for these simulations is dnf.py with slightly modified parameters as noted in the figure caption.

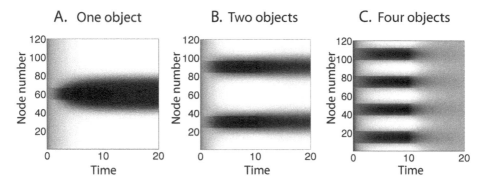

Fig. 10.10 Simulations of the DNF model based on the program dnf.py in which some parameters have been changed. In these simulations 120 nodes are used (nn = 120), the width of the patterns (sig = 2*pi/30) and the inhibition constant (C=0.2) have been reduced, the scaling factor of the weights has been enlarged (w=10*(w-C)), and the width of external simulations have been halved. All these changes are only made to demonstrate better the coexistence of activity packets. The major change to the earlier simulations are the number of areas that are stimulated externally, with (A) one, (B) two, or (C) four areas of external stimulation until time $t = 10\tau$.

For convenience in the discussion, we interpret each memory state in the DNF model in this case as representing an object. In the case of many separate DNF networks, we could thus represent many different objects in the system. However, we are more interested in exploring the interacting case and discuss this in the case of the other extreme, in having a single, large DNF network. In this limit we can have only one activity packet at a time due to the winner-takes-all nature of the network. However, there are several factors in practice which can support the coexistence of several activity packets, at least for a considerable time during a short-term memory phase. These stabilizing mechanisms in DNF models have been discussed in Section 8.3.4. For example, if we make it easier for neurons that are already active to fire again, such as NMDAR activation in recurrent networks, then we can stabilize more than one activity packet. There are other means to stabilize some packets, at least for some sufficient time, and we can even simulate this easily by using a spatially discrete implementation of a DNF model. The discrete nature of the node representations in the computer provide some energetic hurtle for two activity packets within a certain proximity to stay instead of moving toward each other or merge in the continuous case. An example is shown in Fig. 10.10B. However, when presenting four objects to the network, as shown in Fig. 10.10C, the network activity breaks down rapidly.

This simulation demonstrates some interesting properties of competitive networks. When moving from one to two objects in the simulation, the representation of the 'objects' become sharper. This sharpening was already noted by Wilson and Cowan, and is often argued to explain effects such as edge enhancement. Furthermore, while localized activity leads to a strong memory response in the network, diffuse activity can shut off the network activity. It is this principle that could underlie the limited capacity of working memory. Of course, the simulations shown here are very idealized in many ways, such as using equidistant objects which corresponds to a situation of maximal stability. In the brain one needs to consider more distributed representations. For example, neurons can participate in different maps at the same time. When such maps are uncorrelated, then there is little inference between the representations in the maps, since an activity packet in one map would appear as random background in the other map. This idea has been formalized by Alexei Samsonovich as the concept of charts in neural field models. Such charts could, for example, explain how many different place field maps could be accommodated in the hippocampus. In terms of working memory, however, it is possible that overlap in higher-order concepts of the brain will limit the number of charts that can be activated at the same time. Studying the interaction of coupled subnetworks is thus an important area of research.

11 Motor Control and Reinforcement Learning

This Chapter discusses control and decision systems that learn from general guidance in form of environmental feedback. We start with a short overview of classical control systems that describe well basic motor control in the brain. We then move to adaptive control systems that can learn optimal actions from reward feedback. This is somewhat different to the basic supervised learning discussed in Chapter 7 where the teacher would specify precisely the desired response of an agent. It is also different to unsupervised learning as there is still some feedback from the environment in form of reward. The goal of a reinforcement learning agent is to figure out which actions to take in order to achieve optimal returns, often in noisy settings.

11.1 Motor learning and control

Control systems are necessary to guide specific actions in an uncertain environment. For example, it might be possible to pick up a cup of coffee in front of you when looking at it. The motor actions have thereby be initiated by from visual cues, and it is often necessary to incorporate refinements or new sensory information. We can often complete this tasks when our view becomes obscured. It is a fascinating experience when we perturb this system, for example, by using prism glasses that shift the visual appearance of a target systematically away from its actual location, or by changing the dynamics of an arm with a computer-controlled guidance system. Reaching for a target with altered parameters of the controlled system will typically fail within the first few trials. However, we are commonly able to adapt to the changed environment after a few more trials, even without a teacher telling us exactly how we need to modify the control of our muscles.

11.1.1 Feedback controller

The control of mechanical or electrical devices is a major challenge faced regularly by engineers. It is thus not surprising that engineers have contributed a lot of ideas on how limb movements could be controlled by the nervous system. A typical example of a control system is shown in Fig. 11.1.

In the example of this section we designate a signal specifying the desired state as input to the system. This input signal is then converted by a specific module into a motor command that drives the device we want to control. We call this module motor command generator. The generated motor command could, for example, be the signal to activate specific motor neurons in the brainstem that in turn stimulate muscle fibres. The motor command generator can be viewed as an inverse model of the dynamics

Fundamentals of Computational Neuroscience. Third edition. Thomas P. Trappenberg, Oxford University Press. © Oxford University Press 2023. DOI: 10.1093/oso/9780192869364.003.0011

of the controlled object as it takes a state signal and should produce the right motor command so that the controlled object ends up in the desired state. The motor command thus causes a new state of the object that we have labelled 'actual state' in Fig. 11.1.

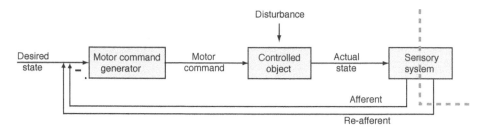

Fig. 11.1 Negative feedback control and the elements of a standard control system.

Of course, a major question is how to find and implement an appropriate and accurate motor command generator. In principle we can utilize a feedforward mapping network that is trained on examples of the motor actions if we would have a supervisor who tells the system what the right motor commands are. However, in reality we never get this detailed feedback. Rather, the feedback is typically at most an indication of 'good' or 'bad', or if things improve or are getting worst. How to learn the motor control generator, also called an actor, from environmental feedback will be the subject of reinforcement learning (RL) discussed later in this chapter. Here we first discuss how such controllers are embedded into control systems.

An important aspect of advanced control systems is that we need to take uncertainty in the environment into account. This includes uncertainty in our observation of the environment, some unpredictability of the environment such as unexpectedly moving objects, and later also reward feedback from the environment. Within the control system discussed here, we have included some of these aspects with a disturbance signal to the controlled object, which can include internal noise, external influences such as different loads on the system, ageing of the system, different temperatures altering physical properties, etc. In such cases we might not reach the desired state and we have to initiate a new movement to compensate for the discrepancy between the desired and actual state of the controlled object. It is then necessary to estimate this discrepancy, which demands a sensory system. For arm movements we could, for example, use visual feedback as mentioned above. The sensory feedback is then generated outside of our body, and we include a dotted line running through the sensory system box to indicate sensory cues originating inside and outside of our body. The visual input about the position can be converted into a feedback signal that we call re-afferent. Sensory feedback can also originate from internal sensors in the body. For example, neural signals are generated by the contraction of muscles that are fed back to the central nervous system, so-called proprioceptive feedback. We labelled this type of sensory feedback afferent in Fig. 11.1.

The sensory feedback can be used in various ways to regulate the system. Fig. 11.1 illustrates the simplest example, that of a negative feedback controller. The sensory signal that indicates the actual state of the system is therein subtracted from the signal that specifies the desired state. This produces a new desired state, which is sometimes called a motor-error signal. This motor-error signal for the correction movement, generated with the help of the feedback signal, generates a new movement that will probably be closer to the desired state. Of course, the sensory feedback has to be converted into the right reference frame to be used by the motor control system (not included in the figure). The basic feedback control systems often work well and are commonly used in mechanical and electrical devices. However, there are several factors that make this simple scheme insufficient for some biological systems. For example, the sensory feedback is usually too slow for many control tasks, and the necessary accuracy is also not without problems. Proprioceptive feedback can be faster but might not be accurate. We therefore turn to more advanced systems that we think are at work in the brain.

11.1.2 Forward and inverse model controller

Two refined schemes for motor control with slow sensory feedback are illustrated in Fig. 11.2. The first one employs some subsystems that mimic the dynamic of the controlled object and the behaviour of the sensory system. These subsystems are called forward models. If these models are good approximations of the real systems they are modelling, then we can use the output of these systems, instead of the slow sensory response, as feedback signal. The models have, of course, to be gauged against the real system during ongoing learning. Thus, the sensory feedback is used to change the behaviour of the forward model. The forward model, which is divided into a dynamic and output component in the figure, influences the sensory feedback to improve performance in the main control loop. This scheme works as long as the changes in the systems that they mimic are much slower than the time scale of the movement that is controlled, which is often the case in biological motor control situations.

The second scheme, shown in Fig. 11.2B, employs an inverse model instead of the forward model in the previous scheme and is therefore called an inverse model controller. The inverse model, which is incorporated as a side-loop to the standard feedback controller, learns to correct the computation of the motor command generator. The reason that this scheme works is similar to that for the previous example. The sensory feedback can be used to make the inverse model controller more accurate while it provides the necessary correction signals in time to be incorporated into the motor command. Both control systems, the forward model controller and the inverse model controller, are robust controllers and could well be implemented in the brain. For example, such models have been discussed as models for the cerebellum, as outlined below. Later we discuss another control system, the adaptive critic, which has been proposed as a model of the basal ganglia.

11.1.3 The actor–critic scheme

In the previous section we have discussed methods to estimate value functions, which can then be used to evaluate policies. When using reinforcement learning for control, we want to change policies to maximize the return for an agent. The full methods do then consist of interleaved procedure, in which policies are changed according to estimated value functions, and then the new policy is evaluated by estimating the

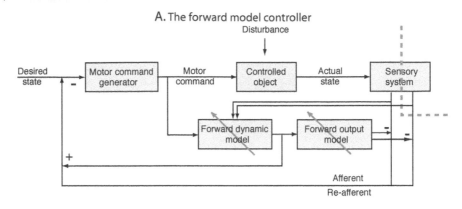

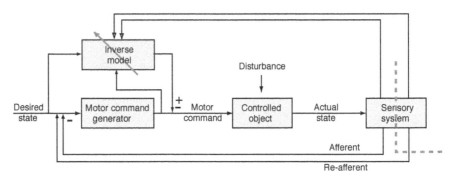

Fig. 11.2 Two advanced control systems which incorporate models for corrective adjustments in the system. These models are trained with sensory feedback, which is indicated by the arrows going through these components.

value function for this policy. Interestingly, it is not necessary to estimate the value function perfectly for a give policy or to find directly the best policy for a given value function. The system can start out with a weakly functional system, and reinforcement learning improves the system incrementally. It can be shown that such a bootstrapping system converges to optimal solutions as long as the system is ergodic, which means that each possible state of the environment is reached in finite time. However, rather than following here the many advanced engineering applications in this area, we will discuss some examples that have been implicated with brain processing.

The most advanced control system called the actor–critic scheme is illustrated in Fig. 11.3. Such a control system represents a fitting framework to discuss brain functions. We provide here the control systems view of such a method, and discuss more details below after we formalized the RL setting.

Note the similarities of this control scheme to the inverse model controller outlined in Fig. 11.2B. The critic is, however, designed to predict the correct motor command for accurate future actions and can thus supervise the motor command generator. The motor command generator is often called actor within this framework. The adaptive critic

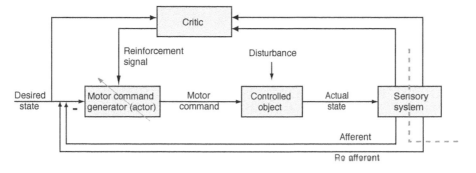

Fig. 11.3 Adaptive critic controller.

estimates value functions and uses them to guide the actions of the agent. This scheme has proven to be very useful in engineering applications such as controlling elevators or adjusting the parameters of a petroleum refinery's operation. Neural implementations and relations to brain processing will be discussed below.

11.2 Classical conditioning and reinforcement learning

In supervised learning we assumed that a teacher supplies detailed information on the desired response of a learner. This was particularly suited to object recognition where we had a large number of labelled examples. A much more common learning condition is when an agent, such as a human or a robot, has to learn to make decisions in the environment without the detailed instructions.

A good example of such a learning tasks for an agent is that of learning to play tennis. In this case the agent might try out moves and get rewarded by points the agent scores rather than a teacher who specifies every muscle movement we need to follow. Or, in the case of a robot, an engineer who designs every sequence of motor activations. One approach that resembles supervised learning is that of a trainer which demonstrates the correct moves. This type of supervised learning a called imitation learning in this context. Much of imitation learning follows the previous discussion so we will concentrate in this chapter on an important learning scenario where the agent only gets simple feedback after periods of actions in the form of reward or punishment without detailing which of the actions has contributed to the outcome. This type of learning scenario is called reinforcement learning (RL).

Learning with reward signals has been studied by psychologists for many years under the term conditioning. In classical conditioning illustrated in Fig. 11.4A, an agent receives reward after a specific cue. For example, in the famous experiments of Pavlov, a dog receives a food reward after a ringing of a bell. The dog thereby learns the cue-reward association that Pavlov demonstrated with measuring the salivation as a response to the ringing of the bell. In a more general term, the agent has to solve the credit assignment problem, that of learning what events correlated with the receiving of the reward. While this is similar to supervised learning in this sense, reinforcement learning does usually also has to solve the temporal credit assignment problem where a reward only appears with temporal delay.

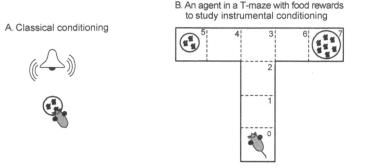

Fig. 11.4 (A) Experimental setting of classical conditioning. Such experiments do not require an action to be taken by the animal (agent). (B) An instrumental conditioning setup where a rodent has to learn to transverse the maze and make a decision at the junction about which direction to go. Such a decision problem necessitates the action of an actor.

In the slightly different setting of instrumental conditioning, the agent has to take an action in order to receive reward. Hence, this forces the agent to make a decision. An example setup is shown in Fig. 11.4B. In the illustrated experiment, a rodent is placed in a T-maze with food of different sizes at the different end of each horizontal arm of the T-maze. The rodent might wander around until it finds some reward. This is an exploration phase. After finding some reward, the agent should then be able to exploit this knowledge in subsequent trials.

We have included two different sizes of reward in the T-maze in order to illustrate a common problem in real-world applications. That is, if we would exploit the reward we find first, how would we ever find better reward. There is hence an interesting exploration-exploitation trade-off that can influence different behaviours.

There are two principle ways we can approach learning such decision systems that we call model-free and model-based RL. In model-free RL we simply exploit a memory of reward in specific states of the environment. In contrast, a model-based approach aims to first learn a model of the world from which is can infer good actions to reach reward states. The word 'model' refers here to a model of the environment and possible actions from which the optimal actions can be calculated. Such a deliberative system seems to have clear advantages in the flexibility and the ability to generalize to new environments with clear goal-directed behaviours. However, it is also clear that such an approach needs a more complex model framework, and calculating optimal responses also needs effort and possibly some time. In contrast, model-free decisions can be fast as it just automates repeating rewarding previous actions without much deliberations. Such decision systems resemble much more habitual decision-making. There is much evidence that both decision systems are realized in the brain.

Much of the reinforcement learning in the AI literature and basic conditioning in the animal learning literature are discussing the model free approach, and it is worth while to outline here already the main idea before diving into the details. The main driver in this theory is temporal difference learning. For this we consider an agent in different possible states s, and the agent want to chose the states with large values. The value $V(s)$ of a state is thereby defined by the immediate reward $r(s)$ plus all the reward in the future. This is also called the return. We could learn the value function

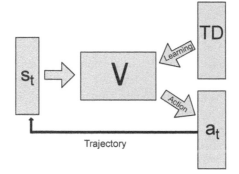

Fig. 11.5 Illustration of model-free RL with a neural network as a approximator for the value function. The training is achieved through Temporal Difference (TD) learning, and the output of this critic is used to guide the behaviour of the agent.

with neural network as shown in Fig. 11.5. The only problem is that the agent does not has a teacher who tells them what the true value of the state is. The teacher only tells them the immediate reward. The main idea is now a form of bootstrapping where the agent estimates the future reward from the value function at the next state that the agents visit. Hence, the learning rule consists of the difference of the (estimated) new value $r(s) + \gamma V(s+1)$ and the value it assumed before the new experience, $V(s)$. This difference is called the temporal difference error

$$TD = r(s) + \gamma V(s+1) - V(s), \tag{11.1}$$

and the network could be trained, for example, by minimizing the mean square of the temporal difference error.

While this captures the principals idea of model-free reinforcement learning, there are many challenges to apply these methods to more complex environments. There has been much recent progress in this field based on additional considerations that we will mentioned further below. However, it is also important to keep in mind that the brain utilizes many more methods than can contribute to good decision-making, including model-based decision-making.

11.3 Formalization of reinforcement learning

We first formalize the learning problem in a Markov decision process and then discuss a variety of related algorithms. We will first discuss RL in a traditional tabular setting where an environment is described with discrete states and the actions are also discrete choices. We will then discuss then describe The second part of this chapter will use function approximators with neural networks which have made recent progress as deep RL.

11.3.1 The environmental setting of a Markov decision process

It is useful to formalize such learning scenarios further with discrete states. We consider an agent that at time t is in a specific state s_t. A state describes thereby the environment such as a location at which the agent could be. Furthermore, we assume that the agent can take an action a_t from each state. In the context of a mobile agent, the action a_t is commonly provided by a motor command from a control program, but we can also think about these actions on a higher level such as turning right or left in the maze. The aim of reinforcement learning is to train a controller, the brain of the agent, to make the decision of which action to take from each state. This function is called the (control) policy in reinforcement learning

$$\textbf{Policy:} \quad \begin{array}{ll} a_t = \pi(s_t) & \text{deterministic} \\ \pi(a_t|s_t) & \text{stochastic.} \end{array} \tag{11.2}$$

We have thereby provided two formulations: a deterministic one with a regular function and a stochastic one by specifying a probability function. In general, it is useful to consider probabilistic settings. For example, even though the controller that executes the policy has the intention to move a vehicle forward, a malfunction in the program executes a tune routine. Hence, in this case, the policy specifies the probability that an action is taken, $\pi(a_t|s_s)$. We will outline most of the discussions in the deterministic setting for simplicity and to minimize notations. We use the probabilistic setting in later sections where appropriate and will continue outlining the formulations of the problem in both settings.

There are two more functions we need to introduce that describe the environment in which the controller has to function. The first one is the

$$\textbf{Transition function:} \quad \begin{array}{ll} s_{t+1} = \tau(s_t, a_t) & \text{deterministic} \\ \tau(s_{t+1}|s_t, a_t) & \text{stochastic.} \end{array} \tag{11.3}$$

which simply specifies the resulting state when an agent takes action a_t from state s_t. Again, it is useful to consider a probabilistic setting since the actual state of an agent could be different than intended due to external factors which are not under the control of the agent. For example, even if the controller executes the forward function for a certain distance, a slope in the road might lead to an overshoot of the desired position. In such a probabilistic setting the transition function specifies a transition probability $\tau(s_{t+1}|s_t, a_t)$ of ending up in state s_{t+1}, when taking action a_t from state s_t.

We restrict the discussion here to the common assumption that the transition function depends only on the previous state and the intended action from the corresponding state. This is called the Markov condition. The series of states with transition probabilities is a Markov chain, and the one for the T-maze example is shown in Fig. 11.4D. A non-Markovian condition would be the case in which the next state depends on a series of previous states and actions, and our agent would then need a memory to make optimal decisions. The situation described by the Markov condition is quite natural as many decisions processes only depend on the current state. The Markov condition is therefore a good scenario and not a real limitation of the reinforcement learning methods we discuss later, but it will simplify some of the notations and discussions.

The second important environmental function encapsulates the assumption that the environment or a teacher provides reward according to the

$$\textbf{Reward function:} \quad \begin{array}{ll} r_{t+1} = \rho(s_t, a_t) & \text{deterministic} \\ \rho(r_{t+1}|s_t, a_t) & \text{stochastic.} \end{array} \tag{11.4}$$

This reward functions returns the value of reward when the agent is entering state s_{t+1} by taking action a_t from state s_t. In most cases, the reward only depends on the state it enters, but therefore it depends on the previous state and the action taken from this state. In the probabilistic setting the reward $\rho(s_{t+1}|s_t, a_t)$ is a probability of receiving reward in the state s_{t+1} when taking action a_t from state s_t.

The environmental functions τ and ρ, together with the specifications of the set of states S and actions A, define the environment in which we want to make decisions. Since we restricted our discussion to Markov chains, the corresponding decision process is called a Markov decision process (MDP). Note that we assume in our notation that the agent knows in which state it is in. While we will see that this is easy in simulations as shown later, this is a major problem in practice when the state needs to be derived from observations. For example, this is a common occurrence in robotics where we have sensors such as cameras or gyroscopes from which we want to estimate the pose of a robot. Moreover, we have to infer the states usually from limited observations. This general setting is commonly referred to as the partially observable Markov decision process (POMDP). We discuss the basic ideas first in the MDP setting, then later discuss DeepRL that can be applied directly to a POMDP setting.

RL faces several challenges. One is called the credit assignment problem. This includes which action (spatial credit assignment) and at which time (temporal credit assignment) of the system should be given credit for the achievement of reward. Another important aspect that is new in contrast to supervised learning is that the agent must search for solutions by trying different actions. The agent must therefore generally play an active role in exploring options. Even if the agent finds a solution that give it some reward, the question might remain if this is a good solution or if the agent should search for a better solution or stick to the known rewards. This problem is commonly stated as 'exploration versus exploitation trade-off'. Let us assume that the rodent (agent) found the smaller food reward at the end of the left arm of the T-maze. It is then likely that the rodent will turn left in subsequent trials to receive food reward. Thus the agent learned that the action of taking a left turn and going to the end of the arm is associated with food reward. Of course, in this case the rodent could also receive a larger reward when exploring the right arm of the maze, which illustrates again the exploration–exploitation trade-off in such learning settings.

Many of the applications of reinforcement learning now apply deep networks as a learner. However, we will start formalizing the discussion of RL with the more traditional tabular representation of functions which will give us the opportunity of discussing exact examples without function approximation. We will later return to the use of function approximators.

To illustrate the different reinforcement learning schemes discussed in this chapter, we will apply these algorithms to a simplified version of the T-maze example mentioned above. To keep the programs minimal and clean, we concentrate on the upper linear part for the maze as illustrated in Fig. 11.6. States s of the maze are labelled 0 to 4. A reward of value 1 is provided in state 0 and a reward of 2 is provided in state 4. The discrete Q-function has 10 values corresponding to each possible action in each state. In states 1, 2, and 3 these are the actions move *left* or move *right*. The states with the reward, states 0 and 4, are terminal states and the agent would stay in these states if unprompted to move. We coded this with action labelled as 0 in the figure.

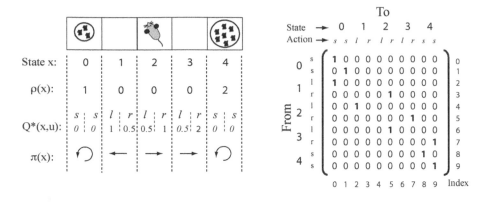

Fig. 11.6 Example experiment with the simplified T-maze where we concentrate on the more interesting horizontal portion of the maze (linear maze). The right hand side shows the corresponding transition matrix for the optimal policy.

In order to start coding these examples, we will define some simple functions as shown below. The first two functions are the environmental functions of the transition function $\tau(s, a)$ and the reward function $\rho(s)$. Note that these functions are usually not known by the agent, but we will come back to this point. In addition, we provide several helper functions, one which calculates the policy from a value function as discussed shortly, and a function $idx(a)$ to transforms the action representation $a \in \{-1, 1\}$ to the corresponding indices $idx \in \{0, 1\}$, which we need for the specific implementation of the actions in this example.

Listing 11.1 RL.ipynb (Part 1)

```
1  ## Reinforcement learning in 1d maze
2  import numpy as np
3  import matplotlib.pyplot as plt
4
5  def tau(s,a):
6      if s==0 or s==4:  return(s)
7      else:          return(s+a)
8  def rho(s,a):
9      return (s==1 and a==-1)+2*(s==3 and a == 1)
10 def calc_policy(Q):
11     policy=np.zeros(5)
12     for s in range(0,5):
13         action_idx=np.argmax(Q[s,:])
14         policy[s]=2*action_idx-1
15         policy[0]=policy[4]=0
16     return policy.astype(int)
17 def idx(a):
18     return(int((a+1)/2))
```

The goal of the agent is to maximize the total expected reward in the future from every initial state. This quantity is called return in economics. Of course, if we assume that this goes on forever, then this return should be infinite, and we have henceforth to be a bit more careful. One common choice is to define the return as the average reward in a finite time interval, also called the finite horizon case. Another common form to keep the return finite is to use a discounted return in which an agent values immediate reward more than a reward to be obtained far in the future. To capture this we define a discount factor $0 < \gamma < 1$. In the example program we will use a value of $\gamma = 0.5$,

Listing 11.2 RL.ipynb (Part 2)

```
1 # Discount Factor
2 gamma=0.5
```

although values much closer to 1 such as $\gamma = 0.99$, are common. For this case we now define a state-action value function. This function gives us a numerical value of the return (all future discounted reward) when the agent is in state s and takes action a and then follows the policy for the following actions,

$$\textbf{Value function (state-action):} \quad Q^\pi(s,a) = \rho(s,a) + \sum_{t=1}^{\infty} \gamma^t \rho(s_t, \pi(s_t)). \quad (11.5)$$

In other words, this functions tells us how good action a is in state s, and the knowledge of this value function should thus guide the actions of an agent. The aim of value-based reinforcement learning is to estimate this function. Here, we consider first the deterministic case and return to another formulation in the stochastic case for finite horizon cases later.

Sometimes we are only interested in the value function even when we follow the policy for the first step in the action sequence from state s. Then, this value function does then not depend explicitly on the action, only indirectly of course on the policy, and is defined as the total discounted return from state $s = s_0$ following policy π,

$$\textbf{Value function (state):} \quad V^\pi(s) = Q^\pi(s, \pi(s)). \quad (11.6)$$

The goal of RL is to find the policy which maximized the return. If the agents knows the

$$\textbf{Optimal value function}: \quad V^*(s) = \max_a Q^*(s, a), \quad (11.7)$$

then the optimal policy is simply given by taking the action that leads to the biggest expected return, namely

$$\textbf{Optimal policy}: \quad \pi^*(s) = \arg\max_a Q^*(s, a). \quad (11.8)$$

This function is implemented here with the python code for `calc_policy`.

The optimal value function and the optimal policy are closely related. We will discuss in the following several methods to calculate or estimate the value function from which the policy can be derived. These methods can be put under the heading of value-search. Corresponding agents, or part of the corresponding RL algorithms, are commonly called critic. There are also methods to learn the policy directly. Such methods are called policy-search and the corresponding agents are called an actor. At the end we will argue that combining these approaches in actor–critic scheme has attractive features, and such schemes are increasingly used in practical applications with the help of neural networks as function approximators. We will work our way towards this exciting area.

11.3.2   Model-based reinforcement learning

In this section we assume that the agent has a model of the environment, which includes both, the knowledge of reward states $\rho(s, a)$ and the transfer functions $\tau(s, a)$. The knowledge of these functions, or a model thereof, is required for model-based RL. The basic challenge in practical applications is to learn these functions from examples of the agent acting in the environment. Here we are more concerned with showing how to calculate optimal policies if we know these functions.

11.3.2.1   The basic Bellman equation

The key to learning the value functions is the realization that the right-hand side of eqn 11.5 can be written in terms of the Q-function itself, namely

$$Q^\pi(s, a) = \rho(s, a) + \gamma \sum_{t=1}^{\infty} \gamma^{t-1} \rho(s_t, \pi(s_t))$$

$$= \rho(s, a) + \gamma \left[\rho(\tau(s, a), \pi(\tau(s, a))) + \gamma \sum_{t=2}^{\infty} \gamma^{t-2} \rho(s_t, \pi(s_t)) \right].$$

The term in the square bracket is equal to the value function of the state that is reached after the transition $\tau(s, a)$

$$Q^\pi(\tau(s, a), \pi(\tau(s, a))) = V^\pi(\tau(s, a)). \tag{11.9}$$

The Q-function and the V-function are here equivalent since we are following the policy in these steps. Using this fact in the equation above, we get the

π **Bellman equation:** $Q^\pi(s, a) = \rho(s, a) + \gamma Q^\pi(\tau(s, a), \pi(\tau(s, a)))$.   (11.10)

If we combine this with known dynamic equations in the continuous time domain, then this becomes the Hamilton–Jacobi–Bellman equation, often encountered in engineering.

As stated earlier, we here assume that the reward function $\rho(s, a)$ and the transition functions $\tau(s, a)$ are known. At this point the agent follows a specified policy $\pi(s)$. Let us further assume that we have n_s states and n_a possible actions in each state. We have thus $n_s \times n_a$ unknown quantities $Q^\pi(s, a)$ which are governed by the Bellman equation. More precisely, the Bellman eqn 11.10 are $n_s \times n_a$ coupled linear equations of the unknowns $Q^\pi(s, a)$. It is then convenient to write this equation system with vectors

$$\mathbf{Q}^\pi = \mathbf{R} + \gamma \mathbf{T}^\pi \mathbf{Q}^\pi \tag{11.11}$$

where T^π is an appropriate transition matrix which depends on the policy. This equation can also be written as

$$\mathbf{R} = (\mathbb{1} - \gamma \mathbf{T}^\pi) \mathbf{Q}^\pi, \tag{11.12}$$

where $\mathbb{1}$ is the identity matrix. This equation has the solution

$$\mathbf{Q}^\pi = (\mathbb{1} - \gamma \mathbf{T}^\pi)^{-1} \mathbf{R} \tag{11.13}$$

if the inverse exists. In other words, as long as the agent knows the reward function and the transition function, it can calculate the value function for a specific policy without taking even a single step. This is an example of a deliberative system where the agent can use the models of reward and the environment to calculate optimal decisions, hence the designation as model-based RL.

To demonstrate how to solve the Bellman equation with linear algebra tools, we need to define the corresponding vectors and matrices as used in eqn 11.13. We therefore order quantities such as ρ and Q with 10 indices. The first corresponds to $(s = 0, u = -1)$, the second to $(s = 0, u = 1)$, the third to $(s = 1, u = -1)$, etc. The reward vector can thus be coded as:

Listing 11.3 RL.ipynb (Part 3)

```
1 print('——> Analytic solution for optimal policy')
2 # Defining reward vector R
3 i=0; R=np.zeros(10)
4 for s in range(0,5):
5     for a in range(-1,2,2):
6         R[i]=rho(s,a)
7         i += 1
```

The transition matrix depends on the policy, so we need to choose one. We chose the one specified on the left in Fig. 11.6 where the agent would move to the left in state $s = 1$ and to the right in states $s = 2$ and $s = 3$. This happens to be the optimal solution, as we will show later, so that this will also give us a solution for the optimal value function. We use this policy to construct the transition matrix by hand as shown on the right in Fig. 11.6. For example, if we are in state $s = 4$ and move to the left, $a = -1$, corresponding to the from-index = 7, then we end up in state $s = 3$, from which the policy says go right, $a = 1$. This correspond to the to-index = 9. Thus, the transition matrix should have an entry $T(7, 9) = 1$. Going through all the cases results in

Listing 11.4 RL.ipynb (Part 4)

```
1 # Defining transition matrix
2 T=np.zeros([10,10]);
3 T[0,0]=1; T[1,1]=1; T[2,0]=1; T[3,5]=1; T[4,2]=1
4 T[5,7]=1; T[6,5]=1; T[7,9]=1; T[8,7]=1; T[9,9]=1
```

With this we can solve this linear matrix equations with the inv() function in the linear algebra package of NumPy,

Listing 11.5 RL.ipynb (Part 5)

```
1 # Calculate Q-function
2 Q=np.linalg.inv(np.eye(10)-gamma*T) @ np.transpose(R)
3 Q=np.reshape(Q,[5,2]); Q[4,0]=0
```

We reshaped the resulting Q-function so that the first row shows the values for left movements in each state and the second row shows the values for a right movement in each state. From this we can calculate which movement to take in each state, namely just the action corresponding to the maximum value in each column,

Listing 11.6 RL.ipynb (Part 6)

```
1 policy=calc_policy(Q)
```

Finally we print the results with

Listing 11.7 RL.ipynb (Part 7)

```
1 print('Q values: \n',np.transpose(Q))
2 print('policy: \n',np.transpose(policy))
```

which gives the output

```
--> Analytic solution for optimal policy
Q values:
 [[0.   1.   0.5 0.5 0. ]
  [0.   0.5 1.   2.   0. ]]
policy:
 [ 0 -1  1  1  0]
```

The agent is moving left in state 1 as this would lead to an immediate reward of 1 and moving right in the other states as this would result in a larger reward, even when taking the discounting for more steps into account. Of course, at this point our argument is circular as we started with the assumption that we use the optimal policy as specified in the transition matrix at the start. We will soon see how to start with an arbitrary policy an improve this to find the optimal strategy. Also note that the transition matrix was perfect in the sense that the intended move always leads to the intended end state. A probabilistic extension of this transition matrix is quite useful in describing more realistic situations.

In the code we save the optimal Q-values for the optimal policy

Listing 11.8 RL.ipynb (Part 9)

```
1 Qana=Q
```

so that we can later plot the differences to the other solution methods.

The Bellman equations are a set of n coupled linear equations for n unknown Q-values, and we have solved these here with linear algebra function to find an inverse of a matrix. Finding the inverse of a function can be implemented with different algorithms such as Gauss elimination. However, it is much more common to use an iterative procedure to solve the Bellman equation. For this iterative algorithm we starts with an estimation of the Q-function, let's call this Q_i^π, and improve it by calculating the right-hand side of the Bellman equation,

$$\textbf{Dynamic programming}: \quad Q_{i+1}^\pi(s,a) \leftarrow \rho(s,a) + \gamma Q_i^\pi(\tau(s,a), \pi(\tau(s,a))). \tag{11.14}$$

The fixed-point of this equation, that is, the values that does not change with these iterations, are the desired values of Q^π. Another way of thinking about this algorithm is that the Bellman equality is only true for the correct Q^π values. For our guess, the difference between the left- and right-hand side is not 0, but we are minimizing this with the iterative procedure above. The corresponding code is

Listing 11.9 RL.ipynb (Part 9)

```
1 print('--> Dynamic Programming')
2
3 Q=np.zeros([5,2])
```

```
4  for iter in range(3):
5      for s in range(0,5):
6          for a in range(-1,2,2):
7              act = np.int(policy[tau(s,a)])
8              Q[s,idx(a)]=rho(s,a)+gamma*Q[tau(s,a),idx(act)]
9
10 print('Q values: \n',np.transpose(Q))
11 print('policy: \n',np.transpose(policy))
```

with output

```
--> Dynamic Programming;
Q values:
 [[0.  1.  0.5 0.5 0. ]
  [0.  0.5 1.  2.  0. ]]
policy:
 [ 0 -1  1  1  0]
```

which is, of course, the same correct solution as found with the explicit matrix inversion. This iterative method is a much more common implementation and it does not require the explicit coding of the transition matrix. Iterative approaches will be used in all further methods discussed later. Note that we have only used three iterations to converge on the correct solution. While here we set the number of iterations by hand, in practice we iterate until the changes in the values are sufficiently small.

11.3.2.2 Policy iteration

The goal of RL is of course to find the policy which maximizes the return. So far we have only discussed a method to calculate the value for a given policy. However, we can start with an arbitrary policy and can use the corresponding value function to improve the policy by defining a new policy which is given by taken the actions from each state that gives us the best next return value,

$$\textbf{Policy iteration}: \quad \pi(s) \leftarrow \arg\max_{a} Q^{\pi}(s, a). \qquad (11.15)$$

For the new policy, we can then calculate the corresponding Q-function and then use this Q-function to improve the policy again. Iterating over the policy gives us the

$$\textbf{Optimal policy}: \quad \pi^{*}(s). \qquad (11.16)$$

The corresponding value function is Q^{*}. In the maze example we can see that the maximum in each column of the Q-matrix is the policy we started with. This is the optimal policy, as we stated earlier.

The corresponding code for our maze example is

Listing 11.10 RL.ipynb (Part 10)

```
1  print('--> Policy iteration')
2
3  Q=np.zeros([5,2])
4  policy=calc_policy(Q)
5  for iter in range(3):
6      for s in range(0,5):
7          for a in range(-1,2,2):
```

```
 8            act = np.int(policy[tau(s,a)])
 9               Q[s,idx(a)]=rho(s,a)+gamma*Q[tau(s,a),idx(act)]
10       policy=calc_policy(Q)
11
12 print('Q values: \n',np.transpose(Q))
13 print('policy: \n',np.transpose(policy))
```

with output

```
--> Policy iteration
Q values:
[[0.  1.   0.5 0.5 0. ]
 [0.  0.5 1.   2.   0. ]]
policy:
[ 0 -1  1  1  0]
```

again leading to the correct result. Note that in this example we again iterated only three times over the policies. In principle, we could and should iterate several times for each policy in order to converge to a stable estimate for this Q^π. However, the improvements will lead very quickly to a stable state, at least in this simple example.

11.3.2.3 Bellman function for optimal policy and value (Q) iteration

Since we are primarily interested in the optimal policy, we could try to solve the Bellman equation immediately for this policy,

$$Q^*(s,a) = \rho(s,a) + \gamma Q^*(\tau(s,a), \pi^*(\tau(s,a))). \tag{11.17}$$

The problem is that this equation now depends on the unknown π^*. However, we can check in each state all the actions and take the one which gives us the best return. This should be equivalent to the equation above in the optimal case. Hence we propose the

Optimal Bellman equation: $Q^*(s,a) = \rho(s,a) + \gamma \max_{a'} Q^*(\tau(s,a), a')$. (11.18)

We can solve this equation again with the iterative method when the transfer function and the reward functions are known,

$$\textbf{Q-iteration:}\quad Q^*_{i+1}(s,a) \leftarrow \rho(s,a) + \gamma \max_{a'} Q^*(\tau(s,a), a'). \tag{11.19}$$

The corresponding code for our maze example is

Listing 11.11 RL.ipynb (Part 11)

```
 1 print('—> Q-iteration')
 2
 3 Q_new=np.zeros([5,2])
 4 Q=np.zeros([5,2])
 5 for iter in range(3):
 6     for s in range(0,5):
 7         for a in range(-1,2,2):
 8             maxValue = np.maximum(Q[tau(s,a),0],Q[tau(s,a),1])
 9             Q_new[s,idx(a)]=rho(s,a)+gamma*maxValue
10     Q=np.copy(Q_new);
11
12 policy=calc_policy(Q)
13 print('Q values: \n',np.transpose(Q))
14 print('policy: \n',np.transpose(policy))
```

with output

```
--> Q-iteration
Q values:
[[0.  1.   0.5 0.5 0. ]
[0.  0.5 1.  2.   0. ]]
policy:
[ 0 -1  1  1  0]
```

In this example we again used only three iterations which are sufficient to reach the correct values. In practice, we can terminate the program if the changes are sufficiently small, which we did not implement here to keep the code short.

There is an interesting difference between this value iteration method and the previous policy iteration method. In the policy iteration method we followed the policy to calculate the updated value function. We call such a method on-policy. In contrast, in the value (Q) iteration, we check out all possible actions from this state for the update of the value function. Such a procedure is called off-policy.

11.3.3 Model-free reinforcement learning

11.3.3.1 Temporal difference method for value iteration

Above we assumed a model of the environment by an explicit knowledge of the functions $\tau(s, a)$ and $\rho(s, a)$. While the Bellman equations have been known since the 1950s, their usefulness has been limited due to the fact that finding the environmental functions can be difficult. This is one of the reasons that such RL techniques have not gained more applications at that point. We could use modelling techniques and some sampling strategies to learn these functions with machine learning techniques and then use model-based RL as described above to find the optimal policy. For example, we can use demonstrations of actions by a teacher as a form of supervised learning for the models. As mentioned earlier, such supervised learning is commonly called imitation learning in the context of robotics and RL. We are not following this line of thought here but will instead combine here the sampling directly with reinforcement learning by exploring the environment. This approach has helped to apply RL to many more applications. Since we do not need to know the environmental functions, this approach is called model-free.

We will start again with a version for a specific policy by choosing a policy and estimate the Q-function for this policy. As in the iterative methods earlier, we want to minimize the difference between the left- and right-hand sides of the Bellman equation. But we cannot calculate the right-hand side since we do not know the transition function and the reward function. However, we can just take a step according to our policy $u = \pi(s)$ and observe a reward r_{i+1} and the next state s_{i+1}. Now, since this is only one sample, we should use this as update of the value function only with a small learning rate α. The corresponding algorithm is

$$\textbf{SARSA:} \quad Q_{i+1}(s_i, a_i) = Q_i(s_i, a_i) + \alpha \left[(r_{i+1} + \gamma Q_i(s_{i+1}, a_{i+1}) - Q_i(s_i, u_i)\right].$$
(11.20)

The name comes from the fact that we are in a state from which we take an action and observe an reward and then go to the next state and take action:

$$s \rightarrow a \rightarrow r \rightarrow s \rightarrow a.$$

The term in the square brackets on the right-hand side of eqn 11.20 is called the temporal difference since it is the difference between the expected value earlier at some point and the new estimate from the actual reward and the following estimate at the next temporal evaluation point. Note that we are following the policy, and the methods is therefore again an on-policy method.

The next step is to use the estimate of the Q-function to improve policy. However, since we are mainly interested in the optimal policy, we should improve the policy by taking the steps that maximizes the reward. However, one problem in this scheme is that we have to estimate the Q-values by sampling so that we have to make sure we trade off exploitation with exploration. A common way to choose the policy in this scheme is the

$$\epsilon\text{-greedy policy:} \quad p\left(\arg\max_a Q(s,a)\right) = 1 - \epsilon. \qquad (11.21)$$

So, we are really evaluating the optimal policy that requires us to make the exploration 0 at the end, $\epsilon \rightarrow 0$.

The corresponding code for the SARSA is:

Listing 11.12 RL.ipynb (Part 12)

```
1  print('-->  SARSA')
2
3  Q=np.zeros([5,2])
4  error = []
5  alpha=1;
6  for trial in range(200):
7      policy=calc_policy(Q)
8      s=2
9      for t in range(0,5):
10         a=policy[s]
11         if np.random.rand()<0.1: a=-a #epsilon greedy
12         a2=idx(policy[tau(s,a)])
13         TD=rho(s,a)+gamma*Q[tau(s,a),a2]-Q[s,idx(a)]
14         Q[s,idx(a)]=Q[s,idx(a)]+alpha*TD
15         s=tau(s,a)
16     error.append(np.sum(np.sum(np.abs(np.subtract(Q,Qana)))))
17
18 print('Q values: \n',np.transpose(Q))
19 print('policy: \n',np.transpose(policy))
20 plt.figure(); plt.plot(error)
21 plt.xlabel('iteration'); plt.ylabel('error')
```

with output

```
--> SARSA
Q values:
[[0.   1.   0.5 0.5 0. ]
 [0.   0.5 1.   2.   0. ]]
policy:
[ 0 -1  1  1  0]
```

Fig. 11.7 shows that the difference between the Q-value of this algorithm and the Q-value of the analytic solution goes to 0 and hence converges to the correct solution.

Sometimes this can take more iterations because exploring off-policy states is not frequent. Of course, this also depends on the exploration strategy.

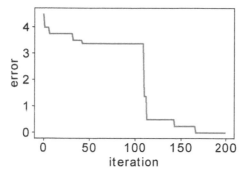

Fig. 11.7 Example learning curve of the SARSA algorithm. The error is the absolute difference between the Q-value of this algorithm and the Q-value calculated analytically above.

Note that we have set the learning rate $\alpha = 1$ for this example, which makes the update rule look similar to the iterative method of the model-based case

$$Q_{i+1}(s_i, a_i) = (r_{i+1} + \gamma Q_i(s_{i+1}, a_{i+1}).\tag{11.22}$$

However, there is a major difference. Previously we iterated over all possible states with the knowledge of the transition function and the reward function; thus an agent does not really have to explore the environment and can just 'sit there' and calculate what the optimal action is. This is the benefit of model-based reinforcement learning. In contrast, here we discuss the case where we do not know the transition function and the reward function and hence have to explore the environment by acting in it. As this is usually associated with a physical movement, this takes times and hence limits the exploration we can do. Thus, it is common that an agent cannot explore all possible states in large environments. Also, a learning rate of $\alpha = 1$ is not always advisable since a more common setting is that reward itself is probabilistic. A smaller value of α then represents a form of taking a sliding average and hence estimating the expected value of the reward.

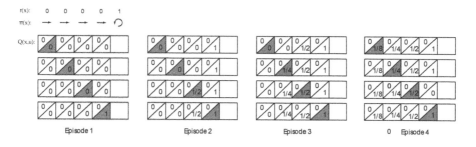

Fig. 11.8 Example of the 'back-propagation' of the reward (not to be confused with the backpropagation algorithm in supervised learning). In this example, an episode always starts in the left-most state and the policy is to always to go right. A reward is received in the right-most state.

It is useful to go through some iterations of the SARSA algorithm by hand for a linear-maze example. In the example shown in Fig. 11.8, we changed the situation to a linear maze in which the state always starts at the left-most state and a reward of $r = 1$ is received in the right-most state. The policy is to always go right, which is also the optimal policy in this situation. At the first time step of the first episode we are in the left-most state and evaluate the value of going right. In the corresponding state to the right there is no reward given, and the value function is also 0. So the value function of this state-action is 0. The same is true for every step until we are in the state before the reward state. At this point the value is updated to the reward of the next state. In the second episode the value of the first and second state remains 0, but the third state is updated to $\gamma * 1$ since the value of the next state following the policy is given by 1, and we discount this by γ. Going through more episodes it can be seen that the value 'back-propagates' by one step in each episode. Note that this back-propagation of the value is not to be confused with the backpropagation algorithm in supervised learning. Also, notice that the values for the Q-function for going left are not updated as we only followed optimal policy deterministically. Some exploration steps will eventually update these values, although it might take a long time until these values propagate through the system.

There is one important additional basic algorithm that we need to mention in this section on temporal difference learning. This final algorithm is to use an alternative way to estimate the value function using an off-policy approach for the estimation step from each visited state. That is, we check all possible actions from the state that we evaluate state and update the value function with the maximal expected return,

Q-learning: $Q_{i+1}(s_i, a_i) = Q_i(s_i, a_i) + \alpha \left[(r_{i+1} + \gamma \max_{a'} Q_i(s_{i+1}, a') - Q_i(s_i, a_i) \right]$

$$(11.23)$$

We still have to explore the environment which usually follows the optimal estimated policy, with some allowance for exploration such as ϵ-greedy or a softmax exploration strategy. The corresponding code for the Q-learning is

Listing 11.13 RL.ipynb (Part 13)

```
1  print('--> Q-Learning:')
2
3  Q=np.zeros([5,2])
4  alpha=1
5  error = []
6  for trial in range(200):
7      policy=calc_policy(Q)
8      s=2
9      for t in range(0,5):
10         a=policy[s]
11         if np.random.rand()<0.2: a=-a #epsilon greedy
12         TD=rho(s,a)+gamma *
13             np.maximum(Q[tau(s,a),0],Q[tau(s,a),1])-Q[s,idx(a)]
14         Q[s,idx(a)]=Q[s,idx(a)]+alpha*TD
15         Q[0]=0;Q[4]=0;
16         s=tau(s,a)
17     error.append(np.sum(np.sum(np.abs(np.subtract(Q,Qana)))))
18
19  print('Q values: \n',np.transpose(Q))
20  print('policy: \n',np.transpose(policy))
```

```
21| plt.plot(error,'r');
22| plt.xlabel('iteration'); plt.ylabel('error')
```

with output

```
--> Q-Learning:
Q values:
[[0.  1.  0.5 0.5 0. ]
 [0.  0.5 1.  2.  0. ]]
policy:
[ 0 -1  1  1  0]
```

11.3.3.2 TD(λ)

The example of the linear maze in the previous section has shown that the expectation of reward propagates backwards in each episode which thus requires multiple repetitions of the episodes in order to evaluate the value function. The reason for this is that we only give credit for making a step to a valuable state to the previous step and hence only update the corresponding value function. A different approach is to keep track of which states have led to the reward and assign the credit to each step that was visited. However, because we discount the reward proportional to the time it takes to get to the rewarded state, we need to also take this into account.

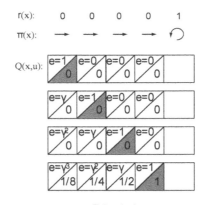

Episode 1

Fig. 11.9 Example of the 'back-propagation' of the reward in the TD(1) algorithm. Compared to the slow back-propagation in the TD(0) algorithm, as shown in Fig. 11.8, the added memory allows for the credit assignment in the whole episode.

To realize this we introduce an eligibility trace that we call $e(s, a)$. At the beginning, this eligibility trace is set to 0 for all the states. For each visited state we set the eligibility state to 1 for this current state, and we discount the eligibility for all the other states by γ. This is demonstrated in Fig. 11.9. In the figure we indicate the eligibility trace at every time step. Note how the eligibility trace is building up during one episode until reaching the rewarded state, at which time the values of all the states are updated in the right proportion. This algorithm does therefore only need one optimal episode to find the correct value function, at least in this case with a learning rate of $\alpha = 1$. Thus to change a TD algorithm to a TD(1), we change the build up the eligibility trace in each step

$$e(s, a) \leftarrow e(s, a)\gamma \quad \text{for all } s,a \tag{11.24}$$

and update all Q-values proportional to the TD error of this step multiplied by the eligibility trace,

$$Q(s, a) \leftarrow Q(s, a) + \alpha TD * e(s, a). \tag{11.25}$$

While this algorithms requires some memory, we see that we only need to store an eligibility trace which indirectly specifies the sequence the agent took. It is also easy to extend this algorithm to a more general form called TD(λ) where we can interpolate between the original TD algorithm with no eligibility trace, called TD(0), with the perfect memory trace of TD(1). An exponential decay of an eligibility trace can be implemented simply by including a factor λ in eqn 11.24,

$$e(s, a) \leftarrow e(s, a)\gamma\lambda \quad \text{for all } s,a. \tag{11.26}$$

This algorithm is implemented for the Q-learning version of temporal difference learning in the code shown in Listing 10.15.

Listing 11.14 RL.ipynb (Part 14)

```
1  print('—> TD(lambda) for Q-learning')
2
3  Q=np.zeros([5,2])
4  alpha=1
5  error = []
6  eligibility=np.zeros([5,2])
7  lam=0.7
8
9  for trial in range(200):
10     policy=calc_policy(Q)
11     s=2
12     for t in range(0,5):
13         a=policy[s]
14         if np.random.rand()<0.1: a=-a #epsilon greedy
15         TD=rho(s,a)+gamma *
16             np.maximum(Q[tau(s,a),0],Q[tau(s,a),1])-Q[s,idx(a)]
17         eligibility *=gamma*lam
18         eligibility[s,idx(a)]=1
19         for si in range(1,4):
20             for ai in range(2):
21                 Q[si,ai]=Q[si,ai]+alpha*TD*eligibility[si,ai]
22         Q[0]=0;Q[4]=0;
23         s=tau(s,a)
24     error.append(np.sum(np.sum(np.abs(np.subtract(Q,Qana)))))
25
26  print('Q values: \n',np.transpose(Q))
27  print('policy: \n',np.transpose(policy))
28  plt.plot(error,'r');
29  plt.xlabel('iteration'); plt.ylabel('error')
```

with output

```
--> TD(lambda) for Q-learning
Q values:
```

```
[[0.         0.99999999 0.49999994 0.49998045 0.        ]
 [0.         0.25       1.         2.         0.        ]]
policy:
[ 0 -1  1  1  0]
```

TD(λ) made famous by Gerald Tesauro in the early 1990s for achieving human level performance in playing backgammon. In addition, Tesauro's solution used neural networks as a function approximator which is important for capturing the high-dimensional state-action space. This will be discussed in the next section.

11.4 Deep reinforcement learning

11.4.1 Value-function approximation with ANN

Up to this point we have outlined the basic ideas behind reinforcement learning algorithms. We will now move on to an important topic to scale these ideas to real-world applications. The previous method we used tabulated the values for the functions. For example, the value function in the above programs were look-up tables or arrays in programming terms that specified the value function for each discrete state and action. Correspondingly, this lead to tables for the policy. Such algorithms are now commonly referred to as tabular RL algorithms. The problem with this approach is that these tables can be very big for large state and action dimensionality. Indeed, the increased computational demand of calculating these quantities in many real-world applications is often prohibitive, in particular in a stochastic setting where we have to sample in the state-action space.

To illustrate this point with a popular example, let us think how tabular RL would look if we implement learning to play a computer game. Let us discuss the example of Atari 2600 games that have been implemented in an arcade learning environment by Michael Bowling and colleagues at the University of Alberta. This environment simulates video input of 210×160 RGB video at 60Hz. An example of these video screens is shown in Fig. 11.10. The state space of these games is equivalent to a state input vector of length 100,800 every 1/60 of a second. Even if each pixel is only allowed to have, say, 8 bit representations, equivalent to $2^8 = 256$ possible values, and all the pixel values are independent, there would be 256^{100800} possible states. Clearly this is impossible to implement with the tabular methods cited earlier. Bellman noticed this practical limitations and coined the phrase 'curse of dimensionality'. The principle idea for overcoming the curse of dimensionality is to use function approximators to represent the functions, and it comes at no surprise that we will specifically use deep neural networks for these function approximations.

Several types of function approximators have been used in the past. Linear function approximation (linear regression) is often discussed in engineering books as this provides some good baseline and is somewhat tractable analytically. However, many real world applications are highly non-linear, and it is the reason we have discussed neural networks. Neural networks have been applied to RL for some time. A nice example of the success of TD(λ) was mentioned above for playing backgammon. We will now show how to implement such basic networks for reinforcement learning.

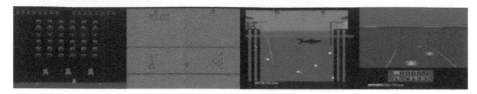

Fig. 11.10 Examples of video screens of the Atari 2600 game simulator.

To illustrate the basic idea of using neural networks with RL, we return to our maze example. The basic form of the implementation of the Q-function with a neural network is to make a neural network that receives as input a state and an action, and which then outputs the Q-values as shown in Fig. 11.11 with network A. In order to train this network with supervised learning we would need examples of the value function, which we of course don't have. However, we discussed how we can estimate such values with temporal differences while exploring the trajectories in the environment. For example, we can start with an arbitrary Q-function, use SARSA to estimate an improved version of Q, and then use this as a desired state in a mean square loss function. That is, we can define the following error term (loss function)

$$E(s_t, a_t) = (r_{t+1} + \gamma Q(s_{t+1}, u_{t+1}; w) - Q(s_t, a_t; w))^2 \tag{11.27}$$

and use back propagation to train the weights of the network that represent the Q-function.

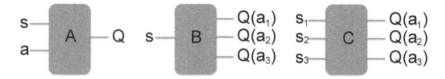

Fig. 11.11 Different ways to implement a function approximator for the value function.

While the neural network approach to SARSA can be applied immediately to a continuous state and action space, many applications have a finite and relatively small set of possible actions, and it is more common to use a Q-leaning (off-policy) strategy in this case. Here we have to compare the Q-values of all the possible actions from a specific state. While we could just iterate over the previous network, we can also learn a network that provides the Q-values for all the possible actions. This approach has been taken by Riedmiller in 2005 with the neurally fitted Q-iteration (NFQ) algorithm. The basic idea is shown in Fig. 11.11 with network B. In this case we can train the network with the following loss-function

$$E(s_t, a_t) = (r_{t+1} + \gamma \max_a Q(s_{t+1}, a; w) - Q(s_t, a_t; w))^2 \tag{11.28}$$

which corresponds to training the connections to the winning node as well as all the connections feeding into it through backpropagation. To apply this strategy to the maze example, we will here represent the state vector as a 1-hot vector. For example, if the agent is in state 2 then we can write the 1-hot input vector to the network as `s=np.array([0,0,1,0,0])`. Such a network is illustrated in Fig. 11.11C. We then have to modify our helper functions slightly to calculate the next state, and we also need a small function to identify if the state is a final state.

Listing 11.15 RLmlp.ipynb (Part 1)

```
1  import numpy as np
2  import matplotlib.pyplot as plt
3  from keras import models, layers, optimizers
4
5  def tau(s,a):
6      if (s[0] and s[4]) == 0 :
7          s=np.roll(s,a)
8      return s
9  def rho(s):
10     return ((s[0]==1)+2*(s[4]==1))
11 def terminal_state(s):
12     return (s[0]==1 or s[4]==1)
13
14 gamma=0.5
15 invT = 1
```

The variable `invT` represents the inverse temperature for the exploration. It is set very high at the beginning, but we will later decay this value. So there is a lot of exploration at the beginning but much less later.

We then define a small dense network with five inputs for the state vector, ten hidden nodes, and two output nodes, each representing the Q-value for each possible action, that of going left or right.

Listing 11.16 RLmlp.ipynb (Part 2)

```
1  # the network
2  inputs = layers.Input(shape=(5,))
3  h = layers.Dense(10, activation='relu')(inputs)
4  outputs = layers.Dense(2, activation='linear')(h)
5
6  model = models.Model(inputs=inputs, outputs=outputs)
7  RMSprop = optimizers.RMSprop(lr=0.01)
8  model.compile(loss='mse', optimizer=RMSprop)
```

To train the network we repeat several trials where we start the agent in state 2 and proceed for maximal 5 time steps. We include in this example a decay of the exploration rate (`invT`) as already mentioned so that the final estimates are closer to the analytical values. From the current state we use the network to predict the corresponding Q-value and then move one step ahead to calculate the target for the gradient learning as $r + Q(next\_s)$. The network is then updated right away.

Listing 11.17 RLmlp.ipynb (Part 3)

```
1  for trial in range(400):
2  s= np.array([0, 0, 1, 0, 0])
3  for t in range(0,5):
4  if terminal_state(s): break
5  if trial > 30 and invT > 0.1: invT -= 0.001
6  prediction=model.predict(s.reshape(1,5), steps=1, verbose=0)
```

```
 7    aidx=np.argmax(prediction)
 8    if np.random.rand() < invT : aidx=1−aidx
 9    a=2*aidx−1
10    next_s = tau(s,a)
11    if terminal_state(next_s):
12    y = rho(next_s)
13    else:
14    y = gamma*np.max(model.predict(next_s.reshape(1,5),steps=1,verbose=0))
15    prediction[0,aidx]=y
16    model.fit(s.reshape(1,5), prediction, epochs=1, verbose=0)
17    s = np.copy(next_s)
```

After the exploration we can evaluate the final policy and value functions.

Listing 11.18 RLmlp.ipynb (Part 4)

```
 1  for trial in range(400):
 2      s= np.array([0, 0, 1, 0, 0])
 3      for t in range(0,5):
 4          if terminal_state(s): break
 5          if trial > 30 and invT > 0.1: invT −= 0.001
 6          prediction=model.predict(s.reshape(1,5), steps=1, verbose=0)
 7          aidx=np.argmax(prediction)
 8          if np.random.rand() < invT : aidx=1−aidx
 9          a=2*aidx−1
10          next_s = tau(s,a)
11          if terminal_state(next_s):
12              y = rho(next_s)
13          else:
14              y = gamma *
15              np.max(model.predict(next_s.reshape(1,5),steps=1,verbose=0))
16          prediction[0,aidx]=y
17          model.fit(s.reshape(1,5), prediction, epochs=1, verbose=0)
18          s = np.copy(next_s)
```

The resulting values should reflect the right solution. While this program seems to be overkill in this simple case, RL with function approximation opens up a whole new world of possibilities. In particular, it gets us away from tabular methods which somewhat alleviate the curse of dimensionality as we can now deal with a finite set of parameters even in an infinite (continuous) state space. Also, while we use a simple model here, we can now combine this with the advancements in deep learning.

11.4.2 Deep Q-learning

At the time of TD-Gammon, the MLP with one hidden layer has been the state of the art, more elaborate models with more hidden layers have been difficult to train. However, deep learning has now made major progress based on several factors, including faster computers with specialized processors such as GPUs, larger databases with lots of training example, the rediscovery of convolutional networks, and better regularization techniques. The combination of deep learning with reinforcement learning has recently made mayor breakthroughs in AI. These breakthroughs have been demonstrated nicely by learning to play Atari games and winning the Chinese board game Go against a grandmaster by the deep RL learning system called AlphaGo by Google DeepMind. The Atari games are a great example of learning directly from sensory data in an environment that is much more complex than typical low-dimensional environments to which RL systems have been applied before. Mastering the game Go is relevant as it has been considered one of the most challenging examples for AI and was thought to require deep intuition by the players. Before AlphaGo, computer versions of Go players have only been able to play on an advanced novice level.

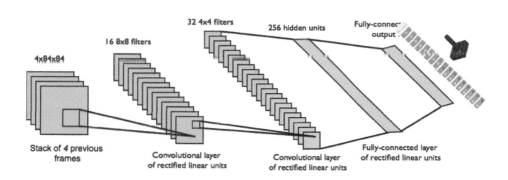

Fig. 11.12 Outline of the DQN network used to learn playing Atari games. Adapted from *Nature* 518 (7540), Volodymyr Mnih, Koray Kavukcuoglu, David Silver, Andrei A. Rusu, Joel Veness, Marc G. Bellemare, Alex Graves, Martin Riedmiller, Andreas K. Fidjeland, Georg Ostrovski, Stig Petersen, Charles Beattie, Amir Sadik, Ioannis Antonoglou, Helen King, Dharshan Kumaran, Daan Wierstra, Shane Legg, and Demis Hassabis, Human-level control through deep reinforcement learning, pp. 529{533, fig. 1, doi.org/10.1038/nature14236, Copyright © 2015, Springer Nature.

DQN (deep Q-learning network) is the basic network that has been used by Mnih (2014/15) to learn to play Atari games from the Arcade Games Console benchmark environment. The network is basically a convolutional network as shown in Fig. 11.12 which takes video frames as input and outputs Q-values for the possible joystick actions. While we have already outlined the basic strategy of using the TD error with back propagation to train such networks in such an RL task, which basically represents the NFQ approach, Mnih et al. have made several important additions that achieve these results. In particular, an important factor in the original DQN network was the use of experience replay. Experience replay is now a common technique for the following reason. It is common that the learning rate has to be fairly small during learning to prevent single instances from dominating. This means that specific episodes only have a very small contribution and one would need a large amount of episodes. In replay, we memorize a chosen action and use mini-batches of random samples for training.

Another common problem regarding why we would need small learning rates is that we need some time to propagate Q-values and values can fluctuate a lot. A second important factor in the practical use of such networks is the use of a target Q-network. In this technique, we freeze the parameters of the Q-network for the estimation of the future reward. Let us call these weights w'. We then calculate the temporal difference as

$$E = (r + \gamma maxQ(s', a', w') - Q(s, a, w))^2 \tag{11.29}$$

$$\rightarrow \frac{\partial E}{\partial w} = (r + \gamma maxQ(s', a', w') - Q(s, a, w))\frac{\partial Q}{\partial w}. \tag{11.30}$$

The weights of this target network are updated only periodically.

There are a variety of other techniques that are used in conjunction with the basic models. For example, clipping rewards or some form of normalizing the network can help to prevent an extreme buildup of Q-values. There are other techniques to keep the network somewhat stable since small changes in rewards can cause large fluctuations in policies. Another important aspects of even larger applications is to find a good starting position to generate valuable responses. That is, if one starts playing the games with random weights it is unlikely to get to a point were sensible learning can take place. Indeed, AlphaGo used supervised learning on expert data to train the system initially, while the RL procedures could then continue and advance the system to the point where it could outperform human players. A combination of RL with supervised learning in form of imitation learning is therefore a common techniques, in particular in robotics applications. However, instead of looking further into these techniques here, there are two more major techniques that are important and discussed next.

11.4.3 Actors and policy search

So far we have focused on finding a value function and we derived from this the greedy policy as the action that leads to the state with the largest return. The value function can be seen as a critic to adapt the policy. Another approach, especially when using function approximators, is to consider a parameterized policy directly and to search for good parameters of the policy. Such an approach is called an actor. We need to find parameters that maximize the payoff. We illustrated such a setting in Fig. 11.13. It is now time to think about the implementation of this actor as deep neural network which takes observations such as pictures from a camera and produces outputs such as motor commands for a mobile robot.

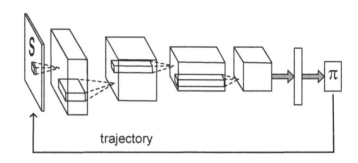

Fig. 11.13 Illustration of an actor that is implemented with a deep neural network.

We will discuss this approach in a stochastic setting with finite horizon episodes that is commonly used for the policy search discussed in the following. In a stochastic setting, the reward is stochastic so that we need to sample over trajectories. A trajectory is the list of all state and action taken in an episode,

$$x = \{s_0, a_0, s_1, a_1, ..., s_T, a_T\}. \tag{11.31}$$

Since the policy and the transitions are also probabilistic, we can write the probability if a trajectory $p(x) = p(s_0, a_0, s_1, a_1, ..., s_T, a_T)$ as

$$p(x|; \mathbf{w}) = p(s_0) \prod_{t=0}^{T} \tau(s_{t+1}|s_t, a_t)\pi(a_t|s_t; \mathbf{w}). \tag{11.32}$$

We indicated here which of the probabilities depend on the parameters of the model as it is these we want to learn. In the stochastic case, the reward is stochastic and we need to sample over trajectories. Since we use here the finite horizon case we do not need discounting, and the objective function can simply be written as the average value of the reward over repeated episodes.

Actor value function: $\quad J(\mathbf{w}) = E[\sum_{t=0}^{T} \rho(s_t, \pi(a_t|s_t; \mathbf{w}))]_{x \sim p(x|\mathbf{w})}. \tag{11.33}$

This is an expected value so that we need to sample to find an approximation of this value

$$J(\mathbf{w}) \approx \frac{1}{N_x} \sum_{x=1}^{N_x} \sum_{t=0}^{T} \rho(s_t, \pi(a_t|s_t; \mathbf{w})), \tag{11.34}$$

where N_x are the number of trials in the sample. To find the parameters that maximize this objective function we follow a gradient, as usual. Thus, we have to find the gradient of the expectation value over trajectories,

$$\nabla_w J = \int_x \nabla_w p(x|\mathbf{w})\rho(x)dx. \tag{11.35}$$

Since $p(x|\mathbf{w})$ is the product of several terms, it is useful to take consider the logarithm of this term

$$\nabla_w \log p(x|\mathbf{w}) = \frac{1}{p(x|\mathbf{w})} \nabla_w p(x|\mathbf{w}), \tag{11.36}$$

so that we can replace the gradient term in eqn 11.35,

$$\nabla_w J = \int_x p(x|\mathbf{w}) \nabla_w \log p(x|\mathbf{w})\rho(x)dx. \tag{11.37}$$

If we now expand the log-probability of a trajectory

$$\nabla_w \log p(x|\mathbf{w}) = \nabla_w \log(s_0) + \nabla_w \log \pi(a|s; \mathbf{w}) + \nabla_w \log \tau(s'|s, a) \tag{11.38}$$

and the probability of the first state and the transition probability do not depend the model parameters, $\nabla_w \log(s_0) = 0$ and $\nabla_w \log \tau(s'|s, a) = 0$, we see that we do not need a model to evaluate the gradient. Also, we can now write the gradient of loss function again as an expected value,

$$\nabla_w J = E[\nabla_w \log \pi(a|s; \mathbf{w})\rho(x)]_{x \sim \pi(a|s; \mathbf{w})} \tag{11.39}$$

This nice result for model-free learning of the actor is called the policy gradient theorem. With this theorem we see that we can estimate the gradient by sampling the log-probabilities of the policies and multiplying this with the sample rewards of the trajectories,

$$\nabla_w J \approx \frac{1}{N_x} \sum_{x=1}^{T} N_x \sum_{t=0}^{T} \log \pi(a_t|s_t; \mathbf{w})[\sum_{t=0}^{T} \rho(s_t, \pi(a_t|s_t; \mathbf{w}))]. \qquad (11.40)$$

This concludes the principle idea of training an actor model. This algorithm is called

$$\textbf{REINFORCE:} \quad w_{t+1} \leftarrow w_t - \alpha \langle \nabla_w log(\pi)R \rangle, \qquad (11.41)$$

where R stands for the accumulated reward of a trajectory. Unfortunately, in practice it turns out that the samples for the gradient of the log-policies usually have very high variance so that the sampling becomes prohibitive. One trick to make this variance smaller is to only take the change of R with each sample from the average of some batch or samples $\bar{R}$ into account. This baseline version is given by

$$\textbf{REINFORCE with baseline:} \quad w_{t+1} \leftarrow w_t - \alpha \langle \nabla_w log(\pi)(R - \bar{R}) \rangle, \quad (11.42)$$

and there have been a variety of other tricks introduced in the literature. However, an important other method is introduced in the next section.

11.4.4 Actor-critic schemes

It is now easy to introduce an important architecture for reinforcement learning, that of the actor-critic architecture. The principle idea is to replace the estimate of the accumulated reward of a trajectory with a better estimate of the values of the visited states. We have discussed the estimation of the Q-function at length in the previous sections and we can now combine the two approaches. We simply replace R with Q in the REINFORCE algorithm

$$\textbf{Actor-critic:} \quad w_{t+1} \leftarrow w_t - \alpha \langle \nabla_w log(\pi)Q \rangle. \qquad (11.43)$$

The Q-function itself can be learned with a temporal difference method,

$$w_{t+1} \leftarrow w_t - \alpha(r_t - V(s_{t+1}) - V(s_t))\nabla_w log(\pi). \qquad (11.44)$$

Such actor-critic architectures are now the common implementations of reinforcement learning with function approximation. Implementations of many recent deep Rl algorithms is provided by Matthias Plappert at https://github.com/keras-rl/keras-rl.

As already suggested, training a neural network while exploiting it to suggest actions is dangerous and usually leads to oscillations and instabilities. One reason is that when Q-values are close to each other, then small changes in the Q-values can lead to drastic changes in response actions that can cause problems and inconsistencies in learning. In this respect, actor-based reinforcement learning seems to have some advantages, but building a appropriate parameterization of actions has its own challenges. However, combining actors and critics has been shown to build much more robust systems. The basic scheme is illustrated in Fig. 11.14 on the left, and in the context of using neural networks on the right. Another implementation is DDAC (deterministic deep actor-critic) as shown in Fig. 11.15.

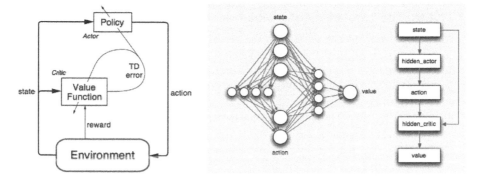

Fig. 11.14 Outline of the actor-critic approach (Sutton-Barto; 1998) on the left and the neurally fitted Q-learning actor-critic (NFQAC) network (Rückstiess, 2010) on the right.

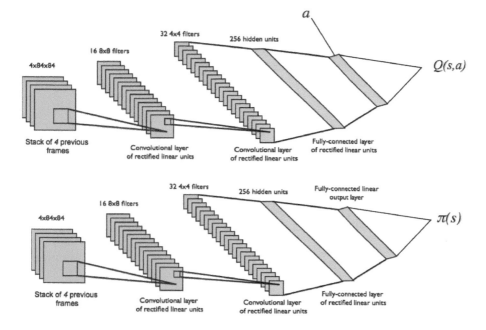

Fig. 11.15 Deep deterministic actor-critic (DDAC) network (from Lillicrap, 2015).

11.4.5 Reinforcement learning in the brain

Several brain areas are associated with adaptive motor control and decision system. For example, the cerebellum has been strongly associated with motor control, and the conditioning of the eyeblink in response to a puff of air is a classic example of condition thought to be mediated by the cerebellum. Another area that has been strongly associated with temporal difference learning is the basal ganglia. We start with a brief discussion of the cerebellum as control system and then focus on the temporal difference learning in the basal ganglia.

11.4.6 The cerebellum and motor control

Are these control schemes used in the brain? There is some evidence that adaptive controllers are realized in the brain and are vital for our survival. The above-mentioned adaptation to the changed physics of the controlled system (for example, arm stiffness) or the variation of the sensory system (prism glasses) hints at an adapting motor control system. Both control schemes, the forward model and inverse model controller, can be realized by mapping networks, and it is a question of identifying characteristic components and signals in order to show which control scheme is realized in the brain.

A brain area that has long been associated with motor control is the cerebellar cortex or cerebellum. The anatomy of the cerebellum displays great regularity and is summarized schematically in Fig. 11.16. Inputs from different sources enter the cerebellum through mossy fibres that contact granule cells and Golgi cells. Granule cells are probably the most numerous cells in the brain, estimated to be in the order of 10^{10}–10^{11}. Granule cells exceed the number of mossy fibres by a few hundred times, which makes this architecture a candidate for expansion re-coding, as discussed in Chapter 9. The granule cells, and some other intermediate neurons, provide a major input to Purkinje cells through parallel fibres, each Purkinje cell receiving as many as 80,000 inputs from different granule cells. Purkinje cells in turn provide the (inhibitory) output of the cerebellum.

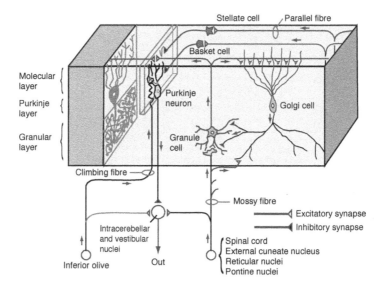

Fig. 11.16 Schematic illustration of some connectivity patterns in the cerebellum. Note that the output of the cerebellum is provided by the Purkinje neurons that make inhibitory synapses. Climbing fibres are specific for each Purkinje neuron and are tightly interwoven with their dendritic tree [adapted from Albus, *Mathematical Bioscience* 10: 25–61 (1971)].

The Purkinje cells also receive input from so-called climbing fibres from the inferior olive, each cell with its own climbing fibre. This one-to-one architecture is unique in the brain, and the climbing fibres have long been speculated to provide a teaching signal to the Purkinje cells. The cerebellum can be viewed as a mapping network, and such networks can learn to predict specific output from input patterns, as discussed in Chapter 7. It is thus possible that the cerebellum implements a forward or inverse model, or another adaptive model that can be used by the motor system in the midbrain or brainstem to guide motor functions.

11.4.7 Neural implementations of TD learning

We have discussed the implementation of TD learning with function approximators such as deep networks, but it is instructive to illustrate a more direct implementation on a neural system level with a small example to appreciate neural architectures specific for RL. We chose the problem simple enough so that the state value function $V^\pi(s)$ can be learned with a simple perceptron as illustrated in Fig. 11.17A.

The input of the node represents a state at time t, $s(t)$, which is conveyed by a specific pattern of rates, $r_i^{in}(s)$ in the input channels. The output of the linear node is

$$V(s) = \sum_i w_i(t) r_i^{in}(s). \tag{11.45}$$

The rate values of the perceptron are, of course, time dependent since the input states s are time dependent. We also indicated explicitly the time dependence of the weight values, $w_i(t)$, since they will change over time as a function of reinforcement signals.

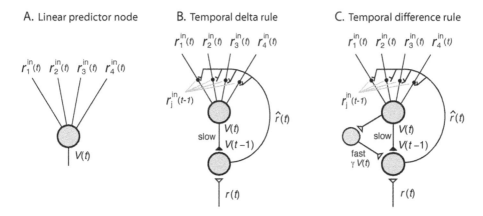

Fig. 11.17 Neural implementation of reward learning algorithms. (A) Linear predictor node. (B) Temporal delta rule with primary reward r. The output of the predictor node is indicated at time $t - 1$ since the connection is considered to be slow. (C) Temporal difference rule with a fast side loop.

Let us no consider that the agent is taking an action in response to policy that is based on this value function. This action results result in a reward at the next time step, $r(t + 1)$, and we want to update the weights at this time of reward to reflect the new knowledge. In this case of receiving reward immediately at the next time step, the actual reward can be used as the desired output, and we can use the delta rule discussed in Chapter 7 to train the linear perceptron,

$$w_i^{t+1} = w_i^t + \alpha * \hat{r}(t + 1) r_i^{in}(s). \tag{11.46}$$

The parameter α is a learning rate, and we introduce in this equation the effective reinforcement signal

$$\hat{r}(t+1) = r(t+1) - V(t). \tag{11.47}$$

The learning rule, eqn 11.46, is sometimes called a temporal delta rule because of the temporal difference between predicted and actual reward. This is analog to the standard delta rule as discussed in Chapter 7 when the reward is supplied at the same time of the corresponding state. However, we keep this time difference to stress some necessary memory in the neural implementation. Thus, the system needs to remember the value $V(s^t)$ for one time step. We include this memory in the model shown in Fig. 11.17B by considering the output channel to be slow such as axonal delay. In addition, the system must remember the input values $(r_i^{\text{in}}(s))$ for one time step because we attribute the cause for the reward to taking the fixed action from the previous state. We can think about this eligibility trace as a short term trace in a synapse as shown in Fig. 11.17B.

The eligibility trace and the axonal delay solves here the temporal credit assignment problem. The weights of the input channels to the node that learns the state value function depend on its delayed output and the primary reward (reinforcement) signal r. The primary reinforcement signal is assumed to have an excitatory effect on a node that mediates learning, whereas the prediction node has an inhibitory effect on the node which mediates training. This training node therefore calculates the effective reinforcement signal of eqn 11.47. This effective reinforcement signal has to be conveyed to all the synapses of the prediction node, where it has to be correlated with an eligibility trace to produce the appropriate weight change proposed in eqn 11.46. The model can produce one-step ahead predictions of a reward signal and corresponds to a particular choice of the state value function. The effective reinforcement signal is zero when the activity of the prediction node matches the primary reinforcement signal.

It is most interesting to point out that his model of reward learning is equivalent to the Rescorla–Wagner theory in classical conditioning. This influential model in behavioural findings in the animal learning literature is in its basic form given by

$$\Delta V = \alpha\beta(\lambda - V). \tag{11.48}$$

This model describes the associative strength between a stimulus and a reward prediction. The term α describes the salience of a stimulus and β is a learning rate. The most interesting part is the expression in brackets that represents the difference between the real reward and the expectation of reward. This model is hence a form of temporal difference model.

The next step is to generalize this implementation to delayed reward situations. This is covered by the more general form of temporal difference learning, which we can write in this context as a modified value for $\hat{r}$ in the learning rule eqn 11.46, namely the temporal difference error

$$\hat{r}(t) = r(t) + \gamma V^\pi(t) - V^\pi(t-1). \tag{11.49}$$

Compared with the temporal delta rule ($\gamma = 0$), we only need the additional value $V^\pi(t)$. Fig. 11.17C shows a possible neuronal implementation of a temporal difference learning, which includes a fast side-loop with a decay factor that conveys the value $\gamma V^\pi(t)$ to the node that calculates the primary reinforcement signal.

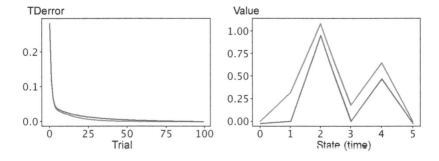

Fig. 11.18 Example experiment of traversing five consecutive states with (red curves) the temporal delta rule ($\gamma = 0$) and with (blue curves) the TD learning algorithm ($\gamma = 3$).

An example of learning value functions when traversing six consecutive states that are encoded with random patterns is shown in Fig. 11.18. Reward is given at state 2 and 4 of size $r(2) = 1$ and $r(4) = 0.5$ (red curves). The value function reflecting the primary reward can be learned with the delta rule (eqn 11.47 with $\gamma = 0$.) (blue curves). When learning the value function with the TD learning algorithm (eqn 11.49 with $\gamma = 0.3$), all states become predictive of the reward and hence even intermediate states carry some value. The learning curves demonstrate that the TD error is declining, although the specific curve depends highly on the specific patterns of representing the states. These simulations were produced with the following TDexperiment1.py.

Programs/TDexperiment1.py

```
1  import numpy as np
2  import matplotlib.pyplot as plt
3
4  gamma=0
5  w=np.zeros(10);
6  Z=np.zeros((100,6)); rhatRec=np.zeros(100)
7  x=np.random.rand(10,6)
8  r=np.array([0,0,1,0,0.5,0])
9
10 for trial in range(100):
11     V=0;
12     for t in range(1,6):
13         Vlast=V
14         V=w@x[:,t]
15         rhat=r[t-1]+gamma*V-Vlast
16         w=w+0.1*rhat*x[:,t-1]
17         Z[trial,t-1]=Vlast
18         rhatRec[trial]=rhatRec[trial]+rhat
19 plt.figure(); plt.plot(Z[-1,:])
20 plt.figure(); plt.plot(rhatRec/5)
```

This experiment shows that temporal difference learning has the ability of transferring the reward response to earlier predictive cues, and such characteristic neural responses where discovered by Wolfram Schulz in dopaminergic neurons in some areas of the midbrain called the Ventral Tegmental Area (VTA) and the Substantia Nigra (SN). This is shown in Fig. 11.19 where the response of the dopamineric neurons first establishes a primary reward association, which is then shifted to an early reward association. They even found that the removal of the reward results in an activity inhibition, in accordance with a negative temporal difference error. Wolfram Schulz, Peter Dayan, and Read Montague related these findings to temporal difference learning and thereby to the behavioural findings summarized by the Rescola-Wagner theory. This is a prime example how computational models can relate behavioural findings with neural mechanisms.

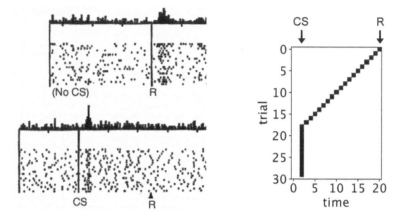

Fig. 11.19 Demonstration of the transfer of neuron activity from signalling primary reward to the prediction of reward with a conditioned stimulus. The recordings are from Schulz, Dayan, Montegeu, 'A neural substrate of prediction and reward', *Science* 275, 1997, and the simulation is a simplified implementation of their model.

Their work is illustrated in Fig. 11.19. On the left is shown recordings of the activity of Dopamineric neurons. First there is no reward prediction and the dopaminergic neuron response to the primary reward. Later in the trial the neuron fires to the prediction of the reward after the conditioned stimulus (CS).

A compact simulation program to demonstrate this ability with TD learning is given below.

Programs/TDexperiment2.py

```
1  import numpy as np
2  import matplotlib.pyplot as plt
3
4  gamma=1
5  w=np.zeros(20); Z=np.zeros((30,21))
6
7  for trial in range(30):
8      x=np.zeros(20); V=0;
9      for t in range(1,20):
10         xlast=np.copy(x)  # np needs copy
11         Vlast=V
12         x[t]=x[t-1] # shift visual memory
13         x[t-1]=0
14         if t==2: x[t]=1  # vis onset
15         print(t,x)
16         V=w@x
```

```
17|        rhat=gamma*V-Vlast
18|        w=w+l*rhat*xlast
19|        Z[trial,t]=rhat
20|      rhat=1-V   # last time gets reward
21|      w=w+l*rhat*x
22|      Z[trial,t+1]=rhat
23| plt.imshow(Z, cmap='binary')
```

An important part of this demonstration is the temporal coding of the signal. The input signal is thereby a vector with components equal to zero except for the components at $t - \Delta t + t_0$. t_0 is thereby the time of the CS, and Δt represents the time since the stimulus onset. In this way, the stimulus codes the states as time steps between CS onset and the reward state. While this temporal coding is certainly a simplifying assumption, the purpose of the simulation is to illuminate the possibility of backpropagation of reward predictions as shown in the results of this simulation on the right in Fig.11.19. Early in the trials, the TD error response to the reward, which shifts backward until the response it to the CS. The experiment demonstrates the backpropagation of the reward prediction, which is one of the signatures of TD learning. It is clear that there can be more elaborate mechanisms at work, including explicit memory or even gated memories such as discussed in Chapter 9.

11.4.8 Basal Ganglia

The substantia nigra that displays the TD error in the brain is part of the a collection of subcortical structures called the basal ganglia. The basal ganglia, which are known to be instrumental in the initiation of motor commands, have many of the structural components required to implement an adaptive critic and to supervise actors that can control the initiation of motor movements. The basal ganglia are a collection of five subcortical nuclei as illustrated in Fig. 11.20. They receive cortical and thalamic input mainly through the putamen and the caudate nucleus, together called the striatum which comprises the input layer of the basal ganglia. The information stream then runs through the globus pallidus (with an internal and external segment) to the major output layer, the substantia nigra pars reticulata. The internal side-loop from the globus pallidus via the subthalamic nucleus is also important for our next discussion. In addition, note that the substantia nigra pars compacta projects back to the striatum with neurons that use dopamine as neurotransmitter.

The information streams within the basal ganglia are thought to be segregated (to a certain extent) within interleaved modules that are called matrix modules and striosomal modules, respectively. A suggested implementation of the actor–critic scheme in the basal ganglia is shown in Fig. 11.21. The input layer of the basal ganglia is rich in spiny neurons (SP), which receive massive cortical (C) connections. The spiny neurons in the striosomal module (SPs) also receive projections from dopaminergic neurons (DA) in the substantia nigra pars compacta (SNc) which synapse on to spines of spiny neurons in the caudate and putamen. It is possible that dopaminergic input is able to alter the efficiencies of specific cortical inputs that are marked with an eligibility trace. The neurons shown in the basal ganglia are also inhibitory so that the dopaminergic neurons in the SNc are inhibited by SPs activity. The subthalamic side-loop, in contrast, disinhibits the DA, which can result in some excitation of DA neurons proportional

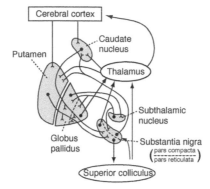

Fig. 11.20 Anatomical overview of the connections within the basal ganglia and the major projections comprising the input and output of the basal ganglia [adapted from Kandel, Schwarz, and Jessell, *Principles of neural science*, McGraw-Hill, 4th edition (2000)].

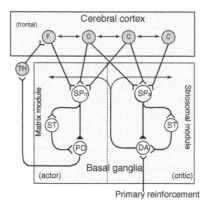

Fig. 11.21 Actor–critic model of the basal ganglia with cerebral cortex (C), frontal lobe (F), thalamus (TH), subthalamic nucleus (ST), pallidus (PD), spiny neurons in the matrix module (SPm), spiny neurons in the striosomal module (SPs), and dopaminergic neurons (DA) [adapted from Houk, Adams, and Barto, in *Models of information processing in the basal ganglia*, Houk, Davies, and Beiser (eds), MIT Press (1995)].

to the inputs from this side-loop and a primary reinforcement signal. If, in addition, the side-loop is faster than the direct SPs–DA influence, then it is possible that the striosomal module implements the critic that minimizes the temporal difference, as discussed above (compare Fig. 11.17C).

The similarities between reward responses of dopaminergic neurons in the SNc and the effective reinforcement signal in temporal difference learning have contributed largely to the hypothesis of reinforcement learning theories of the basal ganglia. This part of the reinforcement system corresponds largely to the critic in the control system. Specific implementations of actors in the basal ganglia have been discussed much less

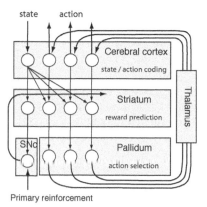

Fig. 11.22 Q-learning scheme of the basal ganglia [adapted from Doya, *HFSP Journal* 1: 30–40 (2007)].

in the literature. One of the earliest suggestions was that the matrix module could implement the actor. Dopaminergic neurons project to these spiny neurons (SPm) and could therefore alter the C–SPm weights in a fashion similar to that in the C–SPs connections. The only difference is that these neurons project to the internal segment of the pallidus and the substantia nigra pars reticulata (SNr), which are thought to be the major output layers of the basal ganglia. The output of the basal ganglia can, in such a way, control the initiation of specific motor actions that are associated with reward.

The classic proposal of an actor–critic implementation in the basal ganglia discussed above leaves many open questions and some questionable assumptions. While there are still many open questions regarding the specific implementation of reinforcement learning in the basal ganglia and the more refined role of the basal ganglia in brain processing, there is a wide consensus that the basal ganglia do contribute to some form of reinforcement learning. More recently, Q-learning has also been mapped on to basal ganglion functions in the work of leading researchers such as Kenji Doya and Peter Dayan. An example is illustrated in Fig. 11.22 where the striatum is hypothesized to calculate a state-action value function, and the dopaminergic neurons in SNc calculate the TD error that is used to update cortico-striatal connections. The state-action value function is then used in the pallidum and thalamus for stochastic action selection. Other researchers, such as Peter Redgrave and Kevin Gurney also pointed out that the basal ganglia might have a large role in discovering novelty actions, which are also essential in establishing task-relevant behaviour. This area is a nice example where theoretical and experimental research strongly benefit from each other.

While we concentrated our discussion of reinforcement learning in the brain on the basal ganglia, it should not be forgotten that there are other areas in the brain that have been associated with reinforcement learning, or at least association of reward contingencies with specific motor actions. Some brain areas that have been implicated with making reward associations are, for example, the prefrontal cortex and the subcortical area called amygdala. Both areas receive projections from many senses and are therefore placed strategically to form associations between different modalities and reward contingencies. Bilateral damage of the amygdala is known to considerably impair such associations. Furthermore, it has been shown that neurons in the orbitofrontal cortex adapt their response to stimuli after changing their reward associations. Dopaminergic neurons also project into the frontal cortex so that reward mechanisms could originate predominantly in the frontal cortex as opposed to the hypothesis of the basal ganglia discussed above. Finally, there are also other neurotransmitters and specific reward systems that might be important in reinforcement learning. For example, serotonin is a neurotransmitter that has been associated with the modulation of such things as mood, appetite, sexuality, and aversive signals, which are all factors that can influence reward values and action selection. Also, human planning, as well as abilities to evaluate long-term goals, are not yet covered with the simple reward associations used in the experiments discussed here.

12   The cognitive brain

We have outlined the basis of neural mechanisms of information processing, the basis of representational learning, short-term memory in dynamic recurrent neural systems, and reinforcement learning as the basis of building decision systems. These subjects are discussed in this book as fundamentals of mechanisms employed in the brain. In this last chapter we want to give some examples of these systems in theories on a higher cognitive level and also a brief introduction to causal networks as one important framework for such models. We start with outlining some hierarchical and attentive vision to give a small example how the brain integrates mechanisms beyond monolithic models such as deep learning. We then discuss a workspace hypothesis that shows how the brain is able to produce novel solutions to new tasks within modular architectures. Finally, we outline models that describe cognitive reasoning with Bayesian causal networks and also give an outlook to more general directions of causal learning.

12.1   Attentive vision

12.1.1   Attentive vision

VisNet includes interactions within each layer to stabilize the sparseness, though the information flow between the layers is strictly feedforward. The next step is to consider top-down information flow in cortical models. Top-down information is crucial in cognitive processes. For example, when asking subjects to search for specific items in a visual scene, such as the top of the Eiffel tower in the example shown in Fig. 12.1. Such a visual search demands the top–down influence of an object bias that specifies what to look for. In contrast, we can ask the subject to identify an object at a particular location, such as identifying the object in the lower right-hand corner of the picture in Fig. 12.1. This demands a spatial attention. Gustavo Deco and collaborators have developed a model that can shed some light on the processes involved in visual search and object recognition. The overall scheme of their model is outlined in Fig. 12.2. The model basically has three important parts: one that is labelled 'V1–V4', one that is labelled 'IT', and one that is labelled 'PP'. We will outline the specific architectures and roles of these parts separately in the following. It is, however, good to keep in mind right from the beginning that the different parts do not work in isolation. Here we are particularly interested in how the different parts influence each other.

Bottom-up input to the model came from visual scenes. In the model this is simulated by taking input images and decomposing them with Gabor functions. This corresponds to representations in the LGN since turning curves in the LGN can be parametrized with Gabor functions. Early parts of the cortical processing are represented with a module labelled 'V1–V4' in the model. In the specific model implementation discussed here, this is only a single layer. However, hierarchical implementation

Fundamentals of Computational Neuroscience. Third edition. Thomas P. Trappenberg, Oxford University Press. © Oxford University Press 2023. DOI: 10.1093/oso/9780192869364.003.0012

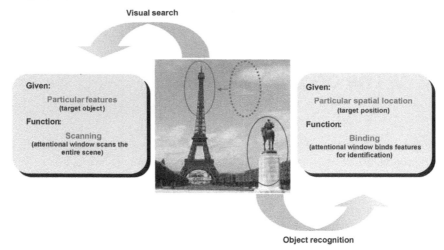

Fig. 12.1 Illustration of a visual search and an object recognition task. Each task demands a different strategy in exploring the visual scene [figure courtesy of Gustavo Deco].

of this model has also been done but is not essential for the following discussion. The principal role of this part of the model is the decomposition of the visual scene into features. This is known to occur at this early stage of visual processing in primates. For example, V1 neurons respond mainly to simple features such as the orientation of edges, and later areas are often specialized to represent other features such as colour, motion, or combinations of basic features.

From the modelling point of view it is not essential that we precisely rebuild all the details of the visual field representation in the brain, as we are primarily interested in other aspects of the visual processing. It is only important here that the feature representation in this part of the model is topographic in that features are represented in sections (shown as boxes in the 'V1–V4' module) which correspond to the location of the object in the visual field, as discussed in Section 1.2.6. Each section represents a feature of a part of the visual field as a vector of node activities. There is no global competition between the modules; only within each section is there an inhibitory pool that keeps the sparseness of the activity in each section roughly constant as discussed in Section 8.5.1.

The representation of the visual field, as decomposed in 'V1–V4', feeds into the module labelled 'IT' in the model. This part is aimed at modelling processes in the inferior-temporal cortex, which is known to be involved in object recognition. This recognition process is modelled as associative memory as outlined in Chapter 9. Point attractors of specific objects are then formed through the Hebbian-trained collateral connections within this structure. The connections between the 'V1–V4' and the 'IT' can also be trained with Hebbian learning. By placing, in turn, an object at all locations in the visual field that are covered by the sections in 'V1–V4', weights between the sections in 'V1–V4' and nodes in 'IT' are basically the same for all sections. This enables the point attractor network to 'recognize' trained objects in test trials at all locations in the visual field, which thus simulates translation-invariant object recognition. However, the attractor network also contributes to the translation

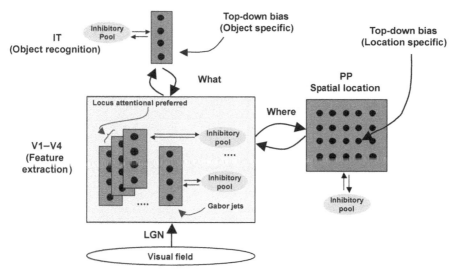

Fig. 12.2 Outline of a model of the visual processing in primates to simulate visual search and object recognition. The main parts of the model are inspired by structural features of the cortical areas thought to be central in these processes. These include early visual areas (labelled 'V1–V4') that represent the content of the visual field topographically with basic features, the inferior-temporal cortex (labelled 'IT') that is known to be central for object recognition, and the posterior parietal cortex (labelled 'PP') that is strongly associated with spatial attention [figure courtesy of Gustavo Deco].

invariance of the object recognition since the attractor network in 'IT' completes a pattern input from 'V1–V4' even if the set of weights between a section in 'V1–V4' and the nodes in 'IT' is weaker than others.

The contribution of the attractor network in 'IT' to translation-invariant object recognition explains some recent experimental findings that showed that the size of the receptive field of inferior-temporal neurons depends on the content of the visual field and the specifics of the task. For example, if a single object is shown on a screen with a blank background, then it was found that the receptive field of a neuron that responds to this object can be very large (as much as 30 degrees or more). An example of the firing rate of one inferior-temporal neuron in a non-human primate engaged in a visual search task is shown by a solid line in Fig. 12.3A. Interestingly, if two objects are presented simultaneously, or if the target object is shown on top of a complex background (which can be viewed as a scene with many objects), then the size of the receptive field shrinks markedly (see dashed line in Fig. 12.3A for the case of an object on a complex background).

A possible explanation of the experimental findings is given by the model discussed in this section, which is based on the attractor dynamics of the auto-associator network in 'IT'. If only one object is shown, then this object would trigger the right point attractor and thus the recall of the object regardless of its location, which corresponds to large receptive fields. If, however, two or more trained objects are shown, then it is likely that the final state of the attractor network is mainly dominated by the object closest to the fovea, which gets the most weight due to cortical magnification.

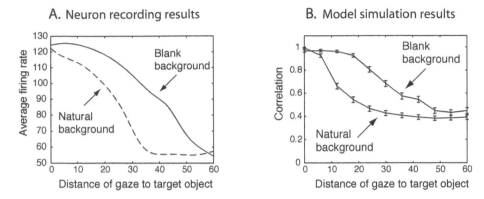

A. Neuron recording results   **B.** Model simulation results

Fig. 12.3 (A) Example of the average firing rate from recordings of a neuron in the inferior-temporal cortex of a monkey in response to an effective stimulus that is located at various degrees away from the direction of gaze [experimental data courtesy of Edmund Rolls]. (B) Simulation results of a model with the essential components of the model shown in Fig. 12.2. The correlation is thereby a measure of overlap between the activity of 'IT' nodes with the representation of the target object that was used during training [adapted from Trappenberg, Rolls, and Stringer, *Advances in Neural Processing Systems* 14, 2002,].

Simulation results, shown in Fig. 12.3B, confirm this hypothesis.

12.1.2 Attentional bias in visual search and object recognition

Visual search can be simulated within the model shown in Fig. 12.2 by supplying an object bias input to the attractor network in 'IT' that tells the system what to look for. Such top-down information is thought to originate in the frontal areas of the brain. Simulations have shown that the additional input of an object bias to 'IT' can speed up the recognition process in 'IT'. The object bias also supports the recognition ability of the input from 'V1–V4' that corresponds to the target object in visual search. Correspondingly, it was found, in simulations as well as in primate experiments, that the receptive fields of target objects are larger than receptive fields of non-target objects.

Parallel conclusions can be drawn in an object recognition task in which top-down input to a specific location in module 'PP' is given. The label of this module suggests processing in the posterior parietal cortex, which is part of the dorsal visual processing pathway ('where' pathway), and hence specifically adapted in spatial representations. This is modelled with a spatially organized neural sheet, which is connected to the corresponding section in 'V1–V4'. This activity in 'PP' can thus enhance the neural activity in 'V1–V4' for the features of the object that are located at the corresponding location in the visual field. Consequently, it will be easier (faster) for the 'IT' network to complete the input patterns for objects, and hence to 'recognize' objects, at the corresponding location.

The attentional biases have different origins in the model shown in Fig. 12.2. The attentional bias used in visual search originates from top-down input to 'IT' and is object-based. The attentional bias in the object recognition task acts on 'PP' and is location-based. However, it may be difficult to separate the different forms of attention in experiments because all parts of the model are bidirectional, in agreement with anatomical findings. For example, an object bias to 'IT' in the visual search task will ultimately trigger some activity in 'PP' that corresponds to the location where the object is, and this activity itself will help the recognition process of that object.

The time elapsed until the activity of a node in 'PP' reaches a certain threshold can be taken as an indication of the reaction time needed to find a specific object in visual search. Deco and colleagues simulated a visual search task in which the visual scene

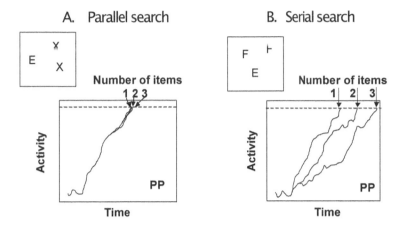

Fig. 12.4 Numerical experiments in which the model simulated a visual search task of a target object (the letter 'E') in a visual scene with visual distractors. (A) In one experiment the distractors consist of the letters 'X', which are visually very different from the target letter. The activity of a 'PP' node that corresponds to the target location increases in these experiments independently of the number of distractors, implying parallel search. (B) The second experiment was done with distractors (letter 'F') that were visually similar to the target letter. The reaction times, as measured from 'PP' nodes, depend linearly on the number of objects, a feature that is also characteristic of serial search. Both modes are, however, present in the same 'parallel architecture' [adapted from Gustavo Deco, personal communication].

had a target (the letter 'E') and a number of distractors. The distractors (the letter 'X') in one experiment were visually very different from the target pattern. The simulated reaction time was in this case independent of the number of objects in the visual scene as indicated in Fig. 12.4A. In contrast, the reaction time increased linearly with the number of distractors when the distractor objects (the letter 'F') were visually similar to the target (see Fig. 12.4B). A linear increase of the reaction time with the number of objects in the visual scene is commonly attributed to a serial search mechanism in contrast to the lack of dependence of the reaction time on the number of objects that indicates parallel search.

Similar findings in psychophysical experiments with humans have often been interpreted as evidence for different search strategies thought to be implemented by different neural mechanisms. However, the simulation results demonstrate that such psychophysical results are consistent with a single parallel neural machinery, and that the apparent serial search is only due to the more intense conflict-resolution demand in the recognition process. The model is able to make many more predictions than can be verified experimentally, on a behavioural level, with brain imaging techniques or with cell recordings. This model is therefore a good example of the type of model that we hope will emerge for many more brain processes.

12.2 An interconnecting workspace hypothesis

It is increasingly clear that complex cognitive tasks can only be solved with the flexible cooperation of many specialized modules. In contrast to most existing models of brain functions, it is highly fascinating to observe how flexible we humans are in coping with the complex world around us. In contrast to most models, which produce very stereotyped behaviour, humans display the ability to master highly skilled functions while still maintaining the ability to produce novel solutions that have not been trained extensively. For example, we can drive a car with such ease that little attention and effort seems necessary to do so. This is despite the fact that we have to react to the unknown environment, for example, in following a road that we have not driven on before. However, when very novel and critical circumstances occur we are able to engage ourselves with many resources applied to this problem, which typically go along with very attentive and often very arduous mental activity.

12.2.1 The global workspace

From a system-level perspective we expect that specialized processors can have a high degree of autonomy while still being able to engage, if necessary, in more global system activities. It is, however, still largely unknown how such flexibility can be achieved in a robust way. In the remainder of this chapter we will review one speculative, yet far-reaching idea as to how this could be achieved in the brain, which was proposed by Stanislas Dehaene, Michel Kerzberg, and Jean-Piere Changeux. In Fig. 12.5 we have reproduced their illustration of the principal idea behind their proposal. In this the authors divided brain functions into five basic subsystems, ranging from a perceptual system, which is our window to the world, to the motor system responsible for executing desired goals. The three remaining subsystems are a memory system, an evaluative system, and an attentional system, all of which are basic ingredients for complex cognitive tasks as viewed by many cognitive scientists. The main point made by Dehaene and colleagues is that these subsystems must be able to work alone or in combinations in a flexible manner, and they speculate that this may be achieved through some form of network between the subsystems. Such an interconnecting network would form a global workspace, which would form the basis of our ability to solve complex tasks in a flexible manner.

In contrast to the more localized basic processing networks that make up the five basic subsystems as illustrated in Fig. 12.5, the workspace has to be a more global computational space in the brain. Projections between cortical areas are indeed abundant, and associated fibres of cortico-cortical connections originate predominantly from pyramidal neurons in layers II and III, as mentioned in Chapter 1. The authors suggest that a large portion of the global workspace could hence be localized within these layers. This suggestion has interesting consequences for the interpretation of anatomical findings concerning these layers. We have mentioned that the extent of layers within the cortex varies considerably. Layers II and III are, for example, elevated

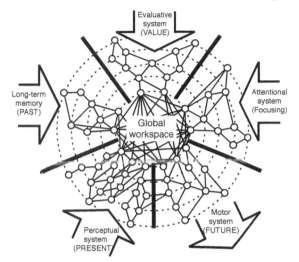

Fig. 12.5 Illustration of the workspace hypothesis. Two computational spaces can be distinguished, the sub-networks with localized and specific computational specialization, and an interconnecting network that is the platform of the global workspace [adapted from Dehaene, Kerszberg, and Changeux, *Proceedings of the National Academy of Science* 95: 14529–34 (1998)].

in the dorsolateral prefrontal cortex, an area that has been implicated in a variety of types of complex mental processing. For example, it was shown to become active in early stages of learning a sequence of numbers, and patients with lesions in this area are thought to have difficulties in switching between different rules in more challenging categorization tasks. It is difficult to record brain activity from specific layers, and direct verifications of the model discussed below are therefore challenging. In such situations it becomes necessary to work out other predictions that can be verified experimentally.

12.2.2 Demonstration of the global workspace in the Stroop task

Dehaene and colleagues demonstrated the principal idea in much more detail with a model that sheds light on the processing of the Stroop task when following the global workspace hypothesis. The Stroop task is illustrated in Fig. 12.6. In a common form it consists of a set of words that name colours, where each word can be printed in a different colour. In the Stroop task a subject is asked to either read the word or name the colour in which the word is written (all relatively rapidly). We are highly trained in reading, so that the display of a word does not render any problems in pronouncing the word. However, the naming of the colour can initially cause some problems as the image of the word prompts us to read the word rather than to ignore the content and to report the colour of the letters. It initially takes some effort to suppress the reading of the word until we have automated our response after a few trials. The explanation offered by Dehaene and colleagues is that the global workspace has to become active to 're-wire' the commonly active word-naming configuration of the brain.

To demonstrate this idea further the authors developed a model that can be tested

image \ task	word naming	colour naming
grey	grey	black
black	black	grey

Fig. 12.6 In a Stroop task a word for a colour, written in a colour that can be different from the meaning of the word, is shown to a subject who is asked to perform either a word-naming or colour-naming task.

on a Stroop task. This is illustrated in Fig. 12.7. The model includes three specialized processors, one that indicates the meaning of the word that is displayed, one that indicates the colour of the word that is displayed, and one that indicates the response of the system. In the more standard word-reading task we can assume that there is a tight coupling between the first input processor and the response processor so that the system could initially report easily the content of the word. The second task, that of naming the colour in which the word is written, then requires a suppression of these connections and the enhancement of the connections between the 'colour' input processor and the response processor. This is achieved by the top-down influence of workspace nodes on the nodes in the specialized processors.

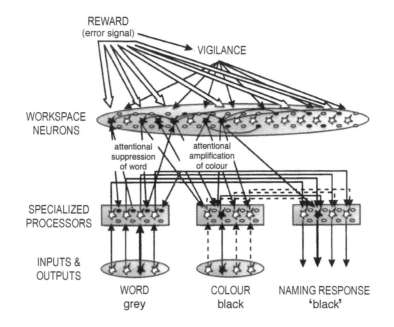

Fig. 12.7 Global workspace model that is able to reproduce several experimental findings in the Stoop task [adapted from Dehaene, Kerszberg, and Changeux, *Proceedings of the National Academy of Sceince* 95:14529–34 (1998)].

What prompts the workspace neurons to become active or to change their behaviour in the first place? Basically, the system has to be told what to do. This is achieved in the form of a reward signal that only indicates a mismatch between the desired response and actual response of the system. The large error signal then triggers a vigilance parameter to increase, which in turn allows the workspace neurons to become active that effectively reconfigure the system to allow a correct response within the required task. The vigilance parameter decreases once the system responds correctly. The authors argue that an increased vigilance (and therefore an increased activity of workspace nodes) could parallel the increased mental effort that is felt by subjects during the initial period after switching the task.

The model makes several predictions, such as increased activity in the workspace network in novel tasks, that can be tested experimentally. The model demonstrates an interesting flexibility to solve different tasks, and we can imagine how this flexibility of coupling specialized subsystems in the brain could be responsible for our ability to cope with the changing environment in which we live.

12.3 Complementary decision systems

We have outlined reinforcement learning in Chapter 11 in conjunction with basic organizations in the brain such as the cerebellum and the basal ganglia. Both of these brain structures have become well recognized in their involvement in some form of conditioning. Here we want to come back to the topic of such decision systems with a brief outline of some emerging hypothesis of complementary decision systems. We concentrate on the example of a complementary decision system in the brain, although there are other examples of complementary systems in the brain such as the already discussed complementary memory systems in Chapter 9. Another often-studied case is that of saccadic eye movements that have several pathways to initiate rapid eye movement.

When we talk about learning and decision-making systems, it is clear that the whole brain is involved, and we have even just argued in the previous section that the brain can recruit diverse areas to flexibly solve tasks. It is obvious that a clear separation of systems will likely run into problems at some level. However, we want to come back to the discussion of model-free (habitual) and model-based (deliberative) decision systems together with some hypothesis of anatomical correlations and supporting structures. This does not mean that these are the only distinguishable decision systems in the brain; we mentioned already before the distinction between Pavlovian (classical) and instrumental conditioning. However, our focus is now on the fascinating fact that there are complementary systems in our brain and that their interactions are an interesting subjects in themselves that also seems relevant in a psychiatric context.

To review, model-free reinforcement learning systems resemble habitual decisions that seem to rely on caching previous experiences, and we saw how temporal difference learning was able to propagate such experiences of reward to memories of states leading up to this. Such a value-action system can then instantaneously and quickly make decisions even faster than a conscious system might be able to comprehend. Such a system can even learn reward-action contingencies very fast with a large learning rate. However, a large learning rate would also mean that decisions can highly fluctuate in a probabilistic environment. The trade-off between such competing objectives is interesting in itself. While we do not know entirely how such learning rates could be adapted themselves in the brain, it is clear that different choices of this trade-off can dramatically alter the behaviour of people. Nevertheless, habitual decision systems are integral in our lives, from being able to efficiently drive a car or operate machinery, to being effective in playing sports. There have been many reports how the dorsolater striatum (DLS) shows many responses related to habitual decision-making. An outline of such anatomical correlates of complementary decision systems is shown in Fig. 12.8.

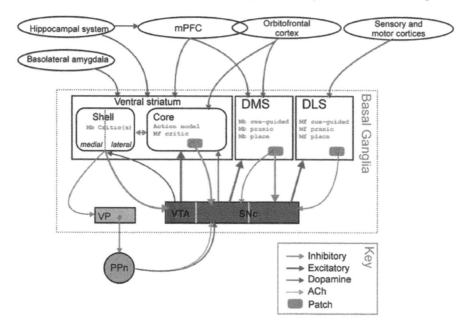

Fig. 12.8 Outline of pathways for habitual and deliberative decision systems [from Mehdi Khamassi and Mark Humpries, *Frontiers in behavioural neuroscience* (2012)].

However, a considerable downside of such habitual systems is their inflexibility to address novel situations and the time needed to reach decisions. To do this better, a model of the causal structure of the world comes in handy. If we understand components of the world together with their possible causal effects, than we can deliberate a new situation before taking risky habitual decisions that might be inappropriate in these circumstances. Of course, creating or learning such a causal model of the world is a whole other beast. Much of this book talked about mechanistic components of such a system such as representational learning, and we will later in this chapter dive a bit more into more abstract cognitive system and questions about causal learning. In Chapter 11 we have seen one example where we knew about the world by knowing all values and possible transitions in the world and saw how this can be used algorithmically. It is clear that this is useful for building deliberative decision systems from a causal world model.

Primates seems to have both of these decision systems. A clear testimony of habitual systems is the large volume of experiments with instrumental conditioning in the animal learning literature. On the other hand, it is easy for us to testify that humans can make deliberative decisions. There is also evidence in non-primate animals of deliberations. For example, it has long been recognized that rodents sometimes halt at decision points such as a junction in a maze. Interestingly, during these times of apparent rest, the hippocampus show a dramatically different firing pattern than during the locomotion phase. We have outlined in Chapter 9 a theory of the hippocampus as a cognitive map, including a spatial-temporal map with place fields. It has been suggested that the hippocampus could therefore supply the necessary simulated exploratory context for deliberate decision-making. This also fits nicely into the observation that hippocampal input feeds via the medial preforntal cortex into the dorso-medial striatum which, together with the orbitofrontal cortex, has been strongly associated with a deliberative decision system as shown in Fig. 12.8.

Furthermore, actor-critic schemes have been discussed in Chapter 11. There is now increasing evidence that specific parts of the ventral striatum called the shell and the core are nicely mapping to this framework. Of course, the complexity of the brain and interactions within brain regions including their dynamics might be more complicated as captured by Fig. 12.8, but sifting through lots of evidence to discover organizations and possible brain functions is an important part of computational neuroscience.

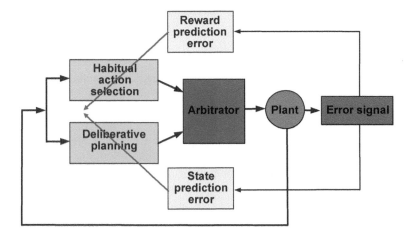

Fig. 12.9 This figure outlines a system that was implemented in a simple robotic arm to study the interaction between habitual and deliberate decision systems. The pathways with the crossing arrows for the decision systems indicate their adaptability (learning) [from Fard & Trappenberg, *Frontiers in neurorobotics* (2019)].

One issue of having complementary decision systems is the question of how to mediate between their decisions. It seems then necessary of having some form of an arbitrator as shown in Fig. 12.9. In the proposal shown in this figure, the arbitrator gives the habitual system the advantage unless this system shows a strong uncertainty in from of the prediction error. It has been noted before that uncertainty should be a strong factor in activating the deliberative decision system. Such an activation could also be triggered by cues that indicate dangers or by attentional systems. Some areas like the prefrontal cortex and the anterior cingulate cortex have been associated with a

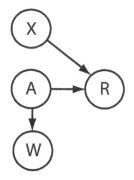

Fig. 12.10 A Bayesian network with four random variables (R, rain; A, atmospheric pressure; W, weather report (forecast); X, other causal factors of rain).

possible involvement in arbitration.

12.4 Probabilistic reasoning: causal models and Bayesian networks

12.4.1 Graphical models

Most of the discussions in this book have been about fundamental mechanisms of representational learning and information processing in networks. Of course, ultimately we want to understand how these mechanisms enable causal reasoning. More abstract models in cognitive science are often starting from a given symbolic representations of the world and are modelling cognitive processes on this more abstract level. One of the most influential and enlightening areas is thereby the field of Bayesian reasoning in causal models. This section outlines some of the fundamentals in this field. These models are often represented with graphs that specify the probabilistic relations between concepts, and those models are therefore also called graphical models.

Let us consider the example of forecasting whether it will rain tomorrow. More specifically, we would like to estimate the probability of rain given certain observations. For example, we could measure the trend of atmospheric pressure with a barometer, or see if the weather report on the evening news calls for rain. Since we cannot predict the precise value of these variables at any given time, we treat these concepts as random variables. There are, of course, many factors that influence the weather conditions; the atmospheric pressure being one of them. In contrast, although we think (or at least hope) that there is a high correlation between the weather prediction on the evening news (which takes several factors into account) and the probability of rain the next day, this prediction is certainly not the cause of rain. Rather, it is somewhat indirect in that some causes of rain influence the prediction of rain on the evening news.

The causal relations of the different factors in this example are illustrated with a graphical model in Fig. 12.10. In such Bayesian networks, each circle represents a random variable (R, rain; A, atmospheric pressure; W, weather report (forecast); X, other causal factors of rain). The arrows between them represent conditional probabilities.

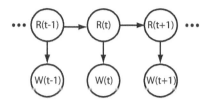

Fig. 12.11 A dynamic Bayesian model with one hidden variable (R) and one observable (W). Each of the variables obeys a first-order Markov condition. Such models are also called hidden Markov models.

Thus, the density function of the whole model can be factorized due to the conditional independence of nodes without arrows between them as

$$P(R, A, X, W) = P(R|A, X)P(W|A, X)P(A)P(X). \qquad (12.1)$$

This expression is much shorter than the general diagnostic statistical model that we would need to evaluate without the knowledge of the causal relationships. Of course, the different conditional distributions need to be estimated from data, but once these quantities are known, one can answer specific questions, such as how likely it is that it rains given that the weather forecast calls for rain.

A useful variant of causal models is the dynamic Bayesian network (DBN), which takes temporal aspects into account. For example, in the model shown in Fig. 12.11, we consider whether it is raining at our favourite vacation destination. Since we are not there, we can only watch the weather channel which reports on that day whether there was rain or not. Thus, only the random variable $W(t)$ at time t is observable, and the random variable $R(t)$ is hidden. The information on the weather network is not entirely conclusive, since the report covers a large area and might not be accurate for our specific vacation destination. The model takes into account that it is more likely to rain when it rained the previous day. Networks with the simple connectivity pattern as shown in 12.11, in which nodes are conditionally independent from other nodes give the parent nodes, are called Markov chains. Also, we usually consider models in which the laws (conditional probabilities) do not depend on time (are stationary). Models with these conditions, and with the structure of Fig. 12.11 that includes one hidden variable and one observable variable, are called hidden Markov models. Efficient algorithms have been found to perform probabilistic reasoning (statistical inference), and such models are increasingly used to describe mental processes.

12.4.2 The Pearl-example

Besides the sheer explosion of parameters with increased probabilistic model complexity, there is another reason why the joined probability function is not exactly what we need to know. The joint density functions of multiple variables describe the co-occurrence of specific values of the random variables, and the joint probability function

$p(X, Y)$ is therefore symmetric in its arguments, $p(X, Y) = p(Y, X)$. What is more relevant in real life is to reason about causal relations. For example, a fire alarm should be triggered by a fire, although there is some small chance that the alarm will not sound when the unit is defective. However, it is (hopefully) unlikely that the sound of a fire alarm will trigger a fire. It is useful to illustrate such casual relations with graphs such as

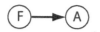

In such graphical models, the nodes represent random variables, and the links between them represent causal relations with conditional probabilities, $p(A|F)$. Since we use arrows on the links, we discuss here directed graphs, and we also restrict our discussions here to graphs that have no loops, so-called acyclic graphs. Directed acyclic graphs are also called DAGs.

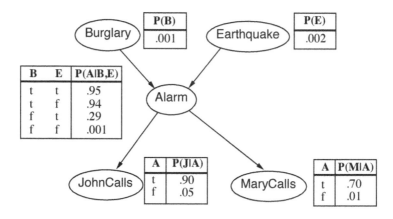

Fig. 12.12 Example of causal model.

Graphical causal models have been advanced largely by Judea Pearl, and the following example is taken from his book *Causality: models, reasoning and inference*. The model is shown in Fig. 12.12. Each of the five nodes stands for a random binary variable (Burglary B={yes,no}, Earthquake E={yes,no}, Alarm A={yes,no}, John calls J={yes,no}, Mary calls M={yes,no}). The figure also includes conditional probability tables (CPTs) that specify the conditional probabilities represented by the links between the nodes.

The joint distribution of the five variables can be factored in various ways following the chain rule (generalized Bayes's rule) of probability theory, for example as

$$p(B, E, A, J, M) = P(B|E, A, J, M)P(E|A, J, M)P(A|J, M)P(J|M)P(M).$$
(12.2)

However, the causal model represents a specific factorization of the joint probability functions, namely

$$p(B, E, A, J, M) = P(B)P(E)P(A|B, E)P(J|A)P(M|A),$$
(12.3)

which is much easier to handle. For example, if we do not know the conditional probability functions, we need to run many more experiments to estimate the various conditions ($2^4 + 2^3 + 2^2 + 2^1 + 2^0 = 31$) instead of the reduced conditions in the causal model ($1 + 1 + 2^2 + 2 + 2 = 10$). It is also easy to use the casual model to undertake inference (drawing conclusions), for specific questions. For example, say we want to know the probability that there was no earthquake or burglary when the alarm rings and both John and Mary call. This is given by

$$P(B = f, E = f, A = t, J = t, M = t)$$
$$= P(B = f)P(E = f,)P(A = t|B = f, E = f)P(J = t|A = t)P(M = t|A = t)$$
$$= 0.998 * 0.999 * 0.001 * 0.7 * 0.9$$
$$\approx 0.00062.$$

Although we have a casual model where parent variables influence the outcome of child variables, we can also use child evidence to infer some possible values of parent variables. For example, let us calculate the probability that the alarm rings, given that John calls, $P(A = t|J = t)$. For this, we should first calculate the probability that the alarm rings as we need this later. This is given by

$$P(A = t) = P(A = t|B = t, E = t)P(B = t)P(E = t) + \ldots$$
$$P(A = t|B = t, E = f)P(B = t)P(E = f) + \ldots$$
$$P(A = t|B = f, E = t)P(B = f)P(E = t) + \ldots$$
$$P(A = t|B = f, E = f)P(B = f)P(E = f)$$
$$= 0.95 * 0.001 * 0.002 + 0.94 * 0.001 * 0.998 + \ldots$$
$$0.29 * 0.999 * 0.002 + 0.001 * 0.999 * 0.998$$
$$= 0.002516442.$$

We can then use Bayes's rule to calculate the required probability,

$$P(A = t|J = t) = \frac{P(J = t|A = t)P(A = t)}{P(J = t|A = t)P(A = t) + P(J = t|A = f)P(A = f)}$$
$$\approx \frac{0.9 * 0.0025}{0.9 * 0.0025 + 0.05 * 0.9975}$$
$$\approx 0.0434.$$

We can similarly apply the rules of probability theory to calculate other quantities, but these calculations can get cumbersome with larger graphs. It is therefore useful to use numerical tools to perform such inference. A Python toolbox for Bayesian networks is introduced in the next section.

While inference is an important application of causal models, inferring causality from data is another area where causal models revolutionize scientific investigations. Many traditional methods evaluate co-occurrences of events to determine dependencies, such as a correlation analysis. However, such a correlation analysis is usually not a good indication of causality. Consider the example in Fig. 12.12. When the alarm rings, it is likely that John and Mary call, but the event that John calls is mutually independent of the event that Mary calls. Yet, when John calls it is also statistically more likely to observe the event that Mary calls. Sometimes we might just be interested in knowing about the likelihood of co-occurrence, for which a correlation analysis can be a good start, but if we are interested in describing the causes of the observations, then we need another approach. Some algorithms have been proposed for structural learning, such as an algorithm called inferred causation (IC), which deduces what the most likely causal structure behind given data is.

12.4.3 Probabilistic reasoning in Python using LEA

There are several tools for working with probabilistic models and Bayesian graphical models. A very prominent general probabilistic programming toolbox is Stan (https://mc-stan.org), but we will here give an example using the LEA3 (https://bitbucket.org/piedenis/lea) which is a simpler tool for working with discrete probabilities in Python. In particular, LEA has direct support for Bayesian models. This brief section is not meant to be a thorough introduction to this tool but merely to give an example in order to demonstrate the usefulness of such tools. We will show an example program for the burglary/earthquake example.

The main part of the program is to define the graph structure and the associated conditional probability tables. The corresponding code is fairly self-explanatory.

Listing 12.1 LeaExample.ipynb (part 1)

```
import lea

burglary   = lea.event(0.001)
earthquake = lea.event(0.002)
alarm = lea.joint(burglary, earthquake).switch({
    (True ,True ): lea.event(0.950),
  (True ,False) : lea.event(0.940),
  (False,True ) : lea.event(0.290),
  (False,False) : lea.event(0.001) })
johnCalls = alarm.switch({True: lea.event(0.90),
                          False: lea.event(0.05) })
maryCalls = alarm.switch({True: lea.event(0.70),
                          False : lea.event(0.01) })
```

This notation includes the specification of the discrete probability tables, and it contains the relations between the variables so that there is no need for a separate specification of the network graph.

Once the graph is specified it is possible to use some inference engines that build the heart of such tools. We have seen earlier that the continuous application of Bayes's rule for variable elimination leads to the analytic answer for specific queries. Such exact computations for variable elimination can be implemented so that inference can be achieved by simple function calls. For example, if we want to know what the probability is that Mary calls given that there is an alarm, we can write in LEA

Listing 12.2 LeaExample.ipynb (part 2)

```
P(maryCalls.given(alarm))
```

The answer is 0.7, which can, of course, be directly read off the conditional probability table. A less obvious example is the probability of an alarm when John calls,

Listing 12.3 LeaExample.ipynb (part 3)

```
1  P(alarm.given(johnCalls))
```

which recovers the 4 per cent that we calculated analytically in the last section. An even more advanced query of a joint probability is

Listing 12.4 LeaExample.ipynb (part 4)

```
1  P(~burglary & ~earthquake & alarm & johnCalls & maryCalls)
```

which is only a small probability of around 0.6 percent.

While exact methods for Bayesian inference are possible, a known factor is that these methods are slow and scale very badly for larger Bayesian networks. There are therefore various approximate inference techniques such as believe propagation, which is based on some message between the nodes in the graph and a minimization of the consistency of the samples. This discussion is, however, beyond the scope of this book.

12.4.4 Expectation maximization

In the example above we showed how to do probabilistic reasoning with given networks of random variables. Of course, this requires knowing about the distributions with associated parameters. Therefore, estimating distribution parameters from data is essential. We discussed how functions can be learned before, in particular with supervised learning as in Chapter 7. Before leaving the probabilistic modelling discussion here, we would like to mention one more techniques that is often used to fit distributions to data in some unsupervised way. Indeed, such a strategy was used already in the predictive coding discussion in Chapter 7. We assume here that the general form of a distribution is given, and the remaining problem is to estimate the parameters of the corresponding models in a self-supervised way.

A widely applicable technique of parameter estimation in such situations is expectation maximization (EM). To introduce the idea behind EM, we follow an example of density estimation in a very simple world. In this simple world, data are generated with equal likelihood from two Gaussian distributions, one with mean $\mu_1 = -1$ and standard deviation $\sigma_1 = 2$, the other with mean $\mu_2 = 4$ and standard deviation $\sigma_2 = 0.5$. These two distributions are illustrated in Fig. 12.13A with a dashed and a dotted lines, respectively. Let us assume that we know that the world consists only of data from two Gaussian distributions with equal likelihood, but that we do not know the specific realizations (parameters) of these distributions. The pre-knowledge of two Gaussian distributions encodes a specific hypothesis which makes up this heuristic model. In this simple example, we have chosen the heuristics to match the actual data-generating system (world), that is, we have explicitly used some knowledge of the world. As argued above, we can think of the brain as a flexible dynamic system, the parameters of which can be adjusted to match world distributions, and it is also possible that, through evolution, this system has evolved to parameterize common concepts in our world.

Learning the parameters of the two Gaussians would be easy if we had access to the information about which data point was produced by which Gaussian, that is, which cause produced the specific examples. Unfortunately, we can only observe the data without a teacher label that could supervise the learning. We choose therefore a

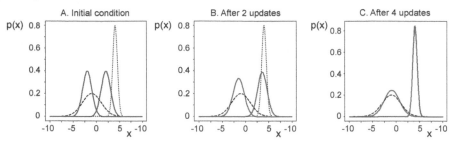

Fig. 12.13 Example of the expectation maximization (EM) algorithm for a world model with two Gaussian distributions. The Gaussian distributions of the world data (input data) are shown with dashed and the dotted lines. (A) The generative model, shown with the coloured solid lines, is initialized with arbitrary parameters. In the EM algorithm, the unlabelled input data are labelled with a recognition model, which is, in this example, the inverse of the generative model. These labelled data are then used for parameter estimation of the generative model. The results of learning are shown in (B) after two iterations, and in (C) after four iterations.

self-supervised strategy. We start thereby with arbitrary values of the model parameters and then repeat the following two steps until convergence:

E-step: We make assumptions of the training labels (or the probability that the data were produced by a specific cause) from the current model (expectation step); and

M-step: use this hypothesis to update the parameters of the model to maximize the observations (maximization step).

In the example shown in Fig. 12.13A we used as starting values $\mu_1 = 2$, $\mu_2 = -2$, $\sigma_1 = \sigma_2 = 1$. These distributions are shown with colored solid lines. Comparing the generated data with the environmental data corresponds to hypothesis testing.

The results of this initial guess are not yet very satisfactory, but we can use the generative model to express our expectation of the data. Specifically, we can assign each data point to the class which produces the larger probability within the current world model. Thus, we are using our specific hypothesis here as a recognition model. In the example we can use Bayes's rule to invert the generative model into a recognition model as detailed in the simulation below. If this inversion is not possible, then we can introduce a separate recognition model (expectation), Q, to approximate the inverse of the generative model. Such a recognition model can be learned with similar methods and interleaved with the generative model as we have seen with predictive coding.

Of course, the recognition with the recognition model early in learning is not expected to be exact, but estimation of new parameters from the recognized data in the M-step to maximize the expectation can be expected to be better than the model with the initial arbitrary values. The new model can then be compared to the data again and, when necessary, be used to generate new expectations from which the model is refined. This procedure is known as the expectation maximization (EM) algorithm. The distributions after three and nine such iterations, where we have chosen new data points in each iteration, are shown in Figs 12.13B and C. The program EM.py was used to produce Fig. 12.13.

Programs/EM.py

```
1  # 1d example EM algorithm
2  import numpy as np
3  import matplotlib.pyplot as plt
4
5  def gaussian(x, mu, var):
6      return np.exp(-(x-mu)**2/(2*var))/np.sqrt(2*np.pi*var)
7
8  x0=np.arange(-10,10,0.1)
9  var1=1; var2=1; mu1=-2; mu2=2;
10 for iteration in range(10):
11     # plot distribution
12     plt.figure()
13     plt.plot(x0, gaussian(x0,-1,4),'k—')
14     plt.plot(x0, gaussian(x0,4,.25),'k:')
15     plt.plot(x0, gaussian(x0,mu1,var1),'r')
16     plt.plot(x0, gaussian(x0,mu2,var2),'b')
17     # data
18     x=np.array([np.random.normal(-1,2,50),np.random.normal(4,0.5,50)])
19     # expectation (recognition)
20     c=gaussian(x,mu1,var1)>gaussian(x,mu2,var2)
21     # maximization
22     mu1=np.sum(x[c>0.5])/np.sum(c)
23     var1=np.sum((x[c>0.5]-mu1)**2)/np.sum(c)
24     mu2=np.sum(x[c<0.5])/(100-np.sum(c))
25     var2=np.sum((x[c<0.5]-mu2)**2)/(100-np.sum(c))
```

We produce thereby new random data from each distribution in each iteration. Recognition of this data is done in Line 16 by inverting the generative model using Bayes's formula,

$$P(c|\mathbf{x}; G) = \frac{P(\mathbf{x}|c; G)P(c; G)}{P(\mathbf{x}; G)}. \tag{12.4}$$

In this specific example, we know that the data are equally distributed from each Gaussian so that the prior distribution over causes, $P(c; G)$, is $1/2$ for each cause. Also, the marginal distribution of data is equally distributed, so that we can ignore this normalizing factor. The recognition model uses the Bayesian decision criterion, in which the data point is assigned to the cause with a larger recognition distribution, $P(c|\mathbf{x}; G)$. Using the labels of the data generated by the recognition model, we can then use the data to obtain new estimates of the parameters for each Gaussian.

We only showed a simple demonstration of the EM algorithm. In practice we have often have also to estimate the priors, which is easy to do when counting the number of data points in each class from the recognition model. We can also make better estimations of the parameters, for example by weighting each mean with the probability that the corresponding data point belongs to this class. Finally, note that when testing the system for a long time, it can happen that one of the distributions is dominating the recognition model so that only data from one distribution are generated. The model of one Gaussian would then be explaining away data from the other cause. More practical solutions must take such factors into account.

12.5 Structural causal models and learning causality

In the previous section we, introduced Bayesian networks that nicely specifies probabilistic reasoning through causal networks. Those networks are specified by a modeller through identifying the semantic components of the network, and usually also the causal relations. While such networks can explain a lot of human behaviour, the question is how those networks can be realized in the brain. This includes causal learning which has in itself two components, that of learning the semantic entities, and that of learning their causal relations. In this last section we outline some exciting research directions in casual representations and learning.

12.5.1 Out-of-distribution generalization

Before we present the formalization of causal systems, it is useful to reflect on the benefits of such causal learning. We have seen that neural networks can learn from examples, and we have shown how this leads to some form of generalization. For example, we have trained on some handwritten images of numbers from the MNIST data and showed how examples not previously seen by the network can be correctly classified. However, this is only one form of generalization where we basically have one set of samples from an underlying distribution. Technically, we refer to this as IID data which stands for independent and identically distributed data. The generalization is within this distribution.

A much harder form of generalization is out-of-distribution (OOD) generalization. These are circumstances where knowledge has to be applied to new circumstances, either due to shifting environments, or to new environments with somewhat different characteristics. Central for such abilities is to learn about processes that can be applied to different situations. For example, if one learns that a hammer can be used to drive a nail into wood, the principle of applying force to a specific area can also be used to knock a hole into a wall. Or learning about wheels on a car and their use for mobility helps to recognize their use in trains. Such causal inference seems clearly a key component in the ability of animals to live in the world, while most machine learning methods have limited generalization of this type.

Learning meaningful or semantic representations has thereby multiple facets. We just gave the example of understanding what a wheel is. While this is just one component of a car, we can distinguish further sub-components such as a tire or a valve when necessary. It seems therefore useful to have hierarchical representations. This not only entail components that are taken together to form more complex objects, but also different levels of abstractions. For example, we could talk about generic cars when planning a traffic system in the city, or we can picture specific examples when we are buying a car.

While we have mostly talked about static elements, an important aspect of information processing and causality in particular seems to be time or the sequence of events happening. This is well known from vision where static pictures can be ambiguous given possible occlusions of objects. Such ambiguities can often be resolved from a series of views. Also, segmenting objects from motion is a common technique that demonstrates the importance of the temporal domain. This has been further developed in slow feature analysis by Laurenz Wiskott. Temporal Bayesian networks such as hidden Markov models (HMM) have also been very useful in many applications. Exploiting temporal information for causal reasoning is only beginning to emerge.

12.5.2 Structural causal models

While we have already introduced the basis of (causal) Bayesian networks, it is possible and useful to refine this notion somewhat more. The Bayesian networks specifies a factorization of a joined probability function such as:

$$p(x, y) = p(x|y)p(x).$$ (12.5)

Using a probabilistic formulation is useful to represent uncertainty, and we have argued that the representation with directed graphs gave us superior models. A general limitation of a probabilistic framework is that measurements of co-occurrences does not specify the causality. Useful refinements of such causal models are therefore structural causal models (SCMs). In SCMs we separate the deterministic causal structure from the stochastic components describing the uncertainty. In such models, the variables X_i are thereby determined by a deterministic function of the parent nodes, $\mathbf{Pa}_i$ and a stochastic variable U_i describing the uncertainty,

$$X_i = f(\mathbf{Pa}_i, U_i).$$ (12.6)

The function f is thereby a deterministic function, although the dependence on a noise term makes the resulting variable itself stochastic. However, separating the deterministic causal structure from the uncertainty helps to specify causal relations better.

A complete causally sufficient graph thereby requires that all the uncertainties U_i are independent of each other. This has the consequence that the causal units of a variable with their parents have only local effects if some of the parents or the uncertainty of the associated processes change. Such a causal network is therefore often described as a disentangled factorization. Probing a disentangled factorization can then be checked with some intervention which should lead only to local changes. It seems that active hypothesis testing, for example by manipulating objects, can thereby help to learn causality.

12.5.3 Learning causality and explainable AI

Learning causality is a new area in AI and cognitive science. So far, only some examples have been discussed in the literature for specific model systems. But I want to finish this chapter with a comment on the related issue of explainable AI that is currently often discussed.

Artificial neural networks have often been dubbed a black box in that there is usually no easy way to explain why the network came up with specific answers. The danger of this characterization is that it give the impression that we do not know what goes on inside. However, most neural networks are deterministic and we can say exactly what is going on. The problem is rather that reporting this knowledge in terms of rules is very cumbersome and would involve a lot of rules. It would mean that we say that '... because this and that neuron fired, and the connectivity is so and so with specific delay, etc, this is why these specific output neurons were active'. Even though this is possible, our problem is that the amount of rules needed to explain simple facts seems overwhelming.

Of course, this is not much different in real neural networks. We cannot observe all the neurons as we can do in our computer simulations of the artificial neural networks, but even if we could we would not be satisfied with such explanations of specific neuron's firings. Rather, we expect humans to articulate explanations. Drawing on semantic entities and causal relations is thereby what humans would accept as explanations. This is another example of a causal deliberative system representing a world model.

Just a final thought on the previous discussion of model-free and model-based decision-making. Even in the case when decisions have clearly been made by the model-free decision system, it has been documented how we will invent explanatory stories after the fact. Such an ability can help to integrate the different decision systems in a conscious one.

12.5.4 The way forward

We hope the material and the discussions provide enough background in computational neuroscience to follow up on more specific issues of your interest in the research literature. Also, we hope we have convinced you that analytical and computational studies of the brain can advance our understanding of how the brain works, by quantifying hypotheses that can lead to more precise predictions, which, in turn, can be verified experimentally. Even if you concentrate on experimental techniques, it is vital to connect them to more quantitative endeavours. For those concentrating on theoretical techniques, we hope that we have made it clear that theoretical studies must be rooted in experimental knowledge. A closer cooperation between theoreticians and experimentalists is currently emerging, and we strongly believe that such collaborations can considerably advance our understanding of brain functions.

Many aspects of brain function are still unknown. There are still many very fundamental questions which are unanswered, including many details of the information-processing mechanisms of the brain. However, there have also been quite specific proposals, such as the brain as an anticipatory memory system that can learn a casual model of the world. We hope this hypothesis can guide further experimental investigations.

Some brain areas have been targeted by modellers, and major progress in understanding these areas is expected. The cerebellum has been a promising area due to its elaborate architecture, but strong hypotheses have also been advanced for the hippocampus, the basal ganglia, and others. A current challenge in computational neuroscience is the multitude of models with diverse aims. This multitude of models is expected, and desirable, since each model is designed to answer specific questions, but it is also necessary to extract principal knowledge from such studies, which can be compared to other types of investigations. The progression of our understanding of brain functions will also certainly lead to more convergence in modelling approaches.

A better understanding of brain processes will ultimately lead to the development of new health-care applications such as advanced rehabilitation treatment after brain damage. In fact, the study of the consequences of specific brain damage alone, is an important application area. Studying rehabilitation techniques takes a lot of effort with patients, and modelling studies can provide flexible and cost-efficient investigations of specific questions. Such modelling efforts could at least narrow down more specific questions to be answered in complementary studies. Computational psychiatry is now a very active and promising field within computational neuroscience where we hope to shed more light on the origin of mental disorders. It is hence an exciting time to be part of the computational neuroscience community.

Index